ALCOHOLISM TREATMENT

Alcoholism Treatment
Context, Process, and Outcome

RUDOLF H. MOOS

JOHN W. FINNEY

RUTH C. CRONKITE

New York   Oxford
OXFORD UNIVERSITY PRESS
1990

Oxford University Press

Oxford New York Toronto
Delhi Bombay Calcutta Madras Karachi
Petaling Jaya Singapore Hong Kong Tokyo
Nairobi Dar es Salaam Cape Town
Melbourne Auckland

and associated companies in
Berlin Ibadan

Copyright © 1990 by Oxford University Press, Inc.

Published by Oxford University Press, Inc.,
200 Madison Avenue, New York, New York 10016

Oxford is a registered trademark of Oxford University Press

All rights reserved. No part of this publication may be reproduced,
stored in a retrieval system, or transmitted, in any form or by any means,
electronic, mechanical, photocopying, recording, or otherwise,
without the prior permission of Oxford University Press.

Library of Congress Cataloging-in-Publication Data
Moos, Rudolf H., 1934–
Alcoholism treatment : context, process, and outcome /
Rudolf H. Moos, John W. Finney, and Ruth C. Cronkite.
p.   cm.
Includes bibliographical references.
ISBN 0-19-504362-6
1. Alcoholism—Treatment.   I. Finney, John W.
II. Cronkite, Ruth C.   III. Title.
[DNLM: 1. Alcoholism—therapy.   2. Outcome and Process Assessment
(Health Care).   WM 274 M825a]
RC565.M67 1990
616.86′106—dc20
DNLM/DLC   for Library of Congress   89-16343   CIP

9 8 7 6 5 4 3 2 1

Printed in the United States of America
on acid-free paper

Preface

This book reports a long-term effort to try to understand the context, process, and effects of alcoholism treatment. When this work began, the dominant model for evaluating interventions was the experimental design espoused by Donald Campbell and his colleagues at Northwestern University. This approach provides a sound basis for estimating the average effects of treatment. However, here we adopted a naturalistic design because we were interested in other issues as well. We wanted to learn more about the process through which treatment might exert its effects, and we wanted to study patients' life contexts and how they can affect treatment outcome. In this regard, we followed in the footsteps of Sir Ronald Fisher, who developed a mechanism (the experimental design) to evaluate the effects of interventions on agricultural crops and then became intrigued by other contextual factors (e.g., weeds, insects, absence of field hands) that influence the ultimate yield of a parcel of land.

Moreover, we wanted to understand the ramifications of remission and relapse. Toward that end, we studied a matched group of normal-drinking families who lived in the same census tracts as the alcoholic patients and their families. This enabled us to determine if remitted patients were functioning in other life areas as well as their neighbors, and what the full costs were of continuing alcohol abuse. Because alcohol abuse exacts a heavy toll on family members of afflicted individuals, we also studied the spouses and children of remitted and relapsed patients and compared them with the spouses and children of the matched community controls.

The research was generously supported by Grant AA02863 from the National Institute on Alcohol Abuse and Alcoholism, by Department of Veterans Affairs Medical Research funds, and by Health Services Research and Development Service funding of the Far West Field Program. The duration of support allowed us to think more deeply about the research and its implications than would otherwise have been possible.

A number of people helped to carry out this project. First, we would like to thank the patients and their families who participated in the study, and the staffs of the treatment programs who allowed the research to take place and, in some cases, actively facilitated it by collecting data.

Evelyn Bromet, Ph.D., played an important part in getting the research off the ground. She was instrumental in securing the participation of the five residential treatment programs, developing the data collection procedures used at treatment intake and at the 6-month follow-up, and reporting the results of the early analyses. Later on, Andrew Billings, Ph.D., collaborated on the research comparing the children of the patients and community controls.

Many research assistants contributed their skills and effort to the project. Fredric Bliss did yeoman work in organizing and conducting the initial data collection and the 6-month follow-ups. James Kulik and Jean Otto helped in this process. Christopher Wuthmann and Bernice Van Dort set up the data files and conducted the initial analyses on the patient sample. Barbara Mehren worked on a study of the residents in the Salvation Army program.

Vivien Tsu took major responsibility for collecting data from family members at the 6-month and 2-year follow-ups. Ron Mewborn, Elizabeth Lee, and Wendy Max collected the first wave of data from the matched community controls and their families, and Ron Mewborn set up the initial patient and family data files and conducted statistical analyses. Suzy Schleuning worked on the follow-up of this sample and analyzed data. Darrow Chan and Wendy Gamble also collected data and performed statistical analyses comparing patients and controls, and their spouses; Sarah Buxton, Diane Denzler, and Ruth Lederman assisted in the analyses. Dani Lawler and Rena David set up computer files for the later waves of data.

Mary Giamarino, with the help of Laurie Plautz, conducted the ten-year follow-up of the patients and their spouses, while Heather Weiss was responsible for the long-term follow-up of the matched community controls and their spouses. Heather Weiss and Purnima Mankekar set up the ten-year follow-up data, which were analyzed primarily by Rena David, Carol Suzuki, and Colleen Moore. Bernice Moos helped to organize data files and conduct statistical analyses throughout the project.

Adrienne Juliano had what often seemed an insurmountable task: word processing the manuscript, providing editorial input, and tracking references. She performed these with her usual high level of competence and good cheer. Ann Margulies taught us to write in a more direct and comprehensible style and thereby helped set the overall tone of the book. Drs. Richard Longabaugh and Alan Marlatt reviewed a draft of the manuscript and made many helpful comments.

PREFACE

We hope that our efforts to understand the process of treatment, the long-term course of alcohol abuse and factors that affect it, and the impact of alcohol abuse on the family will benefit alcoholic patients and their family members.

Palo Alto, California R.H.M.
September 1989 J.W.F.
  R.C.C.

Contents

1. Evaluating and Improving Alcoholism Treatment Programs 3
   Aims of the Research 5
   The Biopsychosocial Perspective 6
   Traditional and Expanded Paradigms for Treatment Evaluation 7
   Stress and Coping Theory 10
   The Book in Brief 12

Part I   A Systems Evaluation of Alcoholism Treatment

2. Objectives, Methods, and Assessment of Treatment Implementation 17
   Research Objective and Methods 17
   Assessing Treatment Implementation 25

3. Short-Term Outcome and Patient Prognosis 36
   Multidimensional Measures of Intake and Follow-Up Functioning 36
   Changes in Functioning between Intake and Follow-Up 38
   Relationships between Drinking and Other Outcome Indices 41
   Prognostic Importance of Pretreatment Factors 43
   Difficulty of Follow-Up 46
   Conclusions 51

4. The Process and Effects of Treatment 52
   An Expanded Evaluation Paradigm 52
   Relative Effectiveness of the Treatment Programs 53
   Program Components and Outcome 58
   Length of Treatment and Outcome 61
   Participation in Aftercare 62
   The Salvation Army Program 63
   The Relative Strength of Treatment 66
   Future Directions 71

5. Gender and Marital Status in Treatment and Outcome   73
    Prior Research on Gender and Marital Status   74
    Gender and Marital Status Subgroups   76
    Overview and Implications for Treatment   82

Part II   Extratreatment Factors and the Recovery Process

6. Life Stressors, Social Resources, and Coping Responses   89
    Life Stressors and Social Resources   90
    Characteristics of Family Settings   91
    Characteristics of Work Settings   98
    Appraisal and Coping Responses   104

7. Context, Coping, and Treatment Outcome   109
    Expanding the Paradigm: Context and Coping Factors   109
    Patients in Family Settings   111
    Homogeneity and Stability of Treatment Outcome   112
    Life Stressors, Coping Resources, and Treatment Outcome   116
    Examining the Conceptual Model   125
    A Unified Model of Remission and Relapse   129

8. The Process of Recovery and Relapse   134
    Comparing Alcoholic Patients with Community Controls   135
    Two-Year Adaptation among Stably Remitted and Relapsed Alcoholics   140
    Long-Term Adaptation of Patients and Controls   146
    Toward a Theory of Recovery and Relapse   150

Part III   Alcoholism and the Family

9. Spouses of Alcoholic Partners   157
    Perspectives on Spouses of Alcoholics   158
    Spouses of Remitted and Relapsed Alcoholics   160
    A Stress and Coping Model of Spouse Functioning   166
    An Integrated Perspective on Spouses of Impaired Partners   174

10. Children of Alcoholic Parents   179
    The Family Context of Children's Adaptation   181
    The Family Context of Children of Depressed Parents   189
    Comparing Children of Alcoholic and Depressed Parents   191
    A Paradigm of Family Functioning   194
    The Broader Social Context   196

Part IV   Practical Applications

11. Improving Treatment, Work, and Family Settings   201
    Monitoring Program Development   201
    Enriching Treatment Environments   207
    Enriching Work Environments of Health Care Staff   210
    Enriching Family Environments   212
    General Perspectives on Improving Social Settings   216

CONTENTS

12. Implications for Treatment and Program Evaluation 220
    The Major Findings 220
    Implications for Diagnosis and Treatment 226
    Implications for Theories to Guide Treatment Evaluations 231
    The Methodology of Evaluation Research 238
    The Expanded Paradigm and Research on Patient-Treatment Matching 242
    The Utility of Treatment Evaluations 245
    Conclusion 248

References 249

Index 275

ALCOHOLISM TREATMENT

1

Evaluating and Improving Alcoholism Treatment Programs

The consequences of alcohol abuse are a heavy drain on society. In economic terms, the annual cost of alcohol abuse in the United States may be as high as $120 billion, including both direct costs for treatment and medical care for alcohol-related illnesses and injuries and indirect costs associated with crime and violence, property losses due to automobile accidents, and losses of productivity from alcohol-related morbidity and mortality. Alcohol plays a role in 10% of all deaths in the United States and is the leading cause of death through accidents among young people of ages 15 to 24 (Cahalan, 1987; NIAAA, 1987; Saxe et al., 1983). A major societal response to the growing awareness of alcohol abuse and its costs has been to expand specialized alcoholism treatment services. In fact, over the course of a generation—from 1942 to 1976—alcoholism treatment services increased twentyfold in the United States (Room, 1980). The annual cost of alcoholism-related health care services is estimated to be more than $15 billion (NIAAA, 1987).

An estimated 18 million Americans 18 years old and older experience problems resulting from alcohol abuse. Alcohol abuse exacts a pernicious toll on these individuals and their families. Alcoholism is associated with premature death; medical complications of virtually all organ systems; neuropsychological deficits; social problems such as divorce, child abuse, and loss of employment; and various forms of psychological distress (NIAAA, 1987). As the physical, psychological, social, and economic costs rise, more alcohol abusers turn to specialized treatment programs for help. Over 1 million people enter treatment for alcoholism each year in the United States alone (Saxe et al., 1983).

Alcoholism treatment plays a prominent role in both the society's and the individual's response to alcohol abuse. In the last 25 years many evaluations have been conducted to try to gauge the effectiveness of treatment programs and, in some cases, to improve them (Emrick, 1975; Hill & Blane, 1967; Mandell, 1979; May & Kuller, 1975; Miller & Hester, 1986; Nathan & Skinstad, 1987; Saxe et al., 1983). In general, these studies suggest that treatment programs are only modestly effective. Thus, the alcoholism treatment field is ripe for improvement; however, program evaluations have had little if any influence on improving treatment.

Simply put, program planners do not perceive evaluations as useful. One way of documenting this point is to ask treatment providers about the information they use when they want to establish or change a program. Treatment providers usually turn to their own clinical experience, data from other programs, or theories about alcoholism and its treatment. Findings from treatment evaluations are the least likely source to be consulted. Although treatment providers may cite results of evaluations when answering questions from laypeople about the general effectiveness of alcoholism treatment, beyond this, journals reporting treatment research are little more than decorations on many clinicians' bookshelves. Our impressions are consistent with those of Ogborne (1988), who suggested that "many program planners and front-line clinicians find little of value in many research reports" (p. 729), and with Cartwright (1985), who noted the "simplicity and mundane nature" of treatment outcome research from a clinician's point of view.

Another way to gauge how treatment providers perceive evaluations is to consider their typical reaction to learning that their program will be evaluated. Is it anticipation that they will learn more about their program and how it can be improved? Or is it likely to be a more negative response—a mixture of fear and resentment? Our answer to this question is inherent in the way we have framed it; we have not entertained the idea that an evaluation might be initiated by clinicians themselves. Can treatment providers be blamed for fearing and resenting evaluations? Is their reaction irrational? We do not think so. A treatment provider has very little to gain from most evaluations. The evaluation is likely to show that the program is only moderately effective or perhaps not effective at all. More significant, it is likely to provide little if any information on which to base program improvements. Why do evaluations contribute so little to the process of improving treatment?

We believe that the most significant problem is the atheoretical, outcome-oriented research paradigm that has guided many of these evaluations. This paradigm does not encompass new developments in our understanding of the probable etiology and nature of alcohol abuse. It has not provided the information clinicians need to develop a better understanding of alcoholism and to improve its treatment.

In this book, we outline an expanded research paradigm that accommodates contemporary theories of alcoholism and program evaluation, and we describe our long-term study of alcoholism treatment, which is an effort to apply this expanded paradigm of evaluation research. We examine treatment more intensively than is usually done, and we focus on factors outside of treatment, such as life stressors, social resources, and coping responses. We also examine the impact of alcohol abuse on spouses and children.

AIMS OF THE RESEARCH

Our research, which spanned more than a decade, had two basic aims: to examine the implementation, process, and effects of residential alcoholism treatment and to learn more about the nature and course of alcohol abuse. To meet the first aim, we studied diverse programs and focused not only on treatment outcome, but also on the specific treatment provided to individual patients, including its quantity and quality and how it was related to treatment outcome. We tried to answer questions such as:

> How can evaluators determine the readiness of a program for evaluation? That is, without data on treatment outcome, what are appropriate criteria for determining that a viable alcoholism program is being offered?
>
> How can the complexity of alcoholism treatment environments be described so they can be understood, improved, and related to multiple measures of treatment outcome?
>
> How much do patient and treatment characteristics contribute to treatment outcome? When treatment components, length of stay, and treatment environment are measured, do they account for more variation in outcome than does a global index of treatment program? Do patients who are harder to follow up experience poorer treatment outcome?
>
> How do women, compared with men, fare in alcoholism treatment programs? Do they benefit less from treatment? Are certain treatment experiences more helpful for women than for men?

To learn more about the nature and course of alcoholism, our second basic aim, we focused on how patients' functioning after treatment was influenced by factors outside of treatment, such as stressful life conditions and family and work environments. We also examined how alcohol abuse affects the spouses and children of patients. The particular questions we addressed include:

> How well can functioning 2 years and 10 years after treatment be predicted by the patient's characteristics when entering treatment, the different kinds of treatment provided in the program, and factors outside of treatment? For example, how important to recovery is a cohesive family environment?
>
> How does the psychological, social, and occupational functioning of remitted patients compare with that of relapsed patients and of peo-

ple who do not have drinking problems? Is remission in terms of drinking associated with better life contexts and better functioning in other areas?

How stable is the course of alcohol abuse or remission over a 10-year period after treatment? If a patient is in remission 2 years after treatment, how likely is he or she to continue recovery during the next 8 years?

What effect does remission have on the patient's spouse? Is the spouse more likely to suffer from this change in family equilibrium or to improve in functioning?

How do patients' remissions and relapses affect their children? Do children's problems continue when their parent is recovering, or does their functioning improve as well? Can the family environment moderate the influence of the parent's alcoholism?

As suggested by these questions, the broad scope of our research and its extended time frame afforded us a unique opportunity to learn more about the processes of remission and relapse, about the role of treatment in the recovery process, and about the impact of families on changes in alcohol abuse following treatment. The breadth of the research flows, in part, from a multifactorial perspective on the nature of alcohol abuse.

THE BIOPSYCHOSOCIAL PERSPECTIVE

In the years following World War II, the disease perspective of alcoholism became the dominant view of the disorder. According to this perspective, physiological and psychological vulnerability to alcohol causes some people (alcoholics) to lose control over their drinking. A person either is or is not an alcoholic; once the condition has developed, it is irreversible. The only significant environmental factor is alcohol itself. Treatment effectiveness is gauged primarily in terms of whether that environmental factor is avoided—that is, by whether or not patients abstain from drinking. Evaluations guided by the disease perspective as an etiologic theory had no need to isolate specific determinants of alcohol abuse because these were presumed to be internal and irreversible. Evaluations could focus simply on determining the proportion of patients who were abstinent following treatment. Thus, an exclusively outcome-oriented evaluation paradigm was appropriately matched to this etiological theory.

Ideas about the nature of alcohol abuse have evolved over the years, however. Most researchers now adopt a multifactorial biopsychosocial perspective, according to which a combination of biological, psychological, and social factors initiates and maintains alcohol abuse, a disorder that affects both excessive drinkers and those whose lives they touch (Kissin & Hanson, 1982). Zucker and Gomberg (1986) have proposed that the etiology of alcoholism is best understood within the context of a longitudinal and developmental framework that includes psychosocial as well as genetic and biological determinants.

The biopsychosocial perspective is leading to revolutionary new approaches in medicine and psychology (Gentry, 1984). Building on an ecological view of psychosomatic medicine, these approaches utilize a systems model of the causes of medical and psychiatric disorders and emphasize the influence of biological, psychological, and social factors in all health and illness. The biopsychosocial systems model is an important advance beyond the biomedical model because it is more comprehensive and integrative in its approach to understanding the nature and determinants of illness and in its implications for treatment and prevention (Schwartz & Wiggins, 1986). It can also help to focus on common processes that may underlie different disorders.

Although many alcoholism researchers and treatment providers subscribe to a biopsychosocial model, relatively few have tried to implement it in practice. The social and environmental aspects of the model are just beginning to receive more emphasis in diagnostic assessment and treatment. For example, the American Psychiatric Association (APA, 1987) has developed a multiaxial diagnostic system, DSM-III-R, that includes a preliminary consideration of the role of psychosocial stressors in alcohol abuse as well as in other psychiatric and behavioral disorders. An evaluation paradigm should include information about such contextual factors and enable treatment providers to consider a patient's life situation when planning and evaluating treatment.

TRADITIONAL AND EXPANDED PARADIGMS FOR TREATMENT EVALUATION

An expanded paradigm of evaluation research is needed to help treatment evaluations probe and refine a biopsychosocial perspective. Such a paradigm should be able to suggest ways to influence the multiple physiological, psychological, and social factors that contribute to the development or maintenance of alcoholism. In this book, we outline some of the psychosocial aspects of such an approach and present the results of a long-term study of alcoholism treatment that has been guided by and contributed to this expanded paradigm.

The Traditional Evaluation Paradigm

Many studies have used a black-box paradigm, shown in Figure 1.1, to evaluate alcoholism treatment programs. Following this summative paradigm, evaluators assess clients at intake and at one or more follow-ups, but pay little attention to the process of treatment (the black box) or to

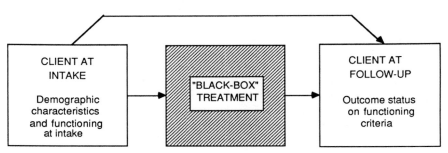

Figure 1.1 The "black-box" evaluation paradigm.

other factors that might affect the client. Such evaluations can gauge the overall outcome of a treatment program, but they reveal little about the process of treatment or about how to improve it.

Researchers who use this approach typically conclude that patients' social background and drinking history have a much stronger impact on outcome than treatment has. In fact, treatment outcome cannot be predicted very well, even by a combination of information about patients and global treatment variables. For example, Polich, Armor, and Braiker (1981) used a combination of patient and treatment-related factors in a 4-year follow-up of alcoholic patients and accounted for only about 4% of the variance in long-term abstinence and just over 9% in drinking problems.

Evaluations based on the black-box paradigm do not examine the influence of specific treatment components on outcome. Accordingly, such studies offer little information about how to make treatment more effective, in part because they do not adequately describe the treatment provided or the associations between specific treatment components and outcome. Instead, attention to treatment often is limited to a description of the treatment modality, the number of outpatient visits, or patients' length of stay in a facility. These studies fail to monitor patients' involvement in different aspects of treatment, the quality of the treatment program, the amount of support provided to patients, and so on.

Moreover, very few studies have considered the influence of factors outside of treatment, even though they may be the primary determinants of remission and relapse among alcoholic patients (Marlatt & Gordon, 1985; Orford, 1985). Stressful life circumstances and a lack of social resources can obscure the benefits of treatment, especially when treatment is brief and there is a long interval between the end of treatment and follow-up. For example, 6 hours of outpatient treatment may have some brief benefits for a client but, because such benefits can be undermined by ongoing life stressors or other factors, there is little reason to expect substantial effects 4 years after treatment. Stable life context factors and recent life changes exert a much stronger influence on posttreatment adaptation than treatment does.

In short, we have learned relatively little in prior evaluations about alcoholism or its treatment. Research using the black-box paradigm leaves many questions unanswered; for example, do patients who are exposed to a specific treatment component experience better outcome? Are patients who are more involved in treatment more likely to have better outcomes? What factors outside of treatment are associated with a positive outcome? Information on these issues provides a basis for improving treatment programs.

An Expanded Evaluation Paradigm

Dissatisfaction with earlier evaluation studies and the emergence of a biopsychosocial perspective are encouraging the use of a broader and more flexible research paradigm. Most important, there is growing recognition that program evaluation is more than just a technical enterprise in which research methods are applied to describe global program effects. Evaluation research can help to formulate conceptual issues; moreover, it produces its greatest yield when it is grounded in a conceptual framework that provides an explanation of how a program generates or fails to generate beneficial effects on patients (Chen & Rossi, 1983; Cronbach, 1982; Finney & Moos, 1989).

The expanded evaluation paradigm shown in Figure 1.2 suggests that the outcome of treatment (Panel V) is influenced by the client's resources prior to intake, including demographic factors, the severity and chronicity of alcohol abuse, and other aspects of functioning (Panel II). Treatment outcome is also influenced by life context factors prior to intake (Panel I) and those that occur during the treatment and posttreatment interval (Panel IV), as well as by the patient's treatment experiences (Panel III). In addition, the paradigm depicts both personal and life context factors (i.e., variables in Panels I and II) as determinants of entry into treatment and of the amount and type of treatment (Panel III).

This expanded paradigm reflects two current trends in program evaluation. First, it encourages the careful study of treatment, including an assessment of how well treatment is implemented and an examination of the associations between specific treatment components and outcome. Second, it explicitly considers factors outside of treatment and how they influence treatment entry, treatment experiences, and treatment outcome. The paradigm highlights the complexity of the treatment and rehabilitation process and puts an intervention program in context as one among many sets of factors that influence outcome. The paradigm is sufficiently broad that it can guide evaluations of pharmacological as well as psychosocial interventions or help to identify processes involved in recovery without treatment.

Program evaluations based on the expanded paradigm can produce valuable insights into the context, process, and outcome of treatment. These evaluations can help program planners to strengthen treatment,

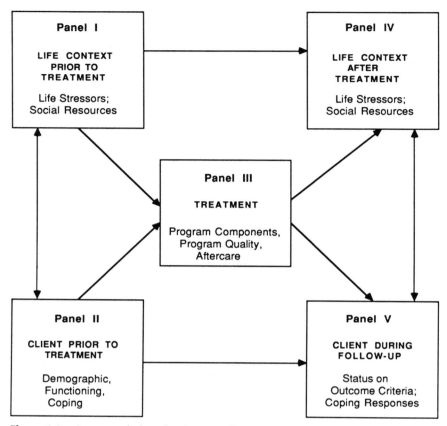

Figure 1.2 An expanded evaluation paradigm.

modify factors outside of treatment to the patient's advantage, and change how people think about alcoholism and its treatment.

STRESS AND COPING THEORY

In order to be more useful, an evaluation should be guided by theory. A biopsychosocial perspective provides a framework for thinking about broad domains or factors that foster and maintain alcohol abuse and for categorizing theories of etiology and relapse. With the exception of a few general systems theory principles (Schwartz, 1982), however, it provides little in the way of explanatory principles that can account for alcohol abuse. It is a perspective rather than a theory (Kissin & Hanson, 1982).

Our research is based on a subset of psychosocial concepts within the biopsychosocial perspective; these concepts are derived from stress and coping theory. The theory posits that adaptation is influenced by the environmental conditions to which a person is exposed, by whether these conditions are appraised as stressors and, if so, by a person's initial reaction to the situation, such as deciding whether it is a challenge or a threat. Adaptation also depends on the personal and social resources available to manage stressors (Lazarus & Folkman, 1984). Although psychosocial stressors are risk factors for alcohol abuse, they do not necessarily foreshadow problem drinking or a decline in functioning. Because stressors are ubiquitous, all people necessarily face situations that can induce problem drinking; their appraisal of the circumstances and their personal and social resources determine whether stressors lead to alcohol abuse.

Alcohol has long been thought of as an effective drug for reducing tension or distress. The Old Testament offers specific prescriptions depending on the severity of psychological distress: "Give strong drink to the desperate and wine to the embittered; such men will drink and forget their poverty and remember their trouble no more" (Prov. 31:6–7). When people today are asked why they drink alcoholic beverages, they often focus on how alcohol helps to reduce stress and forget worries. It is not surprising, therefore, that stressful conditions are often seen as a primary cause of alcoholism. Mulford's (1984) view is typical:

> The developing alcoholic readily learns that alcohol relieves the anxiety and tension of a particular situation, e.g., asking a girl to dance with him. . . . He uses alcohol to cope with an unsatisfactory self-concept and an unpleasant (symbolic) environment, to forget his problems, to get along better with others, etc. He increasingly relies upon alcohol to escape from the everyday problems of living, or for relief from the anxiety and tension they bring until, in a vicious circle, the "morning after" anxiety and guilt only serve to trigger another day of drinking. (p. 37)

Stressors may also play a role in relapse after a period of remission. Relapse is often associated with one of three types of high-risk conditions: negative emotional states, interpersonal conflict, and social pressures. The presence of chronic stressors can make people more vulnerable to these conditions and more likely to resume drinking (Marlatt & Gordon, 1985).

The relationship between stressors and alcohol abuse is complex, however. Many people who experience difficult life circumstances do not turn to or slip back into excessive drinking. In some cases, stressful events motivate an alcoholic to stop drinking. Thus, we need to consider personal and social resources and how they can counteract the potentially negative influence of stressors. In this study, we examine social resources, such as supportive family and work settings, as well as personal resources, such as coping responses, that may protect people from relapse in the face of stressors.

In general, stress and coping theory is consistent with theories that emphasize more specific sets of causal factors in alcohol abuse, such as lack of interpersonal and behavioral skills and maladaptive cognitive and self-regulatory processes (Hull, 1981; Marlatt & Gordon, 1985). However, interpersonal and behavioral theories tend to highlight relatively enduring characteristics of individuals, and cognitive and self-regulatory models typically focus on general and relatively stable patterns of attribution and self-control. In contrast, stress and coping theory concentrates on the environmental precursors of mood and behavior and conceptualizes appraisal and coping responses as somewhat situation-specific ways of managing stressful situations. Stress and coping theory is a dynamic perspective that emphasizes ongoing change and maturation in personal and environmental factors and the current forces that affect an individual's adaptation.

The expanded evaluation paradigm and stress and coping theory have broad applicability. We use them here to analyze the process of treatment and other determinants of outcome. We also use the stress and coping approach to focus on how spouses and children adapt to the stressors involved in living with an alcoholic family member. In addition, stress and coping theory can be used to study remission and relapse among alcoholics who do not receive treatment and to study other types of substance abusers (Orford, 1985) as well as other disorders, such as depression (Moos, in press), whether treated or not.

THE BOOK IN BRIEF

The book is divided into four parts. Part I describes an evaluation of alcoholism treatment. It demonstrates important methods of evaluating the implementation and impact of such programs and their components. In Chapter 2, we describe our research objectives and the five residential treatment programs that participated in our study. These programs comprise diverse treatment approaches, ranging from a Salvation Army center to a for-profit aversion conditioning program. The patients treated at these facilities were correspondingly diverse, varying from skid-row men to middle-class and upper-middle-class men and women. After describing the programs, we summarize the characteristics of the primary sample of over 400 patients whom we followed 6 months after treatment. We then focus on how well treatment was implemented. We review methods of assessing treatment implementation and emphasize the value of tapping both the quantity and quality of treatment.

In Chapter 3, we examine how functioning changes from intake to 6-month follow-up, how different outcome criteria are related to each other, and how intake characteristics help predict short-term outcome. We also address whether outcome for patients who are more easily followed differs from outcome for more difficult to follow patients. Chapter 4 compares the relative effectiveness of the five programs and the effects of different treatment components. Then, using one part of the expanded framework, we consider the independent and combined effects on outcome of several sets of variables, including the patient's social background and symptoms at intake, the type of treatment program, treatment components, the intensity of treatment, and the quality of the program environment. Chapter 5 examines the impact of gender and marital status on treatment and outcome. We compare married and unmarried men and women on drinking history, symptoms at intake, treatment and aftercare experiences, and posttreatment functioning.

Part II examines contextual factors, such as stressful life circumstances and social resources, and their links to treatment outcome. We focus primarily on a subgroup of married patients followed 6 months, 2 years, and 10 years after the end of treatment. In Chapter 6, we present a rationale for examining the influence of life stressors, social resources, and coping responses on the development and course of alcoholism and describe methods for assessing them. We also describe new procedures to evaluate patients' family and work settings and their contribution to treatment outcome. In Chapter 7, we relate life stressors, social resources, and coping responses to treatment outcome among the subsample of persons who returned to their families following treatment. Using the expanded paradigm, we examine how treatment and life context affect outcome. In Chapter 8, we examine whether remitted alcoholics function as well as community controls and whether remitted alcoholics have especially positive life contexts. In addition, we identify the extent to which relapsed patients function more poorly than remitted patients and community controls in areas other than drinking.

Part III focuses on the family. We analyze the impact of alcoholism on patients' spouses in Chapter 9 and on children in Chapter 10. We compare their functioning with that of their counterparts in a community control group. Using a stress and coping framework, we integrate prior research on spouses and children of alcoholics and provide a more complete account of their adaptation than is afforded by focusing solely on the effects of the alcoholic partner's drinking.

Part IV considers practical applications, especially how to improve settings and implications for alcoholism treatment and evaluation research. Chapter 11 focuses on monitoring and improving treatment programs and work and family settings. Chapter 12 concentrates on implications for treatment and for program evaluation. After we summarize our findings and their implications for the diagnosis and treatment of alcohol problems, we describe the role of theory in the expanded paradigm as well as the implications of the paradigm for methodological issues and for studying patient-treatment matching. Overall, we hope to show how evaluations guided by an expanded paradigm can stimulate more effective interventions for more appropriate conceptualizations of alcohol abuse.

I
A SYSTEMS EVALUATION OF ALCOHOLISM TREATMENT

2
Objectives, Methods, and Assessment of Treatment Implementation

The application of the conceptual model guiding any evaluation is specific to the programs studied, the treatment applied, the measurement of relevant variables, and the setting in which the research takes place. In this chapter, we describe our research methods, including the residential programs we studied and the patients in these programs, the measures we used, and our data collection procedures. Then we take the first step in program evaluation: checking the implementation of the treatment programs to assure that each is a good example of the intended intervention.

RESEARCH OBJECTIVES AND METHODS

As described in Chapter 1, our study had many objectives. We wanted to learn more about:

> How residential programs differ in the treatment they provide (Chapters 2 and 3).
> What kinds of people each program serves (Chapters 2 and 4).
> How patient characteristics are related to treatment outcome (Chapters 3 and 4).
> The process of treatment and how treatment components are associated with outcome (Chapter 4).
> The relative effectiveness of different programs (Chapter 4).
> The role of gender and marital status at intake, in treatment, and at follow-up (Chapter 5).
> The influence of factors outside of treatment on remission and relapse (Chapters 6, 7, and 8).

How the patients' alcoholism affects their spouses and children (Chapters 9 and 10).

To study this array of issues, we sought diverse information from a large number of individuals and used a naturalistic longitudinal design; in effect, we followed Cronbach's (1982) maxim that research design should be determined by function, not form.

The expanded evaluation paradigm we discussed in Chapter 1 focuses special attention on treatment experiences and life context factors. Our project was divided into two phases, corresponding to these two areas of interest. Phase I examined the treatment experiences and short-term outcome of 505 alcoholic patients entering one of five treatment programs. We followed 429 of these patients 6 to 8 months after they left treatment.

Phase II concentrated on the life contexts and long-term functioning of 113 of the patients who returned to their families after treatment. We followed these patients and their spouses 6 months, 2 years, and 10 years after treatment. We also studied a demographically matched sample of families that did not have members with a drinking problem; we studied this comparison group over a similar interval. Here we describe the programs, participants, measures, and data collection procedures for Phase I; Chapter 6 provides more details about the family samples and the procedures used in Phase II.

Treatment Programs

The five treatment programs in our study represent the diversity of residential treatment approaches. Three of the programs were nonprofit organizations and two were privately operated, for profit programs. All five programs were located on the West Coast of the United States.

Typical of virtually all residential alcoholism treatment programs, each of our five programs offered a range of therapeutic components such as alcoholism education, individual and group counseling, and on-site Alcoholics Anonymous (AA) meetings. However, the programs differed in the emphasis they put on each component. In addition, some components, such as aversion conditioning and vocational rehabilitation, were specific to some programs.

As Mandell (1979) observed, funding sources and accreditation standards have created "a two-tiered system of [alcoholism] treatment" (p. 320) and a corresponding "social-class bifurcation among the patient populations of treatment agencies" (p. 329). The continued existence of the two tiers is documented by Yahr's (1988) more recent analyses. We studied programs from both tiers. We included three nonprofit programs. A Salvation Army center emphasized educational lectures, films on alcoholism, and part-time jobs. A public, city- and county-funded, hospital-based program provided milieu and group treatment, outpatient services, and vocational rehabilitation. A long-term halfway house offered a therapeutic community orientation in which residents shared household chores and maintained outside jobs.

The two other programs were private, for-profit facilities; these relied exclusively on patient fees, in most cases paid by third parties such as insurance companies. One offered a milieu-oriented program of community, group, and family treatment; the other provided an intensive program of aversion conditioning followed by intermittent outpatient treatment. The following descriptions of each program are based on reports from the program administrators and staff and from preliminary implementation assessments.

Salvation Army Program

The Salvation Army program was a 65-bed treatment center located in an urban skid-row district. Unlike the other programs, the Salvation Army's program was for men only. The center had been in operation for 25 years.

It offered a long-term recovery program that emphasized a milieu orientation, including community meetings, weekly therapy groups, educational lectures and films, AA and fellowship meetings, Sunday worship services, recreational activities, and monthly individual counseling sessions and progress evaluations. The program housed a vocational rehabilitation school that offered training in printing and electronics; residents were regularly placed in part-time jobs in the community. Volunteer house chores were an integral part of the treatment milieu. Residents were expected to pay for the services they received to the extent they could.

The center's staff included a director, five counselors, a psychologist, a part-time psychiatrist, and three vocational counselors. Almost all staff members were men, and 80% held college degrees.

Hospital-Based Program

The second program was a 45-bed, city- and county-funded, public hospital-based facility that had been in operation in a metropolitan area for 4 years. It offered milieu and group treatment during a 4-week program. Antianxiety medications and sedatives were prescribed frequently. The program consisted of daily community meetings, small counseling groups composed of 10 residents and two staff members, AA meetings, films and lectures on alcoholism, and recreational, crafts, and physical activities. The inpatient services were supplemented by outpatient services, a vocational rehabilitation program, and an active volunteer alumni association. Staff consisted of an administrator, 15 to 20 counselors, four nurses, and a rehabilitation counselor.

Halfway House Program

The third program was a halfway house that received some county funds and was located in a residential area of a small city. At the time of our initial contact, this program was a newly established 16-bed, long-term recovery home. Later on, its capacity was increased to 27 beds. It was the only halfway house for alcoholics in the county.

The program had a therapeutic community orientation and offered various types of therapy groups and activities, house meetings, individual counseling, films and lectures on alcoholism, and recreational activities such as exercise and arts and crafts. Tranquilizing medications were not used. The program emphasized each patient's personal responsibility for recovery; consequently, treatment schedules were highly individualized. Residents contributed financially toward the upkeep of the house from their earnings from jobs held in the community.

Staff consisted of two administrators, a program director, two psychiatric counselors, and several part-time group leaders. When the study began, all but one of the staff members were men, and none had extensive prior work experience with alcoholism treatment.

Aversion Conditioning Program

The first of the two private, for-profit programs was a 24-bed aversion conditioning program that had been offering alcoholism treatment for more than 20 years. It was located in a residential community.

This program featured an intensive 2-week program of aversion conditioning sessions in which nausea, induced by Emetine, was paired with various aspects of drinking behavior. In the year following the initial treatment episode, patients received up to seven reinforcement sessions. Patients were routinely administered sedatives and anticonvulsive and antianxiety medications as well as vitamins. There was no formal individual or family-centered psychotherapy, although one weekly group therapy session and two AA meetings were scheduled.

The staff consisted of an administrator and a counselor, both of whom were recovered alcoholics; there were also five full-time nurses and aides and four physician consultants. Most staff members had over 5 years experience in alcoholism treatment.

Milieu-Oriented Program

Located in a rural area, the fifth program was a private, 20-bed facility that provided a 4-week, milieu-oriented program of alcoholism treatment. It had been operating for over 3 years at the time the study began.

The program included community meetings, therapy groups, comprehensive and practical lectures on alcoholism, AA meetings, and recreational activities. A patient government had been established, and longer-term patients helped new arrivals adjust to the facility. A lively, family atmosphere permeated the patient and staff community. Vitamins, antianxiety drugs, and sedatives were frequently prescribed. The staff included two administrators, a medical director, two counselors, a part-time social worker, five nurses, and a recreational counselor.

Participants

The patients in the five treatment programs clearly differed in demographic characteristics and drinking history. Table 2.1 summarizes the data on the Phase I sample of 429 individuals who were followed 6 to 8 months after treatment.

In general, the sample was composed predominantly of men, although about 25% of the patients in the halfway house, aversion conditioning, and milieu-oriented programs were women. Differences between the populations of the two for-profit programs—aversion conditioning and milieu oriented—and the three nonprofit programs are striking evidence of the social class distinction that Mandell (1979) identified and Yahr (1988) confirmed. Compared with patients in the nonprofit programs, patients in the for-profit programs were more socially stable: they were more likely to be married, own their homes, live at the same residence for more than 4 years, and be employed for at least 2 of the past 3 years. In addition, patients in the for-profit programs had higher incomes and more prestigious occupations and were more likely to be college graduates.

Table 2.1 Demographic characteristics and drinking history of patients at the five residential programs prior to treatment (expressed in percentages)

	Nonprofit			For profit	
	Salvation Army ($N = 97$)	Hospital based ($N = 106$)	Halfway house ($N = 59$)	Aversion conditioning ($N = 75$)	Milieu oriented ($N = 92$)
Male	100.0	89.6	74.6	72.0	75.0
Caucasian	93.8	74.5	86.2	94.7	92.3
Married	9.3	16.0	10.2	72.0	71.7
Over age 50	30.9	25.5	25.4	52.7	43.5
College graduate	8.2	15.1	13.6	21.3	27.2
Income less than $3000 past year	67.0	55.8	64.4	3.9	5.7
Own home	1.0	4.8	5.4	71.8	67.4
Same residence for past 4 years	8.2	12.3	6.8	56.0	51.1
Low occupational prestige (Hollingshead index 6-7)	55.3	28.4	33.4	14.3	10.7
Worked at least 24 of past 36 months	38.6	51.7	30.6	87.5	87.3
Prior residential treatment for alcoholism	73.2	59.4	64.4	29.3	33.7
Recognized drinking as a problem after the age of 35	39.2	33.0	22.0	64.0	66.3

Patients in the aversion conditioning and milieu-oriented programs were less likely to have had alcoholism treatment in the past, even though they were older than the nonprofit program patients. As expected, the patients at the two for-profit programs reported that their drinking problem began later in life.

In short, there was a clear difference in social competence, as measured by demographic characteristics and functioning at intake, between patients in for-profit and nonprofit programs. Moreover, patients in for-profit programs sought treatment before their drinking increased and their functioning diminished to levels more typical of patients in the nonprofit programs (Fitzgerald & Mulford, 1981; Mendelson et al., 1982). In Chapter 3, we examine the differences in drinking and psychosocial functioning among the patients in the five programs at intake and, in Chapter 4, we examine how these factors and specific treatment components affect treatment outcome.

Measures and Data Collection Procedures

We obtained data on patient experiences before, during, and 6 to 8 months after treatment.

Pretreatment Measures

Patients were given the Background Information Form (BIF) shortly after admission. The BIF is a structured inventory that can be completed in about 30 minutes. It assesses demographic characteristics, drinking behavior (alcohol consumption and abstinence), physical symptoms (such as indigestion and dry heaves or cold sweats), and psychosocial functioning (depression, social activities, and occupational functioning). In addition, the BIF includes questions about prior treatment for alcoholism. Demographic characteristics and drinking history, as recorded on the BIF, are shown in Table 2.1. An adaptation of the BIF—the Follow-Up Information form (FIF)—was used later to assess outcome. [For copies of these forms, see Moos (1985b).]

Treatment Measures

We designed the Treatment Experiences Form (TEF) to record the quantity of treatment, including patient attendance at program meetings, counseling sessions, and other treatment components, and to document the medications received. At the end of treatment, a staff member summarized this information on a TEF. The TEF has 13 categories of treatment experiences, some of which were not relevant to each program. The categories covered patient attendance at psychotherapy sessions (individual, group, and family), AA meetings, lectures and films on alcoholism, house meetings, recreational activities (arts and crafts, exercise sessions) and, for people in the Salvation Army program, attendance at Sunday worship services and participation in part-time jobs. The TEF also monitored the use of antianxiety medications, sedatives, vitamins, and Antabuse (disulfiram), as well as the number of days the patient was in the program.

We used the Community-Oriented Programs Environment Scale (COPES; Moos, 1988a) to obtain data on patients' and staff members' perceptions of the quality of the treatment environment in each program. The COPES assesses relationship, treatment goal, and system maintenance dimensions of treatment settings. Patients completed the COPES after they had been in treatment long enough (usually 2 to 3 weeks) to become familiar with the program.

Posttreatment Measures

About 6 months after each patient's discharge from treatment, we tried to contact and have the patient complete the FIF, which we used to measure treatment outcome. The FIF includes all the items from the BIF, reworded to cover the period from discharge to follow-up, and an item on abstinence since discharge. The FIF was introduced by a statement reminding each patient of his or her stay in one of the treatment programs, the date treatment ended, the permission secured to recontact the individual, and the independence of the research from the treatment program.

During the process of locating patients and obtaining follow-up information, we kept detailed records on every mail, telephone, or in-person attempt to contact patients (see Chapter 4). We were able to locate and recruit 87% (429 out of 494) of the patients who were still living. The follow-up rates for the five programs varied from 80% for the Salvation Army center to 95% for the halfway house. The initial follow-up took place in virtually all cases between 6 and 8 months after the end of residential treatment.

The Accuracy of Alcoholic Patients' Self-Reports

Although many clinicians and some researchers have expressed reservations about the accuracy of self-report data from alcoholic patients, reviews of the research literature on this topic suggest that, given certain conditions, self-report data are both reliable and valid. For example, Babor and his colleagues (1987) reviewed 17 studies of the test-retest reliability of self-report measures in a variety of groups ranging from adolescents to alcoholic inpatients. Overall, these studies demonstrate acceptable levels of test-retest reliability for many different measures of self-report drinking and alcohol-related behavior. Test-retest reliability estimates for measures of alcoholism severity were high in various samples of alcoholics.

In estimating the validity of self-reports of alcohol use, misuse, and related problems, the most common approach has been to relate self-report data to some criterion—often spouses' or friends' reports of the respondents' behaviors. Although there was some variation associated with patient population and the specific behavior measures, Babor and his colleagues (1987) concluded that all of the studies they reviewed found moderate to good, statistically significant positive correlations. The lack of correspondence that was observed was not due to consistent underreporting by patients—that is, collaterals' reports of patients' alcohol consumption or problems were lower, as well as higher, than the patients' estimates. The correspondence between inpatients' and collaterals' reports was as high for posttreatment alcohol use indices as it was for pretreatment measures. Moreover, Verinis (1983a) found high agreement between patients and collaterals, even when the patients had not been informed that collaterals would be contacted.

We gathered our data under a guarantee of confidentiality, and we were not associated with any of the treatment programs. Also, many of our variables were assessed by multiple items. These conditions are associated with more accurate responses to alcohol use, misuse, and drinking-related adverse consequence questions (Babor et al., 1987; Skinner, 1981a). We note in Chapter 7 that there is a significant and substantial relationship between patient relapse/remission status (obtained from patients' reports of drinking behavior and drinking problems) and spouse reports of whether they had to deal with an alcohol or drug problem in the family during the past year.

We also calculated correlations and t tests on data from our 2-year and 10-year follow-ups to examine the correspondence between alcoholic patients' reports and those of their spouses. Where it was possible to evaluate an environmental factor shared by another person, such as the family milieu, we found significant agreement between the alcoholic patients' and the spouses' reports. The degree of agreement between patients and their spouses was comparable to that shown by the community controls and their spouses. In addition, alcoholic patients did not describe their environments as more stressful or less supportive than did their nonalcoholic spouses. Overall, these findings support the validity of our patient self-report data.

Research Design

Many investigators believe that the basic design of a treatment research project should be an experiment, with persons randomly assigned to varying treatment and/or control conditions. Their belief rests on the assumption that the main objective of such studies is to estimate the effects of treatment. Indeed, the power of experimental designs is focused on rigorously answering the question: How effective is treatment, on average? To use Cronbach's (1982) terminology, experimental designs generally have high "fidelity" but little "bandwidth."

As outlined at the beginning of this chapter, however, we had a broad research agenda. We were interested in a number of questions about the process and context of alcoholism treatment, as well as factors outside of treatment that influence the course of treated alcoholism. Consequently,

OBJECTIVES, METHODS, AND ASSESSMENT

we opted to use a naturalistic design in order to study these processes as they occurred in real-life settings. In our analyses, however, we try to strike a balance between bandwidth and fidelity. We discuss these issues in more detail in Chapter 12. Regardless of whether a study has an experimental or naturalistic design, it should document that treatment was well implemented—a topic to which we now turn.

ASSESSING TREATMENT IMPLEMENTATION

No treatment is so direct or obvious that a researcher should take its implementation for granted. A striking case in point is subcutaneous implants of disulfiram (Antabuse)—a technique used in some countries, but not in the United States. Although it is tempting to assume that surgical implantation exemplifies an implemented treatment, Malcolm, Madden, and Williams (1974) checked blood samples for evidence of disulfiram within one week of implantation and found only 8 of 31 samples were positive. In another study, 30 minutes after 11 chronic alcoholics with disulfiram implants drank alcohol, samples of their blood were tested, and the investigators found no evidence of the expected aldehyde dehydrogenase inhibition and acetaldehyde increase (Bergstrom, Ohlin, Lindblom, & Wadstein, 1982).

Behavioral and psychological treatments may also not be implemented adequately. Sanchez-Craig and Walker (1982) compared halfway house residents who were taught a five-step problem-solving process with groups of residents who experienced only covert sensitization (patients were asked to visualize six alcohol-related scenes, such as drinking in a bar, and pair them with aversive outcomes) or problem-focused discussion. Because problem-solving skills were taught to criterion during treatment (i.e., all patients could list the five skills), there was no variation in implementation of that level across individuals. One month after training, however, only 2 of 15 residents were able to remember all five problem-solving steps. Not surprisingly, the specially trained residents showed no better treatment outcome than the other groups. In another example, Elkins (1980) reported that less than half of the patients who were exposed to covert sensitization (verbal aversion) actually developed conditioned nausea.

A study of how treatment is actually implemented is a prerequisite to evaluating treatment outcome, improving programs, and developing innovative treatment approaches. According to Yeaton and Sechrest (1981), an assessment of treatment implementation should include both the program's strength—"the a priori likelihood that the treatment could have the intended outcome" (p. 156)—and its integrity—"the degree to which treatment is delivered as intended" (p. 160).

Many programs are ineffective because they are not adequately implemented; an implementation check helps researchers avoid evaluating a poor example of the intended intervention. An assessment of treatment strength and integrity makes it possible to gauge prognosis on the basis of information about treatment as well as information about patients. It highlights logical fallacies in the standard pessimistic interpretation of alcoholism program evaluations. A few sessions of outpatient treatment may have a short-term positive influence on an alcoholic patient, but they probably are not strong enough to exert a measurable impact 4 years later (Polich et al., 1981).

Assessing treatment implementation is the first step in illuminating the black box and in carefully studying the treatment process itself. Here we discuss several methods and criteria for assessing treatment implementation. Then we present results of our assessment of the five residential alcoholism treatment programs.

Methods of Evaluating Treatment Implementation

To find out how well a program is implemented, an evaluator must measure the actual program against a standard of what the program should be. Sechrest and his colleagues (1979) identified three sources of information that can be used to define a standard for program implementation evaluation: normative data on conditions in other programs, which allow the evaluator to see how one program compares with others; specifications of an ideal treatment program; and theoretical analyses or expert judgment.

Our implementation assessment criteria were based primarily on normative data from other programs. We also discuss ideal standards briefly here and in more detail in Chapter 11 and consider theory-based standards in Chapter 12.

Assessing Implementation of the Five Programs

To assess treatment implementation in the five programs, we measured both the quantity and quality of program activity. We assessed the quantity of treatment experiences with the TEF, on which the treatment experiences of each patient were recorded; these included the number of therapy sessions attended, the types of medications received, and so on.

Whereas information on treatment components indicates the quantity of treatment activities, treatment "quality" refers to the manner in which such activities are carried out. To assess treatment quality, we used the COPES (Moos, 1988a), a measure of the social climate in each program.

Treatment Quantity

Table 2.2 shows the average quantity of treatment to which patients were exposed in each of the five programs. In general, these data are consistent with the program descriptions presented earlier, which were based on re-

OBJECTIVES, METHODS, AND ASSESSMENT

Table 2.2 Mean treatment experiences for patients in each of the five residential treatment programs

	Nonprofit			For profit	
Treatment variable	Salvation Army (N = 97)	Hospital based (N = 106)	Halfway house (N = 59)	Aversion conditioning (N = 75)	Milieu oriented (N = 92)
TREATMENT DURATION					
Length of stay in days	95.2	29.2	101.5	14.2	29.9
	(78.7)	(8.6)	(79.3)	(2.3)	(7.0)
THERAPEUTIC COMPONENTS					
Individual/group therapy sessions	10.4	12.3	10.9	0.5	17.0
	(9.8)	(7.7)	(9.8)	(1.0)	(4.5)
AA meetings	2.2	1.6	4.7	0.5	11.6
	(5.6)	(2.8)	(5.5)	(0.8)	(2.2)
Lectures/films on alcoholism	11.4	9.7	9.6	0.7	29.2
	(9.8)	(7.7)	(10.4)	(0.8)	(7.0)
House meetings	11.7	13.0	37.3	0.0	0.0
	(9.8)	(8.6)	(33.7)		
Recreational activities (arts and crafts, exercise)	0.7	4.4	5.2	0.0	25.9
	(3.4)	(7.1)	(6.7)		(10.9)
Worship/Spiritual meetings	11.1	0.0	0.0	0.0	0.0
	(10.4)				
MEDICATIONS					
Antianxiety medications (% yes)	6.2	71.7	0.0	90.7	90.2
Sedatives (% yes)	3.1	88.7	0.0	96.0	81.5
Antabuse (% yes)	1.0	24.5	0.0	0.0	44.6

Note. Standard deviations are given in parentheses.

ports from the program administrators and staff and from preliminary evaluability analyses.

These data confirm that we had selected a set of active treatment programs, although there was also variation across programs in intensity of treatment. For example, patients in all programs, except the aversion conditioning program, stayed in the program for an average of a month or longer; in the Salvation Army center and halfway house, they stayed over 3 months. The longer stay is comparable to normative data on conditions in other successful programs; in two groups of programs in which patients had highly successful outcomes at 1- and 2-year follow-ups, the median stay was about 6 to 8 weeks (Costello, 1975a, 1975b). The length of stay in the five programs we studied substantially exceeds the average of 1 week for patients in a group of publicly funded, inpatient alcoholism treatment centers (Polich et al., 1981).

Longer treatment by itself does not necessarily indicate intensive treatment. When we examined patient participation in various treatment components, we found that patients in the milieu-oriented program participated in more therapy sessions, AA meetings, lectures and films on alcoholism, and recreational activities during an average 30-day stay than did clients in the Salvation Army and halfway house programs during average stays of over 3 months. Patients in the aversion conditioning program received relatively little psychosocial treatment; instead, their treatment relied heavily on reinforcement sessions in which drinking was paired with nausea.

The programs varied in their use of medications. Antianxiety drugs and sedatives were used extensively in three programs—the public hospital-based unit and the two for-profit facilities, the aversion conditioning and milieu-oriented programs. About 25% of the public hospital patients and 45% of the milieu-oriented program patients received orally administered Antabuse; this drug was used sparingly, if at all, in the other programs.

Our programs also fared well when compared with a second implementation standard—conceptions of an ideal program. When asked about the treatment components they prefer, patients generally consider individual and group therapy, educational films, and lectures on alcoholism as more valuable treatment components; they report that time-structuring or maintenance activities such as work and manual arts therapy, morning exercise, and art classes are less helpful (Brissett, Laundergan, & Kammeier, 1981; Costello, Baillargeon, & Tiller, 1979; Rollnick, 1982).

Among our programs, only the milieu-oriented facility offered extensive time-structuring and maintenance activities. However, these were offset by an intensive schedule of therapy sessions, AA meetings, films, and lectures. Thus, as measured against patient preferences, our five programs also seem to be well implemented.

Treatment Quality

To measure treatment quality, we evaluated the social context of each treatment program. We used the COPES, which taps 10 dimensions of the treatment environments of psychiatric programs. Social climate scales have been used to assess the quality of social environment of a diversity of psychiatric and substance abuse treatment programs. Such scales have also been used to evaluate other types of intervention programs, such as rehabilitation centers, correctional facilities, and educational settings (Moos, 1987b).

In brief, the 10 COPES subscales have moderate to high internal consistency, are moderately interrelated, and all significantly discriminate among programs. Normative and psychometric information about the COPES is presented elsewhere (Moos, 1974, 1988a).

The 10 subscales, shown in Table 2.3, assess three sets of dimensions: relationship, personal growth or goal orientation, and system maintenance.

The *relationship* dimensions are measured by the involvement, sup-

OBJECTIVES, METHODS, AND ASSESSMENT

Table 2.3 COPES subscales and dimension descriptions

RELATIONSHIP DIMENSIONS

1. Involvement   How active members are in the day-to-day functioning of their program
2. Support   How much members help and support each other; how supportive the staff is toward members
3. Spontaneity   How much the program encourages the open expression of feelings by members and staff

PERSONAL GROWTH DIMENSIONS

4. Autonomy   How self-sufficient and independent members are in making their own decisions and how much they are encouraged to take leadership in the program
5. Practical orientation   The degree to which members learn practical skills and are prepared for release from the program
6. Personal problem orientation   The extent to which members are encouraged to understand their feelings and personal problems
7. Anger and aggression   How much members argue with other members and staff, become openly angry, and display other aggressive behavior

SYSTEM MAINTENANCE DIMENSIONS

8. Order and organization   How important order and organization are in the program
9. Program clarity   The extent to which members know what to expect in the day-to-day routine of the program and the explicitness of program rules and procedures
10. Staff control   The extent to which the staff use measures to keep members under necessary controls

---

port, and spontaneity subscales. These three subscales tap how involved patients are in the program, how much staff support patients and patients support each other, and the amount of openness and expressiveness in the program.

Personal growth or *goal orientation* dimensions are tapped by the autonomy, practical orientation, personal problem orientation, and anger and aggression subscales. Autonomy assesses how much patients are encouraged to be self-sufficient and independent. Practical orientation reflects the emphasis on practical living and job skills and preparation for leaving the program, while personal problem orientation taps how much the program seeks to increase patients' self-understanding and insight. Anger and aggression assesses how much staff encourage patients to express their angry feelings openly.

System maintenance dimensions include order and organization, program clarity, and staff control. These dimensions measure the extent to which the program functions in an orderly, clear, organized, and coherent way.

Average raw scores on the COPES dimensions are converted to standard scores (mean = 50; standard deviation = 10) so they can be compared to normative data from a sample of 54 community-oriented psychiatric treatment programs (Moos, 1988a).

The Salvation Army and Hospital-Based Programs

Figure 2.1 shows the COPES profiles for patients in the Salvation Army and hospital-based programs. Although the patients in these two programs were similar, the treatment environments were quite different. Patients in both programs saw involvement and spontaneity as above average compared with normative data (horizontal dashed line in Figure 2.1). Salvation Army patients reported more involvement than hospital-based patients did. Patients in the Salvation Army program also reported above average emphasis on support, while hospital-based patients did not.

With respect to treatment orientation, patients in both programs appraised independence, concern about personal problems, and the open expression of anger as somewhat above the norm. Salvation Army patients were strongly encouraged to develop practical skills to assist them to adapt to life in the community, but the emphasis on this area was somewhat below average in the hospital-based program.

There were some differences in the perceived structure of the programs. Salvation Army clients saw their program as clear and well organized, whereas this was not true in the hospital-based program. This latter finding is consistent with the constant rescheduling of activities and meetings that we observed in the hospital-based program. Patients in both programs saw staff control as about average.

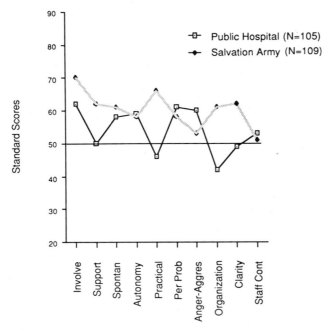

Figure 2.1 COPES profiles for the Salvation Army and public hospital programs.

OBJECTIVES, METHODS, AND ASSESSMENT

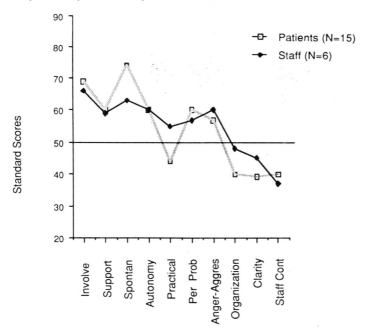

Figure 2.2 COPES profiles for the halfway house program.

Overall, there are some sharp contrasts between these two programs. The Salvation Army program encouraged clients and staff to interact with and support one another. The program emphasized community living skills as exemplified by its training school and the importance given to learning vocational skills. The Salvation Army program was also well organized and clear in its expectations. In contrast, the hospital-based program was just average on support and was below average on practical orientation and organization. These data show that the social climate of a treatment program can be influenced by factors other than the composition of its patient population.

The Halfway House Program

When the COPES was first administered to residents and staff of the halfway house program, it was a newly established, 16-bed, long-term recovery home. Residents and staff had very similar perceptions of it, as shown in Figure 2.2. Both groups saw strong emphasis on the relationship dimensions, especially involvement and spontaneity, and above average emphasis on independence, concern about personal problems, and the open expression of anger. Staff reported somewhat above average emphasis on practical orientation, but patients disagreed. However, staff and patients agreed that organization, clarity, and staff control were below average.

Overall, staff and patients portray a program that is quite well implemented in the relationship and goal orientation domains. On the other hand, the low scores on the system maintenance dimensions reflect partial implementation in this area, perhaps because of the newness of the program. When the program was reassessed 7 months later, the emphasis on the system maintenance dimensions had risen substantially (see Chapter 11).

The Aversion Conditioning Program

Figure 2.3 shows the COPES profiles for the aversion conditioning program. Patients and staff agreed closely in their perceptions of the treatment milieu. Both groups reported high support and spontaneity but little autonomy, which is consistent with the structured schedule patients followed during their 2-week stay. Although there was little concern with a practical orientation or the expression of anger, patients were encouraged to try to understand their personal problems.

The structured treatment schedule is reflected in the emphasis on organization and clarity. At the same time, there was little reliance on staff control. Thus, the aversion conditioning program was highly structured, but nevertheless encouraged patients to feel involved and to share their personal problems.

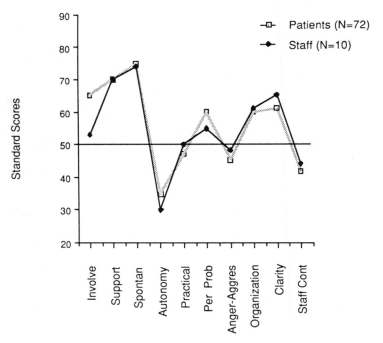

Figure 2.3 COPES profiles for the aversion conditioning program.

OBJECTIVES, METHODS, AND ASSESSMENT

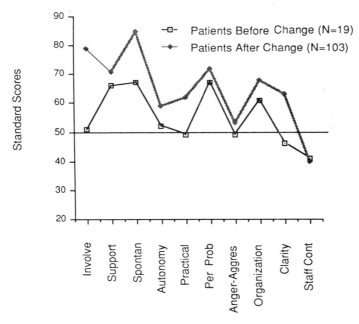

Figure 2.4 COPES profiles for the milieu-oriented program.

The Milieu-Oriented Program

As part of the implementation analysis, we obtained COPES data from a sample of patients and staff in each program to provide initial feedback and elicit cooperation in the evaluation. At that time, the milieu-oriented program was about to undergo a series of changes. This program initially had relied on films and lectures to reeducate alcoholics. Patients spent a great deal of time in their rooms, wore pajamas all day, and had their meals brought to their rooms. Although patients socialized informally, group therapy sessions were not included in the treatment regimen.

Concurrent with the beginning of our project, the program hired a new director who established a therapeutic milieu and family-type atmosphere. Television sets were removed from patients' rooms, and family-style meals were served in the dining room. Patients stopped wearing pajamas during the day, were assigned light housekeeping duties, began running their own film and discussion sessions, and gave personal care and attention to incoming patients. Several types of group treatment were initiated. An alumni organization was started by an active group of recovered graduates of the program to help current patients plan for their life after discharge.

Figure 2.4 shows COPES profiles based on patient data before and after these changes. On the whole, patients were more positive about the program after the changes were made. Patients' involvement increased dramatically, probably because of the new director's effort to get patients invested in program activities. The alumni's efforts to explain the value of the program are reflected in heightened practical orientation and program clarity. Thus, the COPES profiles clearly reflected the changes instituted by the new director. Moreover, the breadth of the innovations was shown by a positive change in 9 of the 10 dimensions.

Comparing the Programs

The COPES profiles, which distinguish the five programs in ways that are consistent with their treatment orientations, complement the information on treatment quantity. For example, they show that required participation in treatment activities does not ensure a highly supportive treatment environment; patients in the hospital-based program participated in a variety of meetings and program activities, but the emphasis on support, as tapped by the COPES, was just average. By contrast, the revamped milieu-oriented program, which maintained an even more active schedule for patients, was substantially above the norm on all three relationship dimensions.

The profiles also reveal that adequate treatment quantity does not ensure positive treatment quality. Treatment climate may be relatively independent of the number of activities, the professional background of the staff, and the patient-staff ratio. Again, comparing the hospital-based and milieu-oriented programs, we found that in spite of their active schedules for patients and similar high staff-patient ratios and staff training, the hospital-based program was disorganized and unclear, whereas the milieu-oriented program was above average on these system maintenance dimensions after the program changes were made.

Conversely, programs that are brief and use very few treatment components can create a positive climate. The aversion conditioning program is a case in point; although the program emphasized the use of conditioning procedures and medications almost to the exclusion of other treatment components, both patients and staff reported good interpersonal relationships and some orientation toward discussing personal problems. These qualities may enhance the effectiveness of behaviorally oriented treatment programs (Etringer, Gregory, & Lando, 1984; Miller, Taylor, & West, 1980). This program also demonstrates that structure is compatible with good interpersonal relationships and the open expression of anger.

A program run by nonmedical staff can develop a very positive social climate, as the Salvation Army program demonstrates. Paraprofessional and minimally trained staff can establish relationships with clients that are just as empathic and helpful as those established by highly trained professionals (Hattie, Sharpley, & Rogers, 1984). In a comparison of programs with and without professionally trained staff, these two groups of programs did not differ on the three relationship dimensions, and the programs without professional staff had somewhat less emphasis on system maintenance (Moos, 1974, 1988a). Results for the Salvation Army are consistent with this pattern, as are AA meetings, which are highly involving, supportive, expressive, and structured, although run by recovering alcoholics who typically do not have professional psychiatric training.

Overall, the patients in these programs apparently developed a unique camaraderie—an interest in sharing experiences and helping each other—that may be facilitated by their shared problem of alcoholism. Such support is not typical of most psychiatric programs, to which patients are admitted for a variety of reasons. The relatively rich staffing in the alcoholism programs also may help to promote a more positive treatment environment.

Our implementation analyses showed us that we were examining five varied but active alcoholism programs. Thus, we proceeded with an impact evaluation, which we describe in Chapters 3 and 4. In addition to its value as a precursor to an outcome study, treatment implementation assessment can detect a short-term deterioration in treatment quantity or quality. If a program is found to be inadequately implemented in either regard, staff can make efforts to improve it. We discuss these issues in Chapter 11.

3
Short-Term Outcome and Patient Prognosis

Many alcoholic patients show short-term improvement after treatment (Riley et al., 1987; Saxe et al., 1983). Unfortunately, treatment research has provided little insight into the range of factors contributing to improvement. Studies using the black-box paradigm have assessed patient pretreatment characteristics more thoroughly than treatment variables. Accordingly, they have found that patient background and intake characteristics are stronger predictors of treatment outcome.

To provide a backdrop for our more intensive investigation of treatment and life context factors in later chapters, we first examine how functioning changes from intake to 6 months after treatment and how well intake characteristics predict short-term outcome. In keeping with a broad perspective on the nature of alcohol abuse, we measured diverse aspects of patient functioning both before and after treatment.

We also address an important but relatively unexamined issue in treatment evaluation: Is outcome for patients who are more easily followed better than outcome for patients who are harder to follow? If patients who are easier to follow do better, then evaluators who follow smaller proportions of patients may draw overly optimistic conclusions about outcome for all patients.

MULTIDIMENSIONAL MEASURES OF INTAKE AND FOLLOW-UP FUNCTIONING

Because abusive drinking is the primary problem presented by most alcoholic patients, the elimination or at least the reduction of drinking behavior was once viewed as the primary treatment outcome criterion. Accordingly, measures of other aspects of individual functioning typically were not included in treatment outcome studies. However, most alcoholic patients have other problems related to their drinking, such as problems in social, psychological, and occupational functioning. These problems may have contributed to the development of alcohol abuse, or they may represent consequences of alcohol abuse that also serve to maintain it. Recognition of patients' multiple problems at intake, and of the role such problems may play in preventing recovery, has led researchers to a multidimensional orientation toward treatment outcome (Babor, Dolinsky, Rounsaville, & Jaffe, 1988; McLellan et al., 1981).

In our study, we measured patients' functioning on multiple criteria both at intake and at follow-up, and we used patient functioning at intake as a baseline for measuring improvement in functioning at follow-up. We used the BIF to assess six areas of functioning, two involving drinking behavior and four addressing other aspects of patient functioning.

1. *Alcohol consumption* during the month before admission to the treatment program; measured in terms of ounces of ethanol—from wine, beer, or hard liquor—that the patient drank on a typical drinking day.
2. *Abstinence* during the month before admission to the treatment program (yes/no).
3. *Physical symptoms,* the mean of 10 items rated on 5-point scales (from never to often): delirium tremens or shakes, memory lapses or blackouts, dry heaves or cold sweats, difficulty sleeping, hallucinations or vague fears, severe hangover, nervous or tense, upset stomach, headaches, and dizzy spells.
4. *Depression,* the mean of seven self-descriptive items rated on 5-point scales reflecting depressed mood: desperate, angry, pessimistic, lonely, unhappy, couldn't get going, and bored.
5. *Social functioning,* the mean of five items rated on 5-point scales: spending time with close friends, attending parties, participating in sports, attending cultural events, and engaging in community activities.
6. *Occupational functioning,* the response to a yes/no question about whether the patient worked part time or full time during the last 6 months.

We used the FIF as a parallel assessment of functioning at the 6-month follow-up. On the FIF, however, abstinence was for the entire time since discharge. Comparing the BIF and FIF on these indices enabled us to measure improvement from intake to the 6-month follow-up.

Overall, our follow-up efforts were quite successful. Eleven of the initial 505 patients died before their scheduled follow-up date. Of the remaining 494 patients, 87% ($N = 429$) completed the FIF, 7% were located but refused to participate, and 6% were not located. The proportion of patients in each program who were followed successfully varied somewhat: Salvation Army, 80%; hospital based, 84%; halfway house, 95%; aversion conditioning, 91%; and milieu oriented, 86%. The follow-up rates across programs were not significantly different, however.

CHANGES IN FUNCTIONING BETWEEN INTAKE AND FOLLOW-UP

Before examining short-term pre- to posttreatment changes in patients' functioning, we describe their "starting points"—that is, the intake functioning of the patients in each of the five programs. The relevant data are shown in Figures 3.1 and 3.2. On alcohol consumption, physical symptoms, and depression, lower scores reflect better outcome. On the remaining criteria, higher scores indicate better outcome.

Using one-way analyses of variance, we found significant differences in intake functioning among the patients in the five programs. Consistent with Mandell's (1979) description of two tiers of alcoholism treatment programs, our for-profit and nonprofit programs differed in patients' intake functioning as well as in their demographic characteristics. On the alcohol-related indices, the for-profit program patients (aversion conditioning and milieu oriented) rated their drinking problem as less severe and reported fewer physical symptoms related to drinking. In addition, patients in the for-profit programs reported fewer symptoms of depression and more positive social and occupational functioning.

Paired t tests within each program indicated that, between intake and the 6-month follow-up, patients improved significantly on the two drinking variables and on physical symptoms and depressed mood. The only exception was a nonsignificant increase in abstinence for the Salvation Army clients. In general, social functioning showed less dramatic changes, although patients in the Salvation Army, halfway house, and milieu-oriented programs improved significantly. We observed significant improvement in occupational functioning for the Salvation Army patients; in contrast, the high rate of employment for the patients entering the milieu-oriented and aversion conditioning programs left relatively little room for improvement in this area.

These findings again confirm the existence of two groups of alcoholism treatment programs; patients in nonprofit programs have more severe symptoms at intake and show poorer treatment outcome, while patients in for-profit programs have fewer intake symptoms and show better outcome. Nathan (1986) noted that 1-year abstinence rates typically range from 25% or less for chronic alcoholics with few personal resources treated at public, inner-city programs to 50% or better for patients with substantial resources who receive treatment at private facilities. These differences in abstinence rates are consistent with the rates we observed for nonprofit (16%) and for-profit (50%) programs.

Overall, the improvement among the patients in our five programs is similar to that obtained in research on other programs of the same type.

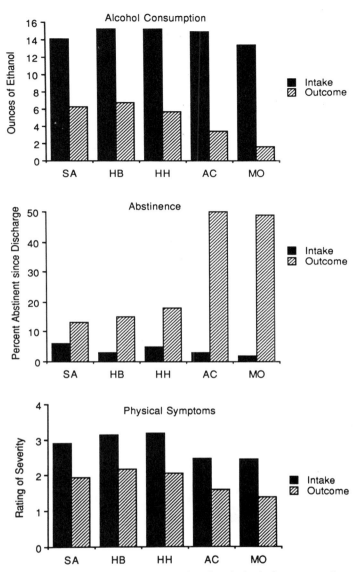

Figure 3.1 Intake and outcome levels of alcohol consumption, abstinence, and physical symptoms by program (SA = Salvation Army, HB = hospital based, HH = halfway house, AC = aversion conditioning, MO = milieu oriented).

For example, Dwoskin and his colleagues (1979) noted that 21% of halfway house residents maintained abstinence during the first 6 months after leaving the program. In our study, 18% of the former residents of the halfway house were abstinent through the 6-month follow-up. For an aversion conditioning program, Neubuerger and his associates (1981) obtained a 1-year abstinence rate of 53% (although minor "slips" were al-

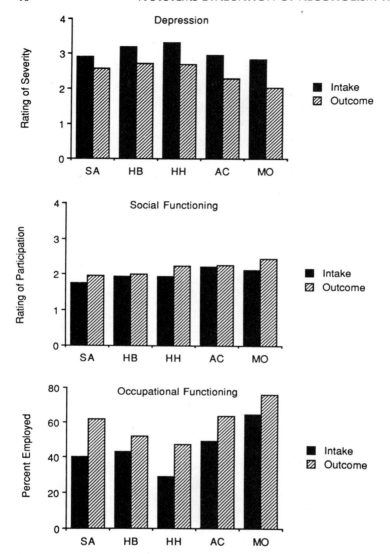

Figure 3.2 Intake and outcome levels of depression, social functioning, and occupational functioning by program (SA = Salvation Army, HB = hospital based, HH = halfway house, AC = aversion conditioning, MO = milieu oriented).

lowed), and Wiens and Menustik (1983) reported a 1-year abstinence rate of 63%; the 6-month abstinence rate (no "slips") for the aversion conditioning patients we studied was 50%.

In the absence of an equivalent no-treatment control group, we do not know how much of the substantial improvement we observed reflects the impact of treatment. However, we can provide a "judgment" of the causal influence of treatment. To us, the most useful basis for judging the causal contribution of treatment is to pose the "counter-factual question" (Einhorn & Hogarth, 1986): Would this group of patients have experienced as much improvement had they not been in treatment? Certainly, one would expect some improvement on the grounds that alcoholic persons may seek treatment when their problems are especially severe. Patients entering treatment may show improvement in the absence of any intervention effect simply because they are reassessed at a later point in their functioning cycles that on average is more positive than the point at which they sought treatment. But would one expect the substantial improvement shown by the patients in our sample? We do not think so. Consequently, we believe that treatment is responsible for at least some of the improvement shown. Similarly, several reviews of the relevant literature have concluded that alcoholism treatment is more beneficial than no treatment (e.g., Miller & Hester, 1980; NIAAA, 1987; Saxe et al., 1983).

RELATIONSHIPS BETWEEN DRINKING AND OTHER OUTCOME INDICES

Because of the linkages between alcohol abuse and problems in other areas of functioning prior to treatment, there is a tendency to assume that if drinking behavior ceases or improves following treatment, one should see improvement in other areas of functioning as well. However, this is not necessarily the case. Abstinence is not consistently associated with improvement in social, psychological, and occupational functioning (Emrick, 1974; Snowden, 1984). As Duckitt and her co-workers (1985) have noted, "outcome is a conceptual and methodological issue in its own right" (p. 153). The relationship between drinking behavior and other aspects of functioning is of special interest.

To learn more about the connections between drinking-related and other outcome criteria, we calculated cross-sectional correlations among the six outcome measures. We found that better functioning in each area was associated with better outcome in all other areas; this conclusion is consistent with the findings of other researchers (Babor et al., 1988; Duckitt et al., 1985; McLellan et al., 1981). Alcohol consumption and abstinence were significantly related to each other ($r = -.41$) and to physical symptoms, depression, social functioning, and occupational functioning (average $r = .32$ and .28, respectively). Physical symptoms and depression were related to each other ($r = .58$) and to the other drinking and nondrinking criteria (average $r = .37$ and .31, respectively). Although occupational and social functioning were essentially independent ($r = .04$), each was significantly related to the other four indices in the expected direction (average $r = .21$ and .20, respectively).

We wondered whether these cross-sectional associations between drinking and other outcome criteria at the 6-month follow-up reflected decreased drinking by patients who, prior to treatment, were functioning better in other areas, or whether they reflected concomitant changes in drinking and other areas of functioning. Because the analysis of change scores is beset by a number of difficulties, we used multiple regression analysis to examine concomitant changes in different outcome domains. More specifically, we calculated partial correlations between outcome criteria at the 6-month follow-up, controlling for the two relevant intake functioning indices, as well as for four background characteristics (gender, age, marital status, and education). Within the limits of linear adjustment techniques, these partial correlations reflect the expected associations among the outcome measures if all patients were functioning at the same level at intake and were identical in background characteristics (see Albrecht & Higgins, 1977). Thus, they provide some indication of the associations among "changes" in different outcome domains.

These "change" correlations were comparable to the cross-sectional correlations for the most part, although the magnitude of the associations was slightly lower. Changes in alcohol consumption and abstinence correlated .30 and .23, on average, with changes in the other four outcome domains. Changes in physical symptoms and depression correlated .54 with each other and showed an average correlation of .32 and .21 with the other four indices. Changes in social and occupational functioning were basically independent of each other, but each was significantly correlated with change in the other four criteria (average $r = .16$ and .15, respectively).

Although drinking behavior is most often seen as the central outcome dimension in studies of alcoholism treatment, McLellan and his colleagues (1981) found that improvement in psychological functioning was related to better outcome on a wider spectrum of indices than was posttreatment drinking behavior. Our data indicate that depressed mood is as central an outcome dimension as alcohol consumption; in fact, depressed mood was associated with one (or, in one analysis, two) more outcome area than was alcohol consumption, and the correlations were of similar magnitude. These findings probably reflect the fact that many alcoholic patients have at least one psychiatric disorder other than alcoholism and that depression is especially common (Hesselbrock et al., 1985).

Both the cross-sectional and longitudinal analyses revealed stronger associations among drinking behavior, physical symptoms, and depressed mood than among drinking and social and occupational functioning. This pattern suggests that reduced drinking is associated with better intrapersonal functioning but less closely tied to better role functioning.

Similarly, Snowden (1984) described two levels of treatment response among problem drinker-drivers. "Reform" reflects general improvement, especially in social and work adjustment, along with a realistic view of oneself as a problem drinker and adoption of reduced consumption as a goal. "Resistance" occurs when patients improve in the social and work domains but are reluctant to designate themselves as problem drinkers and do not decrease their alcohol consumption. Thus, reduced drinking is associated with better role functioning, but there may be an improvement in role functioning without a concomitant decline in alcohol consumption.

Pattison (1976) outlined four reasons (in addition to measurement error) why reduced drinking may not be more highly related to improvement in other areas of functioning. First, for alcoholic patients with little dysfunction in areas other than drinking, such as the aversion conditioning and milieu-oriented patients, there is little room for improvement in these areas. Second, alcoholic patients with major deficiencies in almost all areas of functioning, such as those in the Salvation Army and hospital-based programs, have few personal and social resources to sustain improvement even if they remain sober. Third, some programs, such as aversion conditioning, focus primarily on modifying drinking rather than changing functioning in other areas. Finally, for most alcoholic patients, drinking may not be highly related to functioning in other areas. Problems in all areas of life undoubtedly are multiply determined, and reduction in drinking cannot be expected to result invariantly in improvement across the board. Overall, treatment outcome is composed of a complex array of functioning criteria with different causal systems and varying levels of interconnectedness.

PROGNOSTIC IMPORTANCE OF PRETREATMENT FACTORS

Prognostic indicators can help to identify which alcoholic patients will respond best to treatment or, at a more complex level, which patients should receive what treatment (Caddy & Block, 1985; Nathan, 1986; Ornstein & Cherepon, 1985). Many investigators contend that treatment outcome is influenced most strongly by patients' demographic characteristics and their functioning at intake (Costello, 1980; Nathan, 1986; Neuberger et al., 1981). In essence, sociodemographic factors serve as proxies for some of the personal and environmental assets patients have or lack when entering treatment, such as their motivation and social and coping resources, which tend to be associated with a better prognosis. Thus, higher socioeconomic status and social stability are associated with better treatment outcome. In addition, better levels of initial functioning typically predict better outcome.

We conducted multiple regression analyses to assess the extent to which each of the six treatment outcome criteria could be predicted from relevant patient background and intake characteristics. Two groups of variables were entered in the order reflecting their probable causal sequence. First, we entered sociodemographic characteristics that provide a general profile of an individual's social position; the characteristics were gender, age, marital status, and education. Then we entered the value of the relevant functioning characteristic at intake. Table 3.1 shows the multiple correlations when the demographic variables are used to predict the outcome criteria, as well as the multiple correlations and proportions of outcome variance accounted for by these variables and the measures of functioning at intake.

In general, patients who were older, married, and better educated tended to have better treatment outcome. For alcohol consumption and abstinence, sociodemographic characteristics were better predictors of outcome than were the intake values of these two criteria. Because only a few people in each program had been abstinent in the month prior to entering treatment (see Figure 3.1), the magnitude of relationship possible with later abstinence is limited. Likewise, it might be argued that the month prior to treatment is too short an interval over which to assess stable patterns of pretreatment alcohol consumption for inpatients (Cooper et al., 1980). However, assessing pretreatment drinking behavior over a longer "window" is no guarantee of a stronger association with later drinking behavior. In a sample of outpatients, neither alcohol consumption in the 6 months prior to treatment nor consumption in the 6 months before that was associated with posttreatment consumption (Maisto et al., 1985).

For the other four criteria, intake functioning was more strongly related to outcome than were the background characteristics. Overall, sociodemographic and intake characteristics accounted for 6% to 30% of the variance in treatment outcome.

Even though both demographic and intake characteristics were related to treatment outcome, the majority of the variance in outcome remained unexplained. Moreover, these pretreatment factors explained less than 10% of the variance in alcohol consumption and abstinence at follow-up. These findings show that drinking patterns fluctuate widely over time; they may change in response to treatment and life context factors during and after treatment (Polich, Armor, & Braiker, 1981; Watson & Pucel, 1985). Consequently, prior drinking patterns do not predict 6-month drinking outcome very well.

In sum, we identified improvement in patients' functioning from intake to 6-month follow-up after discharge from a residential treatment program. Demographic and intake functioning factors provide only a limited account of short-term outcome. These findings led us to consider additional issues such as (1) the effects of treatment on outcome (Chapter 4), (2) the stability or change in follow-up functioning over time (Chapter 7), and (3) the influence of life context factors on remission and relapse (Chapters 7 and 8).

Before focusing on these issues, we examine an important question for any study of treatment outcome: Do patients who are more difficult to follow show poorer treatment outcome?

Table 3.1 Associations between sociodemographic and intake characteristics and 6-month treatment outcome ($N = 429$)

	Alcohol consumption	Abstinence	Physical symptoms	Depression	Social functioning	Occupational functioning
Sociodemographic characteristics						
Gender	-.11*	.11*	-.05	-.03	.10*	-.15***
Age	-.15***	.11*	-.19***	-.19***	.07	-.05
Marital status	-.15***	.24***	-.21***	-.24***	.15***	.16***
Education	-.11*	.13**	-.19***	-.05	.16***	.09*
Multiple R	.25***	.29***	.32***	.29***	.23***	.26***
Intake functioning	.09*	-.04	.37***	.46***	.52***	.34***
Overall multiple R	.25***	.29***	.42***	.50***	.55***	.40***
Percentage of variance explained	6.3%	8.4%	17.4%	25.1%	30.1%	15.2%

Note. Gender is coded as 1 = female and 0 = male; marital status is coded as 1 = married and 0 = otherwise.

*$p < .05$. **$p < .01$. ***$p < .001$.

DIFFICULTY OF FOLLOW-UP

One of the major criticisms of treatment outcome studies is that a substantial proportion of patients are not followed successfully (Mackenzie et al., 1987; Polich et al., 1981). The missing patients may be functioning more poorly than patients who are followed, thus leaving an unrepresentative patient sample. Consequently, the conclusions about treatment outcome may be invalid.

Some researchers have attempted to address this issue by comparing successfully with unsuccessfully followed patients on demographic characteristics and functioning assessed at treatment intake or discharge. For example, Polich and his colleagues (1981) found that patients who completed an 18-month follow-up interview had less severe drinking problems and were more stable socially at intake than were patients who were not followed successfully, suggesting that the latter group probably experienced poorer treatment outcome. Penk and his associates (1981) found that psychiatric inpatients who were not successfully followed 2 months after treatment were judged to have been more impaired psychologically at treatment intake than were successfully followed patients. However, Sobell, Sobell, and Maisto (1984) noted that patients who discontinued participation during follow-up were functioning as well as other patients in their cohort, whereas patients who were lost to follow-up were generally functioning poorly prior to being lost. Thus, there may be an important difference between patients who choose not to cooperate in a follow-up and patients who cannot be located.

Although some researchers consider that no difference at intake between patients who are followed and those who are not is evidence of the generalizability of the results on the successfully followed group, intake functioning does not adequately predict treatment outcome. Accordingly, groups of patients who do not differ at intake or discharge may experience quite different treatment outcomes.

A direct examination of these issues requires successful follow-up of a high proportion of a sample and analysis of the association between the amount and type of follow-up effort and treatment outcome. Patients who are more difficult to follow may have better or worse outcomes, depending on a wide range of factors, including the particular outcome criteria used, the intensity and duration of the follow-up effort, and the specific follow-up strategies (Mackenzie et al., 1987).

We examined three aspects of this issue: (1) Does the treatment outcome of alcoholic patients who are harder to follow differ from that of patients who are easier to follow? (2) Does the addition of patients who are increasingly difficult to follow change the overall findings on the outcome of treatment? (3) Do patients who are easy to follow differ in their sociodemographic characteristics and functioning at intake? If so, are there differences in treatment outcome once these factors have been considered?

Follow-Up Effort

About 6 months after discharge, we tried to contact each patient to complete a FIF. During the process of locating patients and obtaining follow-up information, we kept detailed records of every telephone, mail, and in-person effort to reach them. If our initial leads did not locate the patient, we used sources such as telephone directories, the postal service, other treatment programs, and public records. Using these procedures, we located 94% of the surviving patients.

After we located the patients and sent them a FIF, we waited about 2 weeks for them to return the inventory. If they did not do so, we wrote letters and telephoned them to urge their participation. Many patients had moved or were not in contact with the address confirmed initially. For some of the more transient and difficult patients, we had to repeat a process of locating them and urging their cooperation. The follow-up histories of patients varied widely. Some patients were residing at their expected address and completed the FIF right away, whereas many required extensive effort to be located and additional effort to be relocated and urged to cooperate.

Substantial proportions of patients required each of two types of follow-up activity: location and persuasion. For instance, agency contacts (treatment programs, Department of Motor Vehicles, etc.) were needed to locate over one-third of the patients. Although about half of this group (17% of the entire sample) was successfully located by contacting just one or two agencies, the other half (19% of the sample) needed three or four agency contacts. After initial contact was established, 21% of the patients had to be relocated at least once. One-third (34%) of the patients were sent at least one personal letter or an additional FIF urging them to participate, and two out of five patients (42%) had to be encouraged at least once by telephone to complete the FIF.

Treatment Outcome and Difficulty of Follow-Up

We examined the differences in treatment outcome between the more easily located or more cooperative patients and those who required more effort. We used analyses of variance to determine whether these groups of patients differed in treatment outcome; the analyses showed statistically significant differences between patient groups. In every comparison that attained significance, the patients who were more difficult to locate or less cooperative experienced poorer treatment outcome.

There were large differences in outcome for those who were easier versus more difficult to locate (number of agency contacts) or persuade (number of persuasion efforts). Patients who were harder to locate showed worse treatment outcome. Some of the differences were substantial. For example, 36% of the patients who were located without agency contacts were abstinent, whereas this was true of only 13% of patients who needed three or more such contacts. The differences related to number of persuasion efforts were similar, with significant differences in alcohol consumption, abstinence, physical symptoms, and depression for patients who were more and less cooperative. For example, 34% of the patients who participated without any persuasion efforts were abstinent, while this was true for only 15% of those who required two or more persuasion efforts.

A Total Effort Measure of Follow-Up Activity

These results point to the importance of a rigorous follow-up effort for obtaining data from the maximum number of patients possible. We examined this issue further by linking outcome to a general indicator of follow-up effort. We divided the patients into four groups on the basis of the number of different types of follow-up attempts (letters, location efforts, and persuasion efforts) required beyond BIF or agency contacts.

Poorer outcome was associated with more types of follow-up effort (Table 3.2). Specifically, there were significant differences among the four groups of patients on alcohol consumption, abstinence, physical symptoms, and depression. Some of the differences were substantial. For example, while 39% of the persons requiring no additional follow-up effort were abstinent, this was true of only 15% of those requiring all three types of follow-up activities.

We continued our efforts to follow patients for several months. Because more time had elapsed between discharge and follow-up for patients who were more difficult to follow, their poorer treatment outcome might have been due to their longer period at risk. However, when we controlled for the length of time between discharge and follow-up, the findings remained the same. Overall, our results, especially with respect to drinking-related outcomes, would have been significantly different had we stopped our follow-up at none, one, or two additional types of follow-up efforts, resulting in follow-up rates of 41%, 59%, and 77%, respectively, versus the 87% rate we were able to obtain by employing all three types of additional efforts when necessary.

Patient Characteristics at Intake and Difficulty of Follow-Up

We examined differences in the follow-up groups on sociodemographic characteristics and functioning at intake. Analyses of variance indicated that patients who were more difficult to locate tended to be younger and single or separated and to be less well educated and more transient. On

Table 3.2 Relationship between treatment outcome and total follow-up effort

	Number of additional types of follow-up effort				
	0 (N = 203)	1 (N = 90)	2 (N = 86)	3 (N = 50)	F
Alcohol consumption (oz. of ethanol)	3.9^c	4.9	5.6	7.2^c	2.91*
Abstinence (% yes)	39.5^{a,b,c}	25.0^a	11.8^b	14.9^c	10.0***
Physical symptoms (1 = least severe, 5 = most severe)	1.7^{b,c}	1.9	2.0^b	2.2^c	4.8**
Depression (1 = least severe, 5 = most severe)	2.3^{b,c}	2.5^e	2.6^b	2.9^{c,e}	7.6***
Social functioning (1 = least social, 5 = most social)	2.2	2.2	2.2	2.1	<1
Occupational functioning (% employed)	62.6	64.4	54.7	58.0	<1

Note. Pairs that share a common superscript are significantly different ($p < .05$) on the Student-Newman-Keuls test.
*$p < .05$.   **$p < .01$.   ***$p < .001$.

the other hand, there were few differences between more and less cooperative persons in their background and intake functioning.

We wondered whether patients who were more difficult to follow differed in treatment outcome over and above what would be expected from their characteristics at intake. Thus, we conducted analyses of covariance using sociodemographic information (age, gender, marital status, education) and the corresponding intake index as covariates. In general, difficulty of follow-up was still related to poorer treatment outcome even after demographic characteristics and intake functioning were controlled. As expected, patients who required one or more letters urging cooperation still experienced significantly poorer outcome on alcohol consumption, abstinence, and depression. Significant differences also remained on five of the six criteria (all but social functioning) among patients who differed on the number of attempts to relocate and on four of the criteria (alcohol consumption, abstinence, physical symptoms, and depression) among patients who differed on the number of attempts other than letters to obtain cooperation. Thus, the poorer treatment outcome of patients who needed to be relocated was not attributable completely to their characteristics at intake.

Implications

Compared to more accessible patients, patients who were more difficult to locate experienced poorer treatment outcome, which was related only partially to their sociodemographic characteristics and poorer functioning at intake. Patients who needed to be relocated or who were less cooperative experienced poorer treatment outcome, which was not attributable to their characteristics at intake. These findings still held after considering the length of time between discharge and follow-up.

Because some treatment outcome studies report results based on 50% to 70% of the patients in the follow-up cohort (Armor et al., 1978), it is important to know that alcoholic patients who are harder to follow may experience poorer treatment outcome. When there are no differences in sociodemographic characteristics at intake between patients who are and who are not followed successfully, investigators tend to conclude that treatment outcome for the partial follow-up sample is representative of outcome for the entire sample. Our findings imply that this conclusion is incorrect. There apparently are other, untapped differences between the two groups at intake or differences in factors such as their program participation, their motivation, or the life stressors and social resources they experience following treatment.

Patients whom we were unable to locate (6%) probably would have shown somewhat poorer outcome than the patients we found hardest to locate. Patients whom we located but who refused to complete a FIF comprised the remainder of the group not followed (7% of the sample). These patients seemed to be especially concerned about the confidentiality of their alcoholism treatment. As a group, they were more likely to be married and residentially stable, less likely to have been treated previously for alcoholism, and less impaired functionally at intake than the unlocated patients. We do not know whether this group of refusers would have shown poorer treatment outcome. However, in accordance with Sobell and her associates (1984), we assume that they would have been functioning as well as the patients who participated in the follow-up. If possible, it would be useful to obtain some basic information on alcohol consumption and employment from resistant patients who are contacted.

We believe our findings are generalizable. We employed six outcome criteria and an intensive array of follow-up procedures to locate and elicit the cooperation of a high percentage of patients. The five programs represent a broad range of facilities; patients in the follow-up sample were quite heterogeneous and included a substantial proportion of women. On the other hand, La Porte and his colleagues (1981) found no consistent relationship between difficulty of follow-up and indices of 6-month treatment outcome among a mixed group of residentially treated alcoholics and drug addicts. McCrady and her co-workers (1986) also found no difference in outcomes between alcoholic patients who were easily followed and those who were not (but 32% of the sample was lost to follow-up).

Findings on this issue might vary for patients with other types of disorders. Ellsworth (1979) conducted a follow-up of psychiatric inpatients. He identified no difference between the 3-month follow-up functioning of patients who responded to a mailed questionnaire and "reluctant" responders who were subsequently contacted for a telephone interview.

However, 37% of the sample was never successfully followed. In a comparable treatment outcome study of depressed patients, we found that the intensity of our follow-up effort was not related to 12-month outcome (Billings, Cronkite, & Moos, 1985). There may be a stronger association between poorer functioning and difficulty of follow-up among alcoholic patients because alcoholism is more likely than depression to lead to residential instability, homelessness, and social isolation. In addition, depressed patients may be more likely to cooperate once they are located.

Although complex and demanding, follow-up research is a worthwhile and necessary investment of agency resources. The total cost of our follow-up activities was minor when compared with the expense of treating the more than 500 patients we initially studied. Results of treatment evaluations may influence local, state, and national policies on alcoholism treatment. From this perspective, it is well worth the cost to obtain information from as complete and representative follow-up samples of patients as possible.

CONCLUSIONS

We have addressed a number of issues regarding factors associated with the 6-month outcome of treated alcoholic patients, including the extent to which the conclusions of evaluations may be compromised if patients who are not followed experience poorer treatment outcome. Our findings, particularly with respect to drinking-related outcome, would have been unduly optimistic had we stopped our follow-up efforts at earlier stages. Consequently, we believe that the benefits of extensive follow-up efforts outweigh their costs.

We also considered the multidimensional nature of treatment outcome by looking at the associations among six outcome criteria. In general, better outcome in one area was associated with better outcome in other areas; there was more overlap among drinking behavior, physical symptoms, and depression than among these criteria and social and occupational functioning. Such a pattern highlights the distinctiveness of different outcome criteria and shows that a reduction in drinking cannot be expected to result invariably in comparable improvement in every other area of functioning.

A final issue involves the prognostic importance of patient background and intake functioning characteristics. We established that patients as a group improved significantly from intake to 6 months after discharge and that pretreatment factors accounted for 6% to 29% of the variation in treatment outcome. Thus, most of the variance in treatment outcome remains unexplained, suggesting that various aspects of patients' functioning may change over time, perhaps in response to treatment and aftercare. We turn to this issue in the next chapter.

4

The Process and Effects of Treatment

In the previous chapter, we found that patients improved substantially in functioning from intake to 6 months after the end of residential treatment. We also examined the prognostic importance of sociodemographic factors and symptoms at intake and found that these patient characteristics explained a modest portion of the variation in short-term treatment outcome.

In this chapter, we expand our approach and examine the process and effects of treatment. After providing a conceptual model as a guide, we focus on the relative effectiveness of the five programs. Next, we analyze within each program the impact of specific treatment components and length of treatment on outcome, with special emphasis on the unique aspects of the Salvation Army program. Finally, we use the conceptual model to integrate our findings on how patient characteristics and treatment affect outcome. We consider the relative influence on treatment outcome of patient social background and intake functioning, type of treatment program, treatment experiences, and quality of the treatment environment.

AN EXPANDED EVALUATION PARADIGM

In Chapter 1 we described an expanded evaluation paradigm that includes both treatment components and patients' life contexts (Figure 1.2). Here we implement part of the paradigm by examining how factors that vary between and within treatment programs influence outcome. The model in Figure 4.1 shows the connections among five sets of variables that are associated with treatment outcome: patient sociodemographic character-

THE PROCESS AND EFFECTS OF TREATMENT

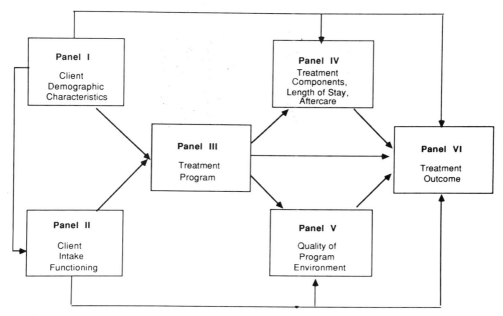

Figure 4.1 An expanded model of the determinants of treatment outcome.

istics (Panel I), patient intake functioning (Panel II), treatment program (Panel III), exposure to treatment components and length of stay (Panel IV), and program environment (Panel V).

We assumed the following causal ordering of variables in the model. Patient social background and intake symptoms determine patient entry into a treatment program; in turn, these variables affect treatment experiences and perceptions of the treatment environment. This model enabled us to examine how each set of variables could affect subsequent sets and be affected by prior sets. For example, part of the influence of intake functioning on outcome may be independent of that of the other sets of predictors; in addition, intake functioning may influence outcome through intervening factors, such as the program a patient enters and the patient's length of stay and treatment experiences.

RELATIVE EFFECTIVENESS OF THE TREATMENT PROGRAMS

Many evaluations of alcoholism treatment have focused on the overall impact of a treatment program, either by itself or as compared with other programs. These black-box evaluations have tended to overlook treatment processes and how specific treatment components influence outcome (see Chapter 1). Consequently, little is known about the relative effectiveness of the specific treatment components offered in multimodal programs. In our evaluation, we first assessed the relative effectiveness of the five programs and then analyzed the influence of several treatment components and length of stay on treatment outcome.

In a naturalistic study such as this one, in which patients are not randomly assigned to programs, preexisting differences in patient background and intake characteristics may explain part of any differences in outcome across programs. As described in Chapters 2 and 3, patients in the for-profit programs (aversion conditioning and milieu-oriented) tended to have higher socioeconomic status and better intake functioning compared with patients in the three nonprofit programs (Salvation Army, hospital based, and halfway house).

Accordingly, our first step was to go beyond the program-by-program improvement analyses presented in Chapter 3 and to examine differences in outcome across the five programs while controlling for patient background and intake characteristics. We did this by conducting an analysis of covariance (ANCOVA) for each of the six outcome criteria. The covariates are sociodemographic factors (gender, age, marital status, and education) and the intake index that corresponds to the outcome criterion.

Similar to the "unadjusted" results presented in Chapter 3, the ANCOVA findings indicate that the five programs differed significantly in treatment outcome on all criteria except occupational functioning, even after controlling for patient demographic characteristics and intake functioning. Figures 4.2 and 4.3 show the outcome pattern as the proportion of a standard deviation from the overall mean, adjusted for the covariates. Thus, a value of .10 reflects a score that is 10% of a standard deviation better than the overall mean adjusted treatment outcome on that criterion. Similarly, a value of −.10 reflects an outcome that is 10% of a standard deviation worse than expected.

For example, the adjusted overall outcome on alcohol consumption is 4.9 ounces, which represents an average decline of 9.7 ounces from the overall mean intake level of 14.6. After controlling for patient characteristics and intake functioning, the adjusted alcohol consumption level for the Salvation Army patients is 5.9 ounces, which is .14 of a standard deviation worse than the expected level of 4.9 ounces. Thus, although the Salvation Army patients showed considerable improvement, it was not quite as much as the average amount of improvement across programs.

It is important to recognize that the adjusted outcome scores are based on controlling only patient background characteristics and pretreatment functioning. They do not take into account all the factors related to treatment selection or allocation (see Chapter 12). For example, since social resources, which did not enter into the calculations of adjusted outcome, are only imperfectly associated with the background characteristics we controlled, programs in which patients had fewer community resources are at a relative disadvantage. The findings can be summarized as follows.

1. *Salvation Army.* Patients improved less than expected on the two drinking criteria, physical symptoms, depression, and social func-

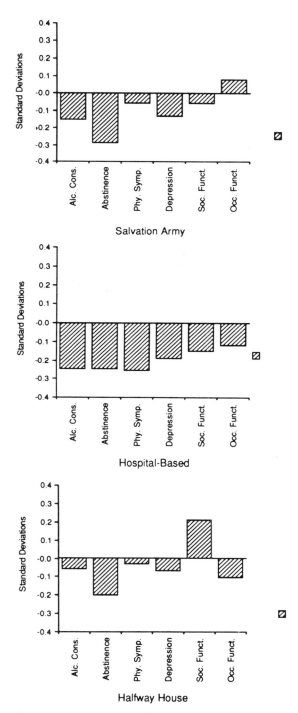

Figure 4.2 Six-month adjusted outcome levels for the Salvation Army, hospital-based, and halfway house programs.

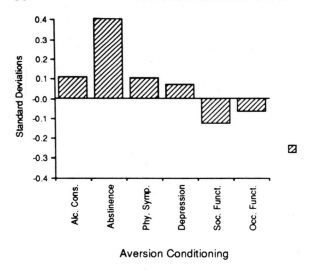

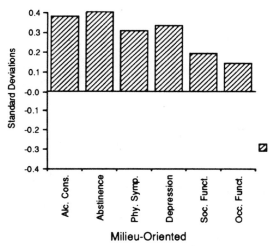

Figure 4.3 Six-month adjusted outcome levels for the aversion conditioning and milieu-oriented programs.

tioning, and slightly more than expected on occupational functioning.
2. *Hospital Based.* Patients improved less than expected in all areas.
3. *Halfway House.* Patients' improvement was slightly lower than expected on the two alcoholism criteria, physical symptoms, depression, and occupational functioning, but higher than expected on social functioning.
4. *Aversion Conditioning.* Patients did much better than expected on abstinence since discharge and somewhat better on alcohol con-

sumption, physical symptoms, and depression. Their scores on social and occupational functioning were slightly lower than expected.
5. *Milieu Oriented.* Patient improvement was better than expected on all outcome criteria.

These findings indicate that, even after controlling for sociodemographic characteristics and intake functioning, patients in the milieu-oriented and aversion conditioning programs improved more than those in the three nonprofit programs. In part, these findings probably reflect the superior treatment offered in the for-profit programs relative to that in at least one of the nonprofit programs—the hospital-based program. The milieu-oriented program had a positive treatment environment in which patients participated actively in a range of treatment components. This program also focused somewhat on the reentry process. An active patient alumni association met with patients while they were in the program and tried to help them plan for community life. The fact that almost half of the patients received Antabuse probably also contributed to good treatment outcome.

The aversion conditioning program also had a cohesive treatment milieu; more important, patients returned to the program for up to seven booster conditioning sessions during the follow-up interval. However, this program had a narrow focus on drinking behavior; it was not family or community oriented. Thus we would expect its beneficial effects to be more circumscribed than those of the milieu-oriented program in all areas except abstinence.

In contrast, the hospital-based program admitted primarily low-bottom alcoholics with minimal economic and social resources. Relative to the deficits of this population, the treatment program was not very intensive. Moreover, there was little emphasis on preparing patients for reentry into the community and virtually no follow-up after discharge from the program. The lack of support aimed at helping low-bottom patients develop a credible position in the community probably explains the worse than expected outcome for this program.

Our findings also show some variations in outcome that may reflect different treatment orientations across the programs. For example, the emphasis on vocational training in the Salvation Army program may promote better occupational functioning. Similarly, the small familylike atmosphere of the halfway house program and the emphasis on group-related and recreational activities probably led to the better than expected social functioning among its residents. In contrast, the aversion conditioning program emphasized only counterconditioning sessions oriented toward abstinence; consequently, the program showed its most positive impact in this area. Thus, information about each program's orientation helps us to understand between-program differences in patterns across the specific outcome criteria. Overall, type of program explained 1.3% to 6.3% of the variance in 6-month treatment outcome.

PROGRAM COMPONENTS AND OUTCOME

As noted earlier, most alcoholism treatment evaluations end at this point—with a comparison of the relative effectiveness of global treatment conditions. Many of these studies find few if any differences between different treatment approaches (Miller & Hester, 1986). Such findings provide no information as to why a program may be more or less effective or how more effective programs might be developed. To address these issues, it is necessary to identify effective treatment components, or what have been referred to as the "active ingredients" of treatment. Accordingly, we related treatment outcome to specific treatment components within each program, while controlling for patient pretreatment factors.

In Chapter 2 we noted that the treatment components offered by the five programs varied. The hospital-based and milieu-oriented programs provided medications in addition to psychotherapy and educational materials, while the Salvation Army and halfway house programs stressed psychotherapeutic and educational interventions. The aversion conditioning program did not share the psychotherapeutic and educational/rehabilitative orientation of the other facilities; it relied almost entirely on the aversion conditioning procedure.

Using data from the TEF (see Chapter 2), we identified three treatment components that were important to most of the programs and comparable across programs and on which the level of patient participation varied within programs (therapy sessions, lectures and films, AA meetings). We related these components to outcome by calculating partial correlations separately for patients within each program; we controlled for patients' sociodemographic characteristics (age, gender, education, and marital status) and their standing on the intake variable that corresponded to the outcome criterion. We also focused on other components emphasized by particular programs: Sunday worship and part-time jobs for the Salvation Army program, recreational activities and Antabuse for the hospital-based program, recreational activities for the halfway house program, and Antabuse for the milieu-oriented program (see Table 4.1). Our findings were the following.

1. *Salvation Army.* Patients in the Salvation Army program who attended more therapy sessions, AA meetings, and Sunday worship services tended to have better 6-month outcome, especially on abstinence and social functioning. Participation in part-time jobs was related to better outcome on four of the six criteria (alcohol consumption, physical symptoms, depression, and social functioning).
2. *Hospital Based.* The therapeutic components of the hospital-based program had negligible associations with outcome except that more involvement in therapy sessions, lectures and films, and recreational activities was associated with better social functioning. More frequent use of Antabuse was related to less alcohol consumption

Table 4.1 Partial correlations between outcome and treatment experiences for patients in four alcoholism treatment programs

	Alcohol consumption	Abstinence	Physical symptoms	Depression	Social functioning	Occupational functioning
SALVATION ARMY ($N = 97$)						
Number of therapy sessions	−.15	.13	−.09	−.02	.18*	.04
Number of lectures and films	−.11	.16	−.08	−.03	.15	.11
Number of AA meetings	−.16	.18*	−.04	−.05	.22*	.02
Sunday worship	−.11	.21*	−.07	−.04	.15	.12
Number of part-time jobs	−.33***	.08	−.22*	−.19*	.23*	−.04
HOSPITAL BASED ($N = 106$)						
Number of therapy sessions	−.15	.06	−.06	.12	.22*	.09
Number of lectures and films	.06	−.01	−.02	.16	.24**	.08
Number of AA meetings	−.09	−.10	−.02	−.07	.12	.02
Number of recreational activities	−.13	−.08	−.03	−.05	.25**	.00
Number of days Antabuse taken	−.23*	.17*	−.11	.01	−.20*	−.10
HALFWAY HOUSE ($N = 59$)						
Number of therapy sessions	−.22*	.28*	−.30*	−.16	.15	.52***
Number of lectures and films	−.06	.36**	−.06	.20	−.09	.23*
Number of AA meetings	.01	.27*	−.01	−.02	.08	.15
Number of recreational activities	−.17	.57***	−.21	.00	−.03	.33*
MILIEU ORIENTED ($N = 92$)						
Number of therapy sessions	−.06	.10	.02	−.11	.17	−.09
Number of lectures and films	.01	−.04	.08	−.19*	.28**	−.07
Number of AA meetings attended	−.13	.12	−.02	−.14	.26**	.11
Number of days Antabuse taken	−.16	.02	−.17	−.21*	.14	.14

*$p < .05$.   **$p < .01$.   ***$p < .001$.

and a greater likelihood of abstinence, but also to poorer social functioning.

3. *Halfway House.* We observed the strongest relationships between treatment experiences and outcome among halfway house patients. In part, these findings reflect the relatively flexible nature of the program and the greater variability in level of participation as compared to that in the other four facilities. In particular, more participation in therapy sessions, lectures and films, and recreational activities was related to better treatment outcome on two or more of the following criteria: alcohol consumption, abstinence, physical symptoms, and occupational functioning. More frequent attendance at AA meetings was associated with a greater likelihood of abstinence.

4. *Aversion Conditioning.* The aversion conditioning program relied almost entirely on the conditioning sessions. The staff did not consider other treatment components to be important. The lack of within-program variability on the treatment components (see Table 2.2) precluded any meaningful partial correlation analyses.

5. *Milieu Oriented.* The Milieu-Oriented program was similar to the

halfway house program in its high overall level of treatment activity. However, there was much less variability in the intensity of treatment among patients in the milieu-oriented program (see Table 2.2). Greater use of Antabuse in the milieu-oriented program was related to less depression. In addition, attendance at educational lectures and films was related to less depression and better social outcome; attendance at AA meetings was associated with better social functioning.

Taken as a whole, our findings show that more intensive participation in psychological treatment and the use of Antabuse are related to better outcome, although the strength of these relationships is modest and varies somewhat across programs. In general, patients in the Salvation Army, halfway house, and milieu-oriented programs who participated more actively in therapy sessions, films and lectures, and AA meetings tend to show better outcome, but we observed only weak associations between these therapeutic components and outcome in the hospital-based program. The variation in the strength of the associations may reflect differences in treatment implementation across programs. For example, patients in the milieu-oriented program participated in more therapy sessions, AA meetings, and lectures and films on alcoholism during their average 30-day stay than did patients in the Salvation Army or halfway house programs during an average stay of more than 3 months.

We also examined the relationships of antianxiety medications and sedatives to outcome. In general, antianxiety medications and sedatives were not consistently related to outcome at the 6-month follow-up. This is as expected because 6 months has elapsed since these medications were taken. In contrast, Antabuse was associated with better overall outcome. Its positive effect is probably due to two factors. First, Antabuse is targeted directly at drinking behavior. Second, Antabuse is typically taken following treatment and thus is more likely to be associated with posttreatment outcome than are medications taken only while in a residential treatment setting.

Most of the relationships between specific treatment components and outcome are modest. Such findings may reflect the weakness of individual components in comparison with the personal and social forces that produce and maintain alcohol abuse. Thus, participating in 5 to 10 individual or group treatment sessions during 1 month in the milieu-oriented program cannot be expected to undo the psychological and social deficits that lead to and follow from prolonged abusive drinking. Another reason for the modest associations between specific components and outcome may be the compensatory influence of other program elements. In a flexibly organized program, a person who chooses to attend only a few AA meetings may participate more in individual or group psychotherapy. Under such conditions, it is difficult to detect a strong association between any single program component and outcome. We address this issue later by looking at the overall impact of multiple treatment components.

Finally, specific treatment components may differ in their influence on different groups of patients. For example, insight-oriented therapy sessions may be more beneficial for socially stable and well-educated patients than for patients who are less socially competent. Sex differences in response to specific treatment components may also reduce the overall magnitude of the relationships between such components and outcome. We address this issue in Chapter 5.

LENGTH OF TREATMENT AND OUTCOME

We also examined the association between length of stay in our five programs and treatment outcome. Clinicians and researchers often assume that patients who remain longer in residential alcoholism programs receive more treatment and therefore experience better outcomes. Empirically, however, a longer stay in inpatient programs has been associated with (1) more positive outcome, (2) better outcome at one follow-up but not at a second follow-up, (3) no better outcome than that from a shorter duration of treatment [most experimental studies fall in this category—see Miller & Hester (1986)], and (4) poorer outcome than a shorter length of stay. [For a review, see Finney, Moos, & Chan (1981).]

One contributing factor in the inconsistency of these results may be the failure in naturalistic studies to control for preexisting differences among patients remaining in treatment for varying periods of time. In our research, we related treatment outcome to length of stay while statistically controlling for pretreatment differences among patients.

We found that longer treatment was associated with better outcome in the halfway house and hospital-based programs, but not in the other programs. Specifically, patients who stayed longer in the hospital-based program drank less at the 6-month follow-up (partial $r = -.24$, $p < .01$). In the halfway house, a longer length of treatment was related to less alcohol consumption ($r = -.23$, $p < .05$) and a greater likelihood of being abstinent ($r = .26$, $p < .05$) and employed ($r = .32$, $p < .01$) at the 6-month follow-up. Although not statistically significant, the relationships between length of stay and outcome criteria for the Salvation Army program are similar to those for the halfway house.

The significant results for the halfway house may be attributable in part to the greater average length of stay. In this latter regard, Sheehan and his colleagues (1981) found that after participation in a 6-month program, 42% to 47% of chronic alcoholic patients were successfully adjusted (abstinent and employed or functioning as a homemaker) at 1- and 3-year follow-ups. They concluded that the typical residential treatment of 1 to 3 months may not be long enough to facilitate stable changes in attitude and behavior among chronic patients. Another factor accounting for the stronger relationship between treatment duration and outcome in the halfway house may be that the treatment was more community oriented, or more closely related to residents' normal life contexts.

Ellis and Krupinski (1964) found that length of stay was related to short-term positive results for first-admission patients but not for patients who had previously been hospitalized for alcoholism. Prior treatment may indicate a drinking problem that is relatively intractable, even with intensive treatment. We examined the relationships between length of stay and outcome separately for patients who had had no treatment for alcoholism in the past 3 years and for repeaters. We found significant partial correlations between length of stay and alcohol consumption ($r = -.46, p < .05$), abstinence ($r = .59, p < .01$), and social functioning ($r = .50, p < .01$) among the 26 first admissions and no significant partial correlations among the 71 repeaters at the Salvation Army center. However, there was no consistent pattern of results for first-admission versus returning patients in the other programs.

PARTICIPATION IN AFTERCARE

It is reasonable to assume that treatment gains are more likely to be maintained when discharged patients have access to and utilize aftercare services. Accordingly, several studies report an association between use of outpatient aftercare services and better treatment outcome (Ahles et al., 1983; Costello, 1980; Gilbert, 1988; Polich et al., 1981; Siegel et al., 1984; Smart & Gray, 1978; Vannicelli, 1978; but see Fitzgerald & Mulford, 1985; Kirk & Masi, 1978). In many of these studies, however, possible differences in background characteristics and pretreatment functioning between aftercare participants and nonparticipants were not controlled. Consequently, it is difficult to interpret the findings with confidence. In addition, it is not clear whether one type of aftercare is more effective than another.

To examine the relationship of aftercare to outcome, we obtained information on whether or not the patient participated in three types of preventive aftercare services during the follow-up interval: AA, outpatient treatment, and aversion conditioning booster sessions. We calculated partial correlations between each type of aftercare and each of the outcome criteria, controlling for patient background characteristics and the intake value of the outcome criterion.

Participation in AA was associated with less alcohol consumption ($r = -.12, p < .01$) and a higher abstinence rate and less depression (both $rs = .08, p < .05$). Similarly, participation in outpatient aftercare was related to better outcome on all of the criteria except occupational functioning (average $r = .12, p < .05$ for all of the remaining five outcome criteria). As might be expected, participation in aversion conditioning sessions was associated with a higher abstinence rate ($r = .15, p < .001$), but not with any of the other outcome criteria.

These findings suggest that participation in aftercare, particularly outpatient services and AA, helps to maintain gains made during residential treatment. Although both of these types of aftercare treatment are beneficial in terms of nondrinking as well as drinking outcome criteria, the benefits of conditioning sessions seem to be specific to abstinence.

THE SALVATION ARMY PROGRAM

There are unique aspects of the Salvation Army center that deserve special attention. About one-fourth of the patients in our study participated in the Salvation Army program. Our follow-up rate of 80% of the original Salvation Army cohort 6 months after discharge is much higher than the 6-month follow-up rates of 34% to 37% reported by Katz (1964, 1966) in two studies of Salvation Army clients. These data gave us an opportunity to focus on the treatment implementation and effectiveness of this program.

The Salvation Army has been looking after alcoholics for more than a century and now treats well over 70,000 clients annually in the United States (Jacobson, 1982). In contrast to the many private, for-profit programs emerging across the country, the Salvation Army treats clients who have few social or personal resources—homeless and indigent people for whom alcoholism is a "total life problem" (Blumberg et al., 1973; Fagan & Mauss, 1986; Halikas et al., 1984; Wiseman, 1979, 1982). Consequently, the Salvation Army provides a self-supporting, broad-spectrum program with a strong emphasis on vocational training. Clients are also provided with an extensive spiritual program, including Sunday worship services, Bible study, and spiritual counseling.

The vocational training aspect of the program allows clients to be partially self-supporting while in residence. The program operates as a self-sustaining business based on the repair and sale of goods donated by the community, with clients providing most of the labor. Despite its unique scope, character, and client population, the Salvation Army program and its impact have rarely been studied (but see Judge, 1971; Katz, 1966).

Treatment Orientation and Outcome

The philosophical orientation of the program is aimed at modifying the client's overall functioning—that is, the underlying processes that accompany and support the alcoholic life-style. The general treatment regimen of Salvation Army clients can be divided into five phases: (1) initial intake where immediate medical and basic living needs are provided and preliminary assessments are made; (2) a 30-day evaluation phase where clients undergo a more extensive medical and psychosocial assessment and begin to participate in spiritual, recreational, educational, AA, and vocational activities; (3) a 2- to 4-month treatment phase with continuation of Phase 2 activities plus specific psychotherapy and other counseling; (4) preparation for return to the community with help in locating housing and employment; and (5) transition from the residential program to independent life in the community (Jacobson, 1982).

The Salvation Army program we studied relied heavily on psychotherapeutic and educational interventions such as group therapy, lectures and educational films, and AA. Clients also participated actively in two treatment experiences that were unique among our five programs: Sunday worship and part-time jobs. Ninety-nine percent of the men went to Sunday worship at least once, and 62% attended six or more Sunday services; 87% of the men worked on at least one part-time job, while 64% worked at five or more.

Treatment outcome at the Salvation Army compared favorably with that in the halfway house and especially the hospital-based program (see Figures 3.1 and 3.2), both of which served demographically similar patients. For example, there was a 22% gain in employment rate from just prior to intake to 6 months after treatment for Salvation Army patients compared to an 18% gain for patients from the halfway house program and 9% for those from the hospital-based program. Two sailent aspects of the program, its social climate and treatment approach, are unique and integral to the Salvation Army and seem to be key factors in its success.

Treatment Environment

The profile presented in Chapter 2 (Figure 2.1) indicates that clients and staff saw the Salvation Army program as average or above average in all areas assessed by the COPES. Involvement, support, practical orientation, organization, and program clarity were emphasized most strongly. These areas reflect the Salvation Army's emphasis on personal control, the rehabilitation of the whole person, milieu therapy, and learning community living skills. The emphasis on practical orientation reflects the training school housed at the facility and the importance of working while in the program.

The COPES profile also reflects an integrated and cohesive social environment. The high agreement between staff and residents indicates that staff have an accurate perception of the program and are in close touch with the residents. The program climate was quite stable over time, as shown in COPES profiles we obtained about 6 months apart. This stability is probably due to the consistent program philosophy, the high agreement between residents and staff, and the clients' relative satisfaction with the program.

Treatment Components

As shown in Table 4.1, of the four treatment components that are significantly associated with outcome among Salvation Army residents, two are unique to the program: Sunday worship and part-time jobs. The other two are therapy sessions and AA meetings. The number of part-time jobs a patient held was associated with improvement in alcohol consumption, physical symptoms, depressed mood, and social functioning, whereas

Sunday worship was related to a higher likelihood of abstinence. Katz (1964) also found that participation in vocational counseling in a Salvation Army program was related to later improvement. Likewise, in an evaluation of a non-Salvation Army rehabilitation program for skid-row alcoholics that focused on the community reentry process, Fagan and Mauss (1986) reported improvements in abstinence and occupational functioning.

The beneficial effects of AA meetings and Sunday worship on abstinence and social functioning for Salvation Army clients are consistent with research on the importance of social support for alcoholics, including skid-row alcoholics (Fagan & Mauss, 1986; Geisbrecht, 1983; Tuchfeld et al., 1983). In Geisbrecht's (1983) comparison of former and current skid-row alcoholics, the two most important predictors of better drinking status were contacts with abstainers or moderate drinkers and religious affiliation. When viewed in relation to establishing reentry into the community, it is easier to provide access to abstainers or moderate drinkers through AA groups or religious organizations than it is to find a steady job, renew contact with family members (if any), or form a close relationship with another person. Consequently, both AA and Sunday worship provide a broad base of opportunities for developing social and personal resources that can be drawn on in the reentry process.

Client Participation and Outcome

A 90-day length of stay in the Salvation Army program is considered desirable because it allows for a detoxification and assessment period and about 2 months of treatment. However, many residents leave prematurely, and the amount or intensity of treatment can vary depending on the client's adjustment and receptivity to treatment. For example, staff may decide that some of the clients are functioning too poorly or lack sufficient motivation for treatment and thus do not offer treatment to them. Some clients reject any help other than food and shelter. To index the overall intensity of program participation, we combined the number of times a client participated in each of six treatment components (therapy, lectures and films, AA, house meetings, Sunday worship, and part-time jobs) by summing the client's standardized scores on these components. The resulting variable measures how actively each client participated in the program.

We used partial correlations to examine the relationship between residents' overall participation and their status on the six outcome criteria, controlling for prior functioning. Three of the six partial correlations were significant ($p < .05$), and all were in the expected direction. In particular, total participation was related to less alcohol consumption ($r = -.22$), a higher likelihood of abstaining ($r = .21$), and better social functioning ($r = .23$).

We also compared the perceptions of the treatment environment of clients who dropped out of the program before the planned time of discharge (26%) with the perceptions of those who completed the program. The dropouts perceived the Salvation Army treatment milieu more negatively than did those who remained. They reported significantly ($p < .05$) less involvement, support, order and organization, and program clarity than did the completers. These findings indicate that clients' early perceptions of the treatment milieu can predict their integration into the program and the likelihood that they will stay until the planned time of discharge. Overall, the findings show that clients' integration and participation in the Salvation Army program are moderately predictive of their status at follow-up.

In sum, the social climate and treatment experiences of the Salvation Army program reflect a relatively successful treatment approach that emphasizes the development of "social margin" or "social credit"—that is, the economic, personal, and social resources needed for chronic alcoholics to reenter successfully and function adequately within the community (Fagan & Mauss, 1986; Wiseman, 1979). The program is also relatively inexpensive, because a substantial proportion of its costs is covered by income from residents' part-time jobs. Salvation Army programs seem to be particularly beneficial for skid-row alcoholics who remain in the program until their planned discharge. However, a lesson from this type of program can be applied to a broader range of alcoholic patients. Treatment programs should be oriented toward changing drinking behavior *and* helping patients develop the personal, social, and economic resources they will need to function better in their normal life situations. We return to this point in Chapter 12.

THE RELATIVE STRENGTH OF TREATMENT

In Chapter 3, we examined the relationship of patient characteristics to outcome; in this chapter, we have broadened our focus and analyzed the role of treatment and its components. Our next step is to integrate these two foci and address the following issues: (1) What are the interrelationships among patient background characteristics, intake symptoms, treatment, and outcome? (2) How do patient characteristics, type of program, treatment intensity, and treatment climate uniquely and jointly affect treatment outcome?

An important issue is the relative influence of patient characteristics and treatment on outcome. Most prior research implies that patient characteristics (Panels I and II in Figure 4.1) are more strongly related to outcome and that treatment (Panels III, IV, and V) has little impact once sociodemographic characteristics and intake functioning are considered (Costello, 1980; Nathan & Skinstad, 1987; Ornstein & Cherepon, 1985). In addition to their relationship to treatment outcome, however, both social background and intake functioning influence the programs patients enter. For example, patients who enter private, for-profit programs tend to be older, married, and better educated. Thus, part of the "influence" of patient characteristics on outcome may be due to the type of treatment patients obtain.

Furthermore, the impact of treatment probably is underestimated by global treatment indices (such as type of treatment program) that do not examine variations in treatment within programs. Thus, we examined treatment not only in terms of which program a patient entered, but also in terms of treatment components and the treatment environment. In our analyses (see Figure 4.1), we assumed that the program a patient enters is the primary determinant of the treatment experiences that the patient receives and the quality of the treatment environment. In addition, patients' characteristics at intake may affect the treatment program they select, the treatment received, and their perceptions of the treatment program. We expected the type of program, the treatment components, and the treatment climate to influence treatment outcome both independently and jointly.

To examine the interrelationships among these variables and to estimate their relative effects on outcome, we constructed composite variables for treatment experiences and treatment environment and conducted regression analyses to estimate the model shown in Figure 4.1. We calculated the amount of variance explained by each of six sets of variables (see Figure 4.1): social background (Panel I), intake functioning (Panel II), program type (Panel III), treatment experiences (Panel IV), treatment environment (Panel V), and outcome functioning (Panel VI). The variables used in these analyses were:

1. *Social Background.* Gender, age, marital status (married, not married), and education.
2. *Intake Functioning.* The intake functioning index corresponding to the outcome criterion.
3. *Treatment Program.* Dummy (0-1) variables representing each of the programs (as is usual practice with dummy variables, four of the five dummy program variables were entered into the regression analysis).
4. *Intensity of Treatment.* The sum of 13 standardized (across programs) treatment components, including the psychosocial treatment components (number of AA meetings, recreational activities, house meetings, lectures and films, therapy sessions, other group sessions, part-time jobs, and Sunday worship meetings), length of stay, and 3 aftercare components (AA sessions, outpatient visits, and conditioning sessions), offered by each program; Antabuse was also included.
5. *Treatment Environment.* The sum of the 10 standardized (across programs) COPES dimensions (anger and aggression and staff control were reverse scored).

We estimated the amount of variance explained by each set of variables when predicting subsequent variables in the model (treatment experiences, treatment environment, and outcome), the amount of variance shared between different sets of variables (patient and treatment factors), and the total amount of variance explained by all of the relevant sets of variables when predicting subsequent variables and treatment outcome.

Relationship of Patient Characteristics to Treatment Factors

Patients of higher sociodemographic status and patients with less severe symptoms were more likely to enter the for-profit programs than the nonprofit programs (see Chapters 2 and 3). However, neither the social background variables nor intake functioning had any strong effects on the intensity of treatment received. On average, patient background and intake characteristics explained only 1.2% of the variance in treatment experiences. In contrast, the treatment program strongly influenced the intensity of treatment. The milieu-oriented, Salvation Army, and halfway house programs offered more intensive treatment, whereas the aversion conditioning and hospital-based programs had less intensive treatment. The average amount of variance in treatment intensity that can be attributed solely to the program is 30.4%; adding the joint and independent effects of patient background and intake functioning raises the total explained variance only slightly to an average of 32.4%. Thus, almost all of the variation in intensity of treatment is related to the type of program a patient enters.

Likewise, neither patient sociodemographic characteristics nor intake functioning account for much of the variation in perceptions of the treatment milieu (average explained variance is 1.4%). While only a small amount of explained variance can be attributed uniquely to patient characteristics, about 4.5% of the variation in perceptions of the treatment milieu is shared between patient and treatment factors. As expected, however, the type of program strongly affects perceptions of the treatment environment. On average, 18.9% of the variation in perceived treatment environment is attributable to program; this is about two-thirds of the average total explained variance of 26.2%. The milieu-oriented, Salvation Army, and aversion conditioning programs had especially positive treatment environments. In contrast, there is virtually no association between intensity of treatment and the perceived treatment environment. Thus, the COPES is a useful tool for obtaining unique, relatively "objective" information about characteristics of alcoholism treatment programs.

Relationship of Patient and Program Factors to Outcome

Table 4.2 shows the percent of variation in the six outcome criteria attributable to each of the five sets of predictor variables (social background, intake functioning, treatment program, treatment intensity, and treatment

Table 4.2 Percent variance in six-month outcome associated with patient and treatment factors

	Outcome criteria					
	Alcohol consumption	Abstinence	Physical symptoms	Depression	Social functioning	Occupational functioning
PATIENT FACTORS	1.9	0.5	8.5***	17.1***	25.8***	12.2***
Social background (Panel I)	1.6	0.4	1.5	0.6	1.5	3.0*
Intake functioning (Panel II)	0.2	0.1	5.1***	14.8***	24.0***	6.9***
Shared between Panels I and II	0.1	0.0	1.9	1.7	0.3	2.3
TREATMENT FACTORS	6.0***	9.0***	6.8***	3.8**	4.2**	2.8
Treatment program (Panel III)	1.8	7.3***	0.9	1.0	0.7	0.9
Intensity of treatment (Panel IV)	2.9***	2.7***	1.7*	0.4	1.7***	1.4*
Treatment environment (Panel V)	0.2	0.0	2.5***	1.0*	0.4	0.1
Shared among panels III, IV, and V	1.1	–	1.7	1.4	1.4	0.4
Shared between patient and treatment factors	4.4	8.0	8.9	8.0	4.4	3.0
Total variance explained	12.3***	17.5***	24.2***	28.9***	34.4***	18.0***

*$p < .05$.   **$p < .01$.   ***$p < .001$.

environment). The total explained variance ranges from 12.3% for alcohol consumption to 34.4% for social activities. We observed some consistent patterns of findings across the different outcome criteria. First, patients' social background accounts for a small amount of variance in outcome (0.4% to 3.0%). In contrast, except for alcohol consumption and abstinence, intake functioning accounts for a larger amount of outcome variance (5.1% for physical symptoms to 24% for social activities). In addition, patient characteristics share some additional outcome variance with treatment factors (3.0% to 8.9%). This shared variance can be interpreted as a joint effect of patient characteristics and treatment on outcome. Patients with better personal and social resources are more likely to enter the for-profit programs, which have better treatment outcome.

Except for abstinence, type of program independently accounts for only a small amount of variance (0.7% to 1.8%) in outcome. Program type explains 7.3% of the variation in abstinence; this is because patients in the for-profit programs were more likely to be abstinent in the 6-month follow-up period. These generally nonsignificant *independent* effects of program, considered together with the larger and significant *total* effects for program found in the analyses of covariance presented earlier, indicate that, except for abstinence, the effects of the treatment programs are mediated by patients' treatment experiences and the quality of the program environment.

In addition to mediating the effects of the programs, treatment intensity had independent effects on all the outcome criteria except depression (accounting for 1.4% to 2.9% additional variance). After patient pretreatment characteristics, type of program, and treatment intensity are taken into account, the quality of the treatment environment explained an additional 1% of the variance in physical symptoms and 2.5% of the variance in depressed mood. Like the partial correlations between individual treatment components and outcome presented earlier, these findings point to the value of looking within the black box of treatment. By taking into account variations in treatment within programs, we explained some additional variation in outcome. Overall, the three sets of treatment variables accounted for between 2.3% (occupational functioning) and 9% (abstinence) of the variance in outcome that was independent of variance explained by patient pretreatment factors.

When we compared the contribution of patient pretreatment characteristics to that of treatment characteristics, a somewhat unexpected finding emerged. Treatment-related variables are much better predictors of alcohol consumption and abstinence than are patient pretreatment characteristics (6.0% versus 1.9% and 9.0% versus 0.5%, respectively—see Figure 4.4). The contributions of patient-related and treatment-related variables are about equal when predicting physical symptoms (8.5% versus 6.8%), whereas patient factors are more important than treatment factors in predicting depression (17.1% versus 3.8%), social functioning (25.8% versus 4.2%), and occupational functioning (12.2% versus 2.8%). These findings suggest that drinking behavior is more responsive to treatment, whereas other outcome criteria are somewhat less responsive. Nevertheless, treat-

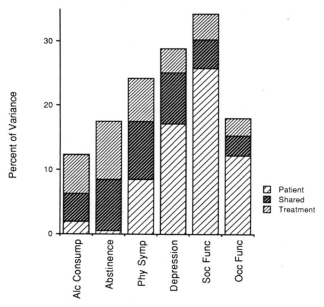

Figure 4.4 Percent of variance in outcome associated with patient and treatment factors.

ment intensity and/or treatment environment contributed to the explained variance on each outcome criterion.

Overall, alcoholism programs seem to have more short-term impact on the presenting problem of drinking behavior than they do on functioning in other life areas. This targeting effect is as expected given the primary focus of these intervention programs. As we will discuss later (Chapter 7), however, unresolved problems in other life areas may account for the eventual high relapse rates among alcoholic patients, particularly those who have fewer personal and social resources (Tuchfeld et al., 1983; Vaillant, 1983).

FUTURE DIRECTIONS

We have focused on the process and outcome of treatment by examining its effects between and within programs. We used an integrated approach to analyze the interrelationships between patient and treatment factors and treatment outcome. We identified differences among the five programs in overall outcome after controlling for pretreatment factors and observed some positive relationships between outcome and specific treatment components, length of stay, and participation in aftercare. We focused special attention on the Salvation Army program, which serves skid-row alcoholics and includes worship services and part-time jobs. The Salvation Army exemplifies the uniqueness of each program and the potential value of matching treatment orientations to the specific needs of patients.

Our conceptual paradigm helps to clarify how patient-related and treatment-related factors influence outcome. Consistent with prior research, intake functioning is a moderately strong predictor of some outcome indices, although it does not predict posttreatment drinking behavior. The relatively strong total contributions of treatment-related factors in explaining outcome on drinking behavior underscore the importance of treatment intensity and treatment environment. In addition, our findings show that patients with more social competence and better initial functioning enter programs that offer a better-quality treatment environment. We draw this conclusion from the finding that 3% to 9% of the variance in outcome is shared between patient-related and treatment-related variables. In prior research, patient characteristics have been credited with these shared effects, which led researchers to underestimate the power of treatment. In fact, some of the "influence" of patient pretreatment characteristics on outcome seems to be mediated by the type and intensity of treatment and aftercare experiences patients obtain.

Prior studies have reported little or no influence of treatment on outcome after patient characteristics are taken into account. By extending our analyses beyond those of the typical black-box approach, we identified substantial combined contributions of treatment-related factors to outcome. In fact, for both alcohol consumption and abstinence, the proportion of variance in outcome uniquely accounted for by treatment-related variables is much greater than that uniquely accounted for by patient-related variables. These findings indicate that alcoholism treatment programs may have stronger influences on short-term treatment outcome than previously thought.

Overall, we were able to explain 12% to 34% of the variance in treatment outcome by the sets of patient- and treatment-related factors taken together. These percentages represent gains of 3% to 9% (mean = 6%) over the variance explained by patient background and intake functioning alone (see Table 3.1). This is a somewhat larger proportion of the outcome variance than that accounted for by treatment in most similar studies (Costello, 1980; Ojehagen, Skjaerris, & Berglund, 1988; Schuckit, Schwei, & Gold, 1986). Our approach embodies a more robust conceptualization of treatment and apportions the predictable variance more appropriately between patient and treatment factors. Thus, we find that treatment has a moderately strong short-term influence on outcome, especially alcohol consumption and abstinence. Even so, most of the variance in outcome remains unexplained.

5
Gender and Marital Status in Treatment and Outcome

In Chapters 3 and 4, we saw that patient demographic characteristics and treatment variables exert only a modest impact on 6-month treatment outcome. Our analyses assessed the main or average effects of those variables. However, the influence of patient and treatment variables may vary, depending on the effects of other patient factors. For example, the prognostic significance of marital status may be different for men and women patients. We address this issue here.

Similarly, a particular treatment component may exert only a modest influence overall because it affects some patients differently than others. Some patients may respond positively, while other patients may be unaffected or even respond negatively. According to the "matching hypothesis," overall outcome should be more favorable when patients are more appropriately matched with treatment. We wanted to know whether men and women might respond differently to different components of treatment programs. Our focus on this issue, and on possible differential implications of marital status depending on patient gender, reflects the recent increased attention to alcohol abuse among women (Wilsnack & Beckman, 1984).

Most comparative studies have focused on gender differences in family history and drinking behavior at the time of intake into treatment. Only a few studies have followed up on intake sex differences and compared the treatment process and outcome for men and women alcoholics. Moreover, although marital status is an important prognostic factor for alcoholism treatment outcome, it has rarely been examined in conjunction with sex differences in treatment outcome.

In this chapter, we examine gender and marital status differences in drinking history, intake symptoms, treatment and aftercare experiences, and treatment outcome. We assess the effects of marital status, treatment components, and aftercare on the treatment outcome of men and women patients. We also discuss how the match between treatment modalities and sex-role expectations can contribute to the process of remission.

PRIOR RESEARCH ON GENDER AND MARITAL STATUS

Gender, Marital Status, and Drinking History and Symptoms

Previous comparisons of the personal histories of alcoholic men and women show that women are more likely than men to (1) come from homes in which a parent or spouse was a heavy drinker, (2) become problem drinkers at a later age, (3) enter treatment sooner, and (4) have fewer drinking-related arrests (Annis, 1980; Beckman, 1975; Beckman & Amaro, 1984; Bourne & Light, 1979; Gomberg & Lisansky, 1984).

Prior to treatment intake, women alcoholics consume less alcohol and are more likely to drink alone or at home, whereas their male counterparts tend to drink with friends or in bars (Beckman, 1975; MacDonald, 1987; Sokolow et al., 1980). There is also some evidence that women are more likely than men to drink in response to stressful life events (Linsky et al., 1985) and that they are more susceptible to social pressure to drink (Gomberg & Lisansky, 1984).

Findings related to gender differences in psychological adjustment among alcohol abusers are contradictory. Some researchers have suggested that due to their greater incidence of mental illness and psychiatric treatment (Leaf & Bruce, 1987; Verbrugge, 1985), women alcoholics are more maladjusted than men alcoholics (Beckman, 1975). However, Douglas and Nutter (1986) found no differences in self-esteem between men and women alcoholics entering a public alcoholism treatment facility.

Although marital status is related to better mental health (Thoits, 1986), few studies have compared married and unmarried alcoholics within each gender group. In general, marital status has been used as an index of social competence and maturity, which reflects the achievement of important social skills and resources. Such personal and social resources may mediate the link between marital status and drinking behavior. Marital status predicts consumption patterns among men, with married men tending to drink less (Parker et al., 1980; Sokolow et al., 1980), but not among women. Some studies find no relationship between alcohol consumption and marital status for women (Parker et al., 1980), while others suggest that married women are more (Sokolow et al., 1980) or less (Wilsnack et al., 1984) likely to abuse alcohol.

Gender, Marital Status, and Treatment

Most studies of treatment effectiveness do not distinguish between the outcome of men and women alcoholics; those that do report contradictory findings (Annis & Liban, 1980; Blume, 1980; Vannicelli, 1984). Sokolow and his co-workers (1980) found that women patients were easier to follow, but there were no sex differences in treatment outcome. Two reviews (Annis, 1980; Vannicelli, 1984) suggest no difference in outcome between men and women alcoholics; some studies that report gender differences show better outcome among women (Kammeier & Conley, 1979), but others show worse outcome (Blume, 1980; Braiker, 1982; Wilsnack, 1982). Overall, men and women seem to show comparable treatment outcome.

Using a somewhat different approach, some studies have suggested that men and women vary in their response to specific treatment modalities. Lindbeck (1975) reported that women patients rated individual therapy as more helpful, while men patients rated group therapy as more helpful. Similarly, Pemberton (1967) observed that men patients tended to support each other, to discuss openly their alcoholism-related difficulties, and to conduct spontaneous therapy groups, while such group-related interactions rarely occurred among women patients. These differences may stem from the higher levels of shame and guilt experienced by alcoholic women and their resulting reluctance to discuss these problems in a mixed-sex group. As a result, women's group-oriented activities and therapy may be more effective for women than mixed-sex groups (Wilsnack, 1982). However, Vannicelli (1984) found little empirical support for the generally held views that (1) women respond better to individual and family therapy and men respond better to group therapy, and (2) women need to be treated separately in segregated rather than mixed-sex groups.

Just as men and women may respond differently to specific types of treatment, variations in treatment environments may have differential impacts on the outcome of one gender group (Chapters 2 and 4). Sokolow and his co-workers (1980) rated the treatment orientation of 17 alcoholism programs. Medically oriented programs were characterized by more physicians, psychiatrists, and nurses, more drug treatment, and a focus on structured patient-staff relationships. Peer group-oriented programs had more staff who were recovered alcoholics and tended to emphasize patient independence and self-government. Women alcoholics were more successfully treated in medically oriented facilities, while men were more successfully treated in peer group-oriented facilities. The investigators concluded that women alcoholics may respond best in treatment settings in which they maintain a more traditional patient role. In contrast, men may do better when there is more emphasis on peer group interaction.

Prognostic Factors and Treatment Outcome

In Vannicelli's (1984) review of prognostic factors in treatment outcome, few consistent findings pointed to specific personal, psychosocial, or treatment factors related to better outcome for women patients. Although Emrick (1975) reached similar conclusions, he suggested that patients with different personal characteristics may respond differently to varying types of treatment. Such personal characteristics could be gender related.

Another set of prognostic factors are life stressors and social resources.

Gender and marital status differences in social contexts may be related to treatment outcome. Alcoholic patients who are more satisfied with their marriages and whose spouses are involved in treatment are likely to participate in treatment longer (Noel et al., 1987). In addition, at least for women, levels of drinking are influenced by the drinking patterns of their spouses and their close friends and siblings (Dahlgren, 1979; Wilsnack et al., 1984). These factors may explain Wiens and Menustik's (1983) finding that married men respond better to treatment than unmarried men, but that this relationship did not hold for women.

We address some of these issues by examining gender and marital status differences in the treatment process and course of alcoholism. For instance, do men and women patients respond differently to treatment overall or to particular treatment components? Are specific aspects of the program environment associated with differences in men's and women's drinking after treatment? Do married and unmarried men and women have differential posttreatment experiences, such as participation in outpatient aftercare and living with a heavy drinker? If so, how do these experiences influence their treatment outcome?

GENDER AND MARITAL STATUS SUBGROUPS

We have described the 429 patients who participated both at intake and at the 6-month follow-up (Chapter 3). Because the Salvation Army program admitted only men, the 97 patients in that program were omitted from the analyses reported here, leaving a sample of 332 patients (262 men and 70 women).

Personal Characteristics and Drinking History

We first compared the demographic characteristics of four gender and marital status subgroups: married women, unmarried women, married men, and unmarried men. As expected, married patients in both gender groups tended to be older, to have higher income levels, and to be more residentially stable than those who were not married. The four groups were roughly comparable in educational level, religious preference, and ethnic background. The only notable gender difference was that women had lower incomes than men.

We found gender differences in drinking history similar to those of prior studies. Women were older than men when they first drank and when they first drank to get drunk; they had fewer arrests, and a larger proportion reported that their mothers and husbands are or were heavy drinkers. Among the currently married, women were more likely to report heavy drinking among other household members than were men (28% versus 13%). With respect to marital status differences, married patients were older when they first drank to get drunk and when they first recognized their drinking as a problem, had fewer arrests, and were less likely to have been hospitalized previously for alcoholism.

Intake Functioning and 6-Month Outcome

Table 5.1 presents means for the four sex and marital status subgroups on five of our functioning criteria at intake and at the 6-month follow-up. On three of the variables (alcohol consumption, physical symptoms, and depressed mood), lower scores represent better outcome; on abstinence and social functioning, higher scores represent better outcome. Overall, all four subgroups improved from intake to follow-up on the drinking-related criteria (alcohol consumption and abstinence) and on physical symptoms. Because most of the married women were not employed, we did not use occupational functioning as an outcome criterion here.

Men and women patients did not differ on any of the functioning indices at intake or follow-up. Thus, men and women showed comparable treatment outcome. However, there were some expected marital status differences. Compared with their unmarried counterparts, married patients were less impaired on all of the criteria except social functioning at both intake and follow-up.

We also identified some interactions between sex and marital status. At intake to treatment, unmarried women consumed considerably more alcohol relative to married women than did unmarried men relative to married men. Moreover, marital status was unrelated to social activities for men, but married women were more active socially than unmarried women.

The interaction effect of gender and marital status on posttreatment abstinence is due to the high abstention rates at follow-up for married men (45%) and unmarried women (42%) relative to unmarried men (18%) and married women (28%). Being married increases the likelihood of abstaining for men patients, but it lowers the likelihood of abstaining for women patients.

In sum, the four sex and marital status subgroups differ in outcome on the drinking criteria, physical symptoms, and depression, even after controlling for intake functioning. This differential improvement may be related to treatment and life context factors. We examine such factors first for the treatment period (treatment experiences and perceptions of the treatment environment) and then for the 6-month follow-up period (outpatient aftercare treatment and living with a heavy drinker).

Treatment Experiences and Perceptions of the Treatment Environment

Two-way analyses of variance (Table 5.2) showed no gender or marital status differences in treatment experiences, except for one main effect for marital status: married patients attended more educational lectures and films than unmarried patients did.

Table 5.1 Sex and marital status differences in functioning at intake and 6-month follow-up

	Unmarried men (N = 141)	Married men (N = 121)	Unmarried women (N = 31)	Married women (N = 39)	F statistics		
					Sex	Marital status	Interaction
FUNCTIONING AT INTAKE							
Alcohol consumption (oz. of ethanol)	15.77	14.34[b]	16.03[c]	10.83[b,c]	3.27	5.18*	4.12*
Physical symptoms (1-5 scale)	3.05[a]	2.56[a]	3.10[c]	2.51[c]	.02	17.92***	.64
Depression (1-5 scale)	3.23[a]	2.82[a]	3.29	3.01	.72	11.06**	.61
Social functioning (1-5 scale)	2.05	2.07	1.86	2.25	.00	1.53	4.96*
FUNCTIONING AT 6-MONTH FOLLOW-UP							
Alcohol consumption (oz. of ethanol)	6.12[a]	3.31[a]	4.08	2.00	2.20	6.28*	.08
Abstinence (% yes)	.18[a]	.45[a]	.42	.28	.07	11.86***	8.83**
Physical symptoms (1-5 scale)	2.04[a]	1.57[a]	1.96	1.56	.06	7.68**	.01
Depression (1-5 scale)	2.65[a]	2.17[a]	2.64[c]	2.18[c]	.35	12.10**	.07
Social functioning (1-5 scale)	2.14	2.26[b]	2.07[c]	2.54[b,c]	2.25	2.40	1.24

Notes. Means that share a common superscript differ significantly ($p < .05$) by the Student-Newman-Keuls test.
Analyses of covariance on functioning at the 6-month follow-up control for intake functioning.
*$p < .05$. **$p < .01$. ***$p < .001$.

Table 5.2 Sex and marital status differences in treatment and posttreatment experiences

	Unmarried men (N = 141)	Married men (N = 121)	Unmarried women (N = 31)	Married women (N = 39)	F statistics		
					Sex	Marital status	Interaction
TREATMENT EXPERIENCES							
Group therapy sessions	10.75	9.33	11.39	9.54	.13	2.64	.04
Lectures and films	10.96	14.64	13.48	15.36	.82	5.55*	2.34
TREATMENT ENVIRONMENT							
Personal problem orientation	7.00	7.41	6.19	6.74	5.84*	3.06	.06
Staff control	4.97	4.39	4.07	4.00	7.70**	6.56*	1.31
POSTTREATMENT EXPERIENCES							
Been outpatient (%)	41[a]	50	68[a]	44	2.17	1.23	6.20*
Nonrehospitalized patients (n = 163)	61	56	67	48	.12	1.04	.53
Rehospitalized patients (n = 167)	33[a]	38	69[a]	36	3.97*	.09	3.87
Been in AA (%)	31	32	31	31	.01	.10	.10
Living with a heavy drinker (%)	6	13[b]	6[c]	28[b,c]	4.52*	8.67**	3.27

Note. Percentages that share a common superscript differ significantly ($p < .05$) by the Student-Newman-Keuls test.
*$p < .05$. **$p < .01$.

Two-way analyses of variance of gender and marital status differences in patients' perceptions of the treatment environment yielded two main effects for gender. Men saw their program environment as providing more personal problem orientation and staff control than women did. Married patients perceived less staff control than unmarried patients did. As described in Chapter 2, a high personal problem orientation reflects a program emphasis on understanding patients' personal problems and feelings. Staff control reflects the extent to which staff use measures to keep patients "in line," for example, by setting rules, scheduling activities, and structuring their interactions with patients.

Posttreatment Experiences

Table 5.2 also presents the results of two-way analyses of variance of gender and marital status differences in experiences during the follow-up period. The first set of results shows the percent of patients in each subgroup who participated in preventive aftercare, such as outpatient therapy or AA. The results for outpatient treatment are presented for the entire sample, and separately for patients who were and were not rehospitalized for alcoholism during the 6-month follow-up interval. The last row shows the percent of patients who were living with a heavy drinker.

Unmarried women and married men were more likely to participate in outpatient treatment than married women or unmarried men. Except for unmarried women, rehospitalized patients were less likely than nonrehospitalized patients to have received outpatient treatment, suggesting that participation in aftercare is related to better outcome. For example, only 38% of the married men and 36% of the married women who were rehospitalized participated in outpatient aftercare, while 56% and 48% of their nonrehospitalized counterparts obtained outpatient aftercare; we found that unmarried women were most likely overall to have been outpatients. There were no gender or marital status differences in AA attendance.

Table 5.2 also shows that married women were most likely to have been living with a heavy drinker during the follow-up period (28%). This finding is consistent with other research indicating that many women alcoholics come from homes where a parent or a spouse is a heavy drinker.

Treatment and Posttreatment Experiences and Treatment Outcome

To assess the relative effects of treatment and posttreatment experiences on outcome and to examine differences in remission processes for men and women, we conducted regression analyses separately for each gender group and for each of the five outcome criteria. The independent variables are: (1) marital status; (2) intake index corresponding to the outcome criterion; (3) treatment experiences (number of group therapy sessions, number of lectures and films); (4) perceptions of program environment (personal problem orientation and staff control); and (5) posttreatment experiences (outpatient aftercare and living with a heavy drinker). These analyses examine the relationship of treatment and posttreatment experiences to outcome while controlling for other prognostic factors.

Unstandardized regression coefficients are presented in Table 5.3 so that the results for men and women patients can be compared. The differential effect of marital status on abstinence is consistent with that of the simpler analyses shown in Table 5.1. Being married is related to a higher likelihood of abstaining for men and a lower likelihood of abstaining for women. In addition, compared to unmarried men, married men consumed 2.32 fewer ounces of alcohol at the 6-month follow-up.

Men and women patients differed in their response to group therapy and lectures and films. For men patients, participation in group therapy is related to less alcohol consumption at follow-up, while attendance at lectures and films is related to more alcohol consumption. In

Table 5.3 Unstandardized regression coefficients indicating the relationship of sex, marital status, and treatment process to 6-month outcome

	Alcohol consumption	Abstinence	Physical symptoms	Depression	Social functioning
MEN PATIENTS					
Married	−2.32*	.17*	−.20	−.20	.06
Intake functioning	.09	.07	.38***	.50***	.52***
Group therapy	−1.90*	−.10	−.11	.08	.04
Lectures and films	1.33*	.04	.09	−.04	.04
Personal problem orientation	−.29	.03	−.05*	−.03	.01
Staff control	.97**	−.01	.11**	.03	−.02
Been outpatient	−2.68**	.15*	−.27*	−.31**	.16
Living with a heavy drinker	1.42	−.13	.07	.15	.05
R	.37	.36	.53	.59	.54
Percent variance explained	13.3	13.0	28.0	35.3	29.5
WOMEN PATIENTS					
Married	−.36	−.36*	−.15	−.22	.12
Intake functioning	−.08	−.18	.19*	.29**	.54***
Group therapy	3.49**	.01	−.04	−.09	.28*
Lecture and films	−2.66***	.06	−.09	−.12	−.01
Personal problem orientation	.21	−.03	.02	−.03	.02
Staff control	−.31	−.07	.08	.11*	−.15**
Been outpatient	.40	−.28*	.11	.36*	−.41*
Living with a heavy drinker	−.63	.16	.26	−.04	−.01
R	.48	.45	.51	.59	.74
Percent variance explained	23.3	20.5	25.7	35.4	55.4

*$p < .05$. **$p < .01$. ***$p < .001$.

contrast, attendance at lectures and films is related to less alcohol consumption for women patients, while participation in group therapy is associated with more alcohol consumption. Group therapy participation is also associated with involvement in social activities for women; those activities may provide more opportunities for drinking. Thus, women show better drinking outcome when they attend more lectures and films and participate in fewer group therapy sessions; the opposite findings hold for men.

For men, perceiving high personal problem orientation in the treatment environment was associated with improvement in physical symptoms and with abstinence ($p < .10$). In contrast, personal problem orientation was not significantly related to any of the outcome measures for women. Although men tend to perceive more staff control in treatment settings than do women, higher staff control is associated with poorer treatment outcome for both groups. Men who report more staff control during treatment show more posttreatment alcohol consumption and physical symptoms. Among women, higher staff control is associated with more depression and fewer social activities.

Outpatient aftercare is an important predictor of better outcome on four of the five criteria for men patients. In contrast, it is associated with a lower likelihood of abstaining, higher depression, and fewer social activities among women patients.

Overall, the proportions of 6-month outcome variance explained by pretreatment, treatment, and posttreatment factors ranges from 13% to 35% for men patients and from 20% to 55% for women patients. In general, the amount of explained variance is somewhat higher for women (average = 32%) than for men (average = 24%). In addition, the increment in the amount of explained variance that can be attributed to environmental factors overall (treatment, aftercare, and living with a heavy drinker) is greater for women (average added explained variance is 17%) than for men (average added explained variance is 5.8%).

OVERVIEW AND IMPLICATIONS FOR TREATMENT

We observed no overall differences in treatment outcome between men and women patients once marital status and intake functioning were controlled. Within each gender group, however, being married relates differently to outcome. Among men patients, being married was an asset—it was related to an increased likelihood of abstinence. For women patients, being married decreased the likelihood of abstinence.

A woman problem drinker's tendency to be influenced by her spouse's drinking behavior (Dahlgren, 1979; Wilsnack et al., 1984) may explain the differential impact of marriage on treatment outcome for men and women alcoholics. Because a higher proportion of women alcoholics are married to heavy drinkers, we would expect less abstinence among women subsequent to release from a treatment program. Although they provide no information on spouse drinking patterns, Sokolow and his colleagues (1980) noted that the proportions of women alcoholics abstinent at two follow-up points (3 months and 8 months after discharge) declined more quickly than did those for men. Price and his colleagues (1981) found that spouses who both smoke tend to resist change in smoking and to reinforce one another's smoking behavior. Furthermore, alcoholic patients are more likely to remain in treatment when their spouse is involved in the treatment process (Noel et al., 1987).

These findings are also consistent with the idea that being married has different role identity implications for women and men. For example, the norms and demands associated with being married (particularly high family role demands) may lead to more social isolation and role strain for women than for men (Aneshensel, Frerichs, & Clark, 1981; Thoits, 1983). A potentially fruitful avenue for future research is to consider the influence of specific combinations of multiple role identities on treatment outcome for men and women patients.

Our findings also led us to focus on the treatment and posttreatment experiences that might contribute to differences in outcome among the subgroups. The analyses of gender and marital status showed that men and women patients responded differently to two treatment components. Group therapy sessions were associated with less alcohol consumption for men, and educational lectures and films were related to less alcohol consumption for women. In addition, men tended to report more emphasis on personal problem orientation in the treatment setting and to respond somewhat more positively to it. These findings are consistent with those of other researchers who have found that women patients report a greater need for educational counseling (Beckman & Amaro, 1986) and that men patients tend to engage in group-related activities and to rate group therapy as most helpful, whereas women rarely form group-related interactions and rate individual aspects of treatment as most helpful (Lindbeck, 1975).

Some of these differences in response to individual and group treatment may be attributed to differences in men's and women's drinking patterns. We found that men are more likely to drink in bars and with friends than women are. Similarly, Harford (1978) noted that it is more acceptable and common for men to drink with others in bars and at social gatherings than it is for women to do so. As a consequence, women alcoholics are more likely to drink alone and to be regarded as more deviant than men alcoholics are (Beckman, 1975; Beckman & Amaro, 1986).

Because men associate group settings with drinking-related behavior, men alcoholics may feel more comfortable than women in group therapy and may be more receptive to treatment aimed at open communication about their drinking problem. In contrast, women alcoholics, who often are "hidden" drinkers, may anticipate disapproval from others and thus feel less comfortable about dealing openly with their drinking problem in group treatment (Beckman & Amaro, 1986). Consequently, they may prefer to deal with problem drinking in a way that minimizes negative sanctions for violating sex-role expectations related to alcoholism, such as through educational lectures and films. This interpretation is consistent with the finding that women experience more opposition to alcoholism treatment from their friends and family than men do. In fact, women alcoholics are more reluctant to utilize treatment facilities than men are (Beckman & Amaro, 1984; Litman, 1986; Thom, 1984).

The high men-to-women ratio in most programs and therapy groups may also contribute to the differential effectiveness of group treatment. In our study, about 25% of the patients in each program were women, so groups were typically composed of more men than women. This imbalance can lead to men emerging as the more active or dominant participants and, in turn, being more satisfied with group interaction. Research on the sex composition of work groups has shown that when women are in the minority, they experience more social isolation and expend more effort to maintain a satisfactory role within the group (Kanter, 1977). Following this line of reasoning, some clinicians have recommended that women patients be treated in all-women groups.

In contrast, Sokolow et al. (1980) reported higher abstinence rates for women treated in facilities with lower proportions of women. Possible explanations for their findings include (1) the positive effects of receiving more attention from men clients when there are fewer women, (2) a tendency for women in facilities with a high proportion of men to "huddle together" and reinforce each other's treatment goals, and (3) possible differences in client composition across facilities that may be associated with the men-to-women ratio. Overall, more research on the association between the proportion of women in a facility and treatment outcome for men and women patients is needed.

The association between men's perceptions of staff control and poorer outcome may be related to sex-role norms regarding the greater power and freedom that men expect to enjoy (Cox, 1987). Men patients may respond adversely to staff efforts to maintain control by enforcing rules, scheduling activities, and so on. Consequently, poorer treatment outcome among men may be associated with a treatment environment that is too stifling to facilitate the recovery process. Although some researchers speculate that women may react positively to structure in the treatment setting (Sokolow et al., 1980), staff control was also associated with more depression and less social activity among women. Thus, the relationship between highly structured treatment environments and poorer treatment outcome (Moos, 1988c) holds for both men and women patients.

We also observed differential associations between outpatient aftercare and posttreatment functioning for men and women. For men patients, outpatient aftercare is associated with lower alcohol consumption, increased abstinence, less depression, and fewer physical symptoms. For women patients, however, outpatient care is associated with decreased abstinence, more depression, and fewer social activities. The fact that much of this outpatient aftercare was provided in groups made up predominantly of men may explain the differential response of men and women to it. It is also possible that outpatient treatment with male therapists is not as helpful for women as for men.

We also found that unmarried women were most likely to participate in outpatient follow-up care and married men were the next most likely group to do so. These differences may be due to sex-stereotyped staff expectations about dependency and vulnerability and their resulting evaluations and aftercare recommendations. Doherty (1978) found that recommendations for discharge or for continued psychiatric treatment were related to ratings of pathology for men patients but not for women patients. Recommendations for further treatment for women were more related to being young, single, and unemployed. Staff may see women with these characteristics as lacking support at home or at work and thus as more vulnerable to an exacerbation of their illness. Along similar lines, Sokolow and his associates (1980) noted that women alcoholic patients were more frequently referred to aftercare than men alcoholic patients were.

A second factor that may account for the differences in aftercare participation rates is the likelihood of being encouraged by others to continue with follow-up visits. Among married alcoholics, Mulford (1977) reported that a man discusses his personal problems with his wife more often than a woman turns to her husband for help. Thus, while married men may rely on and be encouraged by their wives to participate in preventive aftercare (Thom, 1984), husbands of alcoholic women may be less aware of and concerned about their wives' drinking problem and less likely to encourage aftercare treatment. In addition, because of society's greater intolerance of women alcoholics, as well as potential reinforcing consequences of a woman's drinking (e.g., facilitating social and sexual interaction), the husband of a woman alcoholic may be less willing to recognize and accept her need for treatment (Beckman & Amaro, 1984; Hanna, 1978; Johnson & Garzon, 1978). Furthermore, married women alcoholics are most likely to be living with a heavy drinker who is unlikely to encourage follow-up treatment. For all these reasons, married women may be less likely to participate in outpatient aftercare compared to unmarried women.

Overall, we found that environmental factors (treatment and posttreatment) had a stronger influence on women patients than on men patients, thus suggesting that treatment and life context factors may be especially important for understanding the process of relapse and remission among women. These findings are consistent with other research suggesting that women in general are more vulnerable than men to stressful circumstances and more responsive than men to social resources (Cronkite & Moos, 1984).

Clausen (1983, 1986) and Clausen, Pfeffer, and Huffine (1982) obtained some comparable findings in a follow-up of married men and women psychiatric patients. Being married was associated with a much more favorable prognosis for men patients, but it did not connote any such favorable prognosis for women patients. Men patients also enjoyed better family relationships than the women did; in addition, wives were more likely to be supportive of and sympathetic to their ill husbands than husbands were to their ill wives. Husbands were less likely to recognize their wives' symptoms and more often delayed seeking professional help for their wives despite long histories of severe emotional problems. Men patients were more resistant to seeking additional treatment for later episodes of symptoms, but wives helped get their ill husbands back into treatment whereas husbands were less likely to arrange treatment for their symptomatic wives. Thus, our findings are consistent with those on men and women with disorders other than alcohol abuse.

Overall, our findings indicate that patient-program congruence effects are important for understanding the treatment process and posttreatment experiences of gender and marital status groups. Although men and women patients receive relatively uniform treatment within a program, they seem to respond in different ways to specific treatment experiences. They also differ in their aftercare experiences and in the extent to which treatment components and posttreatment environment factors maintain remission. Program planners and clinicians need to find out more about how the match between treatment settings and personal characteristics (in this case, gender and marital status) can contribute to the process of remission among both men and women patients.

Even after taking into account the degree to which gender moderates the effects of marital status and treatment experiences, however, most of the variance in outcome remains unexplained. Accordingly, we tried to identify other important factors that may influence outcome, such as patients' life stressors, social resources, and coping responses. We turn to these issues next.

II
EXTRATREATMENT FACTORS AND THE RECOVERY PROCESS

6
Life Stressors, Social Resources, and Coping Responses

This chapter presents a rationale for examining the influence of life stressors, social resources, and coping responses on the development and course of alcohol abuse; we also present measures to assess these domains and describe their clinical and research applications.

The traditional evaluation paradigm, which focuses on treatment as the main factor affecting outcome, implicitly assumes that patients are exposed only to treatment. In reality, the patient's life context, including stressors and social resources, is more enduring than treatment and, like treatment, shapes mood and behavior. Life context factors can reinforce or nullify the impact of treatment, for example, when family and work factors reinforce abstinence or when co-workers convince a patient to resume drinking. Life context factors can also compensate for a program's lack of impact; for example, patients' spouses can abstain from drinking alcohol, reduce their alcohol consumption, or impart coping skills that patients did not learn in formal treatment.

Multiple sets of psychological and social factors affect the process of developing and overcoming alcohol abuse. Although formal treatment may exert a positive influence on remission, it is neither necessary nor sufficient to sustain recovery, as shown by recent studies highlighting fluctuations in alcohol consumption after treatment and the cycling between short- and long-term abstinence, nonproblem drinking, and episodes of alcohol abuse (Polich, Armor, & Braiker, 1981; Watson & Pucel, 1985). In conjunction with the high prevalence of relapse among alcoholic patients, such fluctuations have spurred investigators to analyze the connection between patients' life contexts and the cessation and resumption of problem drinking.

LIFE STRESSORS AND SOCIAL RESOURCES

Although it is widely acknowledged that life stressors and social resources can influence the development and course of alcohol abuse, systematic research on this issue is sparse. Life context factors have been implicated in the formation of problem drinking among adolescents (Harford, 1984; Jessor & Jessor, 1977), but there is little longitudinal research on their role among adults. Cross-sectional surveys show that persons who are experiencing stressors and who have fewer personal and social resources are more likely to use alcohol or drugs to relieve tension (Timmer, Veroff, & Colten, 1985). An accumulation of life stressors has been associated with more severe hangover symptoms among normal drinkers (Harburg et al., 1981) as well as with first arrests for drunken driving among men over age 60 (Wells-Parker, Miles, & Spencer, 1983). In addition, both experimental and naturalistic studies have shown that individuals' levels of alcohol consumption change predictably in line with contextual resources and stressors (Babor et al., 1980; Choquette, Hesselbrock, & Babor, 1985).

Social conditions that produce stressors also seem to increase alcoholism rates. For example, Linsky and his colleagues (1985) found that aggregate indices of negative life events and chronic social stressors were linked to statewide variations in alcohol consumption and alcohol-related death rates. These associations were somewhat stronger among women than among men and held after demographic factors related to drinking were controlled. In contrast, protective social processes, such as moderate drinking norms and close personal relationships, lessen the chance of problem drinking.

Aspects of a person's family and work settings are especially closely connected to changes in alcohol consumption and drinking problems. As expected, people located in alienated, conflict-ridden families are more likely to develop alcohol-related problems. When serious problems in family relationships are identified at intake to treatment, clients tend to show poorer treatment outcome (Vannicelli et al., 1983). In contrast, recovery can be promoted by positive changes in family relationships, such as reconciling with a supportive spouse who can exert effective social controls on problem drinking (Tuchfeld, 1981).

In the area of job factors, alcohol consumption and adverse consequences of drinking have been associated with lack of job challenge, role conflict and ambiguity, and high work demands. Markowitz (1984) noted that alcohol misuse is linked to a perceived lack of power and job responsibility, perhaps because these stressors arouse a sense of personal frustration and lead to a decline in self-efficacy. Other researchers have found a relationship between work stressors, boredom, and lack of job complexity and psychological dependence on alcohol (Parker & Brody, 1982). Such work-related problems may increase alcohol consumption by mak-

LIFE STRESSORS, SOCIAL RESOURCES, AND COPING RESPONSES

ing an individual more likely to justify drinking as a response to job stressors.

Although stressful life circumstances may foreshadow the development of problem drinking, they also can promote the recovery process. A serious personal illness, the alcohol-related injury or death of a friend, or being fired from a job for alcohol abuse can convince a person to abstain from drinking. Similarly, apparent social resources may have an unexpected effect on outcome; for example, social involvement or integration into a close-knit peer group may prompt an initiation or renewal of problem drinking if the peer group is oriented toward heavy drinking (Cosper, 1979; Seeman & Anderson, 1983). In this regard, Ludwig (1985) highlighted the cognitive processes associated with recovery. Consistent with stress and coping theory, he argues that life events and conditions must be evaluated in light of the person's cognitive appraisal. The coping strategies used to prevent and manage stressful situations are important determinants of recovery and relapse.

Guided by these considerations, we developed methods to measure the characteristics of family and work settings and the coping responses patients use. As noted earlier, the social climate scales focus on family, work, and social group contexts as well as on hospital-based and community-based treatment settings. We used two of these scales, the Family Environment Scale (FES) and the Work Environment Scale (WES), to assess patients' family and work settings and to examine the influence of these settings on posttreatment adaptation.

CHARACTERISTICS OF FAMILY SETTINGS

The Family Environment Scale

The FES is a 90-item scale composed of 10 subscales that measure three domains of family social climate (see Table 6.1). Cohesion, expressiveness, and conflict assess the quality of family relationships or the relationship domain. Independence, achievement orientation, intellectual-cultural and active-recreational orientation, and moral-religious emphasis assess the personal growth domain. Organization and control measure the system maintenance and change domain, that is, the level of structure and openness to change in the family. The family incongruence score measures how much family members disagree about the family climate.

We constructed the FES by using interview and observational methods to obtain a pool of items and to gain an understanding of families. The formulation of three domains of dimensions guided the choice and wording of items. That is, each item had to tap the emphasis on interpersonal relationships (such as cohesion), on an aspect of personal growth or goal orientation (such as achievement), or on family structure (such as organization). For instance, an emphasis on cohesion is inferred from the fol-

Table 6.1 Family Environment Scale dimensions

RELATIONSHIP DOMAIN
1. Cohesion   The commitment, help, and support family members provide for one another
2. Expressiveness   How much family members are encouraged to express their feelings openly
3. Conflict   The amount of anger and conflict among family members

PERSONAL GROWTH DOMAIN
4. Independence   The extent to which family members are assertive and self-sufficient
5. Achievement orientation   How much activities (such as school and work) are cast into an achievement-oriented or competitive framework
6. Intellectual-cultural orientation   The interest in political, social intellectual, and cultural activities
7. Active-recreational orientation   The participation in social and recreational activities
8. Moral-religious emphasis   The emphasis on ethical and religious issues and values

SYSTEM MAINTENANCE AND CHANGE DOMAIN
9. Organization   The importance of clear organization and structure in planning family activities and responsibilities
10. Control   The extent to which set rules and procedures are used to run family life

---

lowing kinds of items: "Family members really help and support one another" and "There is a feeling of togetherness in our family." An orientation toward achievement is inferred from these items: "We feel it is important to be the best at whatever we do" and "Getting ahead in life is very important in our family." An emphasis on organization is inferred from items such as "Activities in our family are carefully planned" and "We are generally very neat and orderly."

The norms for the FES are based on a representative group of 1,125 normal families and 500 distressed families selected to include various sizes, stages of the life cycle, and socioeconomic and ethnic backgrounds. The internal consistencies of the 10 FES subscales range from .61 to .78 and their test-retest reliabilities range from .68 to .86 for a 2-month interval (Moos & Moos, 1986). Moreover, family environments are quite stable over time, as shown by average subscale correlations of more than .60 over 18 months among our alcoholic patients and their spouses.

The FES taps some important family stressors and resources. In part, family resources are a function of the quality of interpersonal relationships. Accordingly, we used the three FES relationship dimensions (cohesion, expressiveness, and lack of conflict) to index the quality of family relationships. Other family resources include an emphasis on independence and organization and a high level of social connectedness, or interest in cultural, social, and religious pursuits. In addition to high conflict, family stressors can be indexed by high family incongruence and control, especially in the context of strong achievement expectations and lack of independence.

Alcoholic Patients' Family Environments

The FES can be used to describe the social environment of a family, to compare an alcoholic patient's views of the family with those of his or her spouse and children, and to track changes in a family during and after treatment. We illustrate such applications here by providing examples of FES profiles of families of alcohol abusers.

A High-Conflict Family

We conducted a case study of Mr. A, a 36-year-old Caucasian man who began heavy drinking in his teens. He had an eighth-grade education and held a steady job as a line foreman for 3 years prior to his admission to the halfway house program. At that time he reported drinking binges during which he consumed 2 to 3 pints of hard liquor in a day. He also described dizzy spells, memory lapses or blackouts, missing meals and work due to drinking, and severe hangovers and withdrawal symptoms.

Mr. A and his wife had been married for more than 10 years and had three young children living at home. The FES profile shown in Figure 6.1 was obtained 6 months after the completion of treatment, at which time the patient was drinking heavily again. Mr. A and his wife reported high family conflict and control and very little cohesion and expressiveness. The lack of emphasis on intellectual, recreational, or religious pursuits was consistent with the patient's disinterest in social activities and his professed lack of religious beliefs. Moreover, there was little emphasis on achievement or independence, and both partners saw the family as quite disorganized. This profile depicts a family in which high conflict was not mitigated either by cohesion or by a shared value orientation. It also shows that spouses in a conflict-oriented family can be quite congruent in their perceptions.

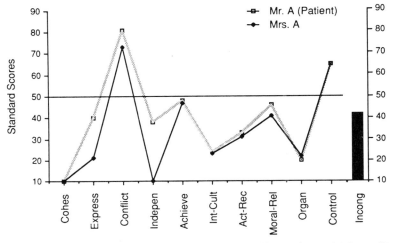

Figure 6.1 FES profiles for an alcoholic man and his wife in a high-conflict family.

Consistent with expectations, this patient did not show any improvement in his drinking pattern 18 months later. He and his wife separated and reconciled during this interval, but his views of the family were virtually identical to those shown in Figure 6.1. Sensing the hopelessness of her husband's drinking problem, Mrs. A began to develop interests outside the home. This change was reflected by a rise in her perceptions of independence, achievement, and intellectual and social emphasis, as well as a decline in conflict. By gradually withdrawing emotionally from her husband, Mrs. A started to gain some independence and to establish her own identity and life-style.

A Structured Religious Family

The second example is of Mr. S, a 49-year-old Hispanic father of two children who had been stably married for over 15 years. He began to drink in his teens but, unlike Mr. A, did not engage in heavy drinking or develop a serious alcohol problem until he was well into his thirties. Mr. S had held a steady job for 5 years as a warehouse clerk for a manufacturing company; he had not had any alcoholism treatment in the 3 years prior to entering the hospital-based program. At that time, he reported consuming more than a pint of hard liquor per day. He complained of hangovers, missing meals, and varied physical symptoms.

As shown in Figure 6.2, Mr. S saw his family as quite cohesive and well organized. Although he reported little emphasis on cultural or social pursuits, family independence and achievement were about average; concern about moral-religious issues was well above average. Mr. S and his wife showed little conflict and virtually complete agreement in their views of their family. Consistent with the FES profile, Mr. and Mrs. S reported

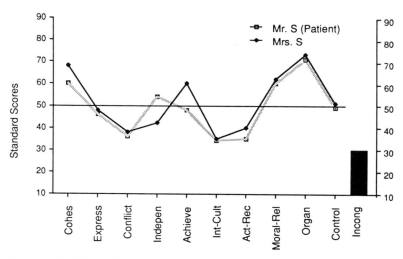

Figure 6.2 FES profiles for an alcoholic man and his wife in a structured religious family.

LIFE STRESSORS, SOCIAL RESOURCES, AND COPING RESPONSES

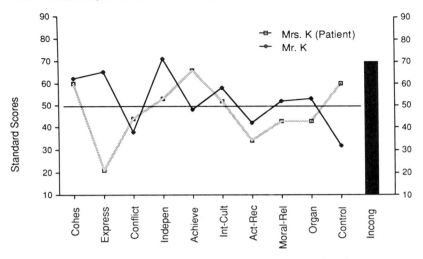

Figure 6.3 FES profiles for an alcoholic woman and her husband in an incongruent family.

that they attended church often and were involved in community activities.

The FES profile was obtained 6 months after Mr. S was released from the hospital-based program. At this point, Mr. S reported that he had abstained from alcohol completely for 6 months. Although Mrs. S had been a moderate social drinker, she decided to stop drinking completely. Eighteen months later both spouses reported a stable family environment as well as no drinking and no problems due to alcohol. Together with his ongoing active religious orientation, a cohesive, well-structured family seems to have facilitated a full recovery for Mr. S.

An Incongruent Family

The third example is of Mrs. K, a 57-year-old Caucasian woman who had been stably married for more than 30 years. Although Mrs. K was a college graduate and had no children, she was a homemaker and did not work outside her home. Mrs. K began to drink in her early twenties, but her history of alcohol abuse did not start until her middle thirties. When she entered the aversion conditioning program, she reported frequent heavy drinking of up to 2 pints of hard liquor a day. She complained of anger, depression, and boredom and noted that she drank to relax and escape from her problems.

The FES profile shown in Figure 6.3 was obtained during a temporary period of sobriety several months after Mrs. K had been discharged from the aversion conditioning program. Mr. and Mrs. K saw their relationship as quite cohesive and low in conflict. However, Mrs. K reported high family control and little expressiveness; her husband reported above average expressiveness and little control. Moreover, Mrs. K saw considerable emphasis on achievement, average independence, and relatively little concern with social or religious pursuits. In contrast, Mr. K reported high independence and average achievement. Thus, there was considerable incongruence between the spouses. The FES profile implies that Mrs. K felt trapped and controlled by her husband but was unable to share these feelings with him. Her drinking may have been a way of coping with this situation.

These ideas were supported by the FES profile obtained 18 months later, when Mrs. K was drinking heavily again. Although her appraisals of family cohesion and conflict remained stable, Mrs. K now felt that expressiveness and independence were well above average. She also saw control as well below average, whereas her husband perceived it just as before. Mr. K's view of the family remained constant irrespective of whether or not his wife was currently drinking. However, Mrs. K experienced a much more positive family climate when she was drinking than when she was sober. The spouses agreed quite closely about the family when Mrs. K was drinking. Thus, excessive drinking by one spouse can serve an adaptive function for the family.

A Typology of Family Environments

To facilitate the interpretation of FES profiles, we developed a typology of family environments based on data drawn from a representative community sample. In essence, we formulated a set of classification rules that are relatively parsimonious and can be applied without the use of a computer or other complex scoring methods. Families are grouped according to their most salient aspects, considering personal growth, then relationship, and then system maintenance characteristics. We used this procedure to identify seven family types: independence oriented, achievement oriented, moral-religious oriented (see Figure 6.2), intellectual-cultural oriented, support oriented, conflict oriented (see Figure 6.1), and disorganized. By classifying a family as representative of a more inclusive type, a clinician can compare it to a group of similar families and formulate more accurate prognoses and interventions. (For the classification rules and FES profiles of each type, see Billings & Moos, 1982a.)

Clinical Studies of the Family

The FES has been used widely in clinical research on families. We illustrate some applications by providing a brief overview of three areas of relevant work (for more details, see Moos & Moos, 1986).

Family Environment and Substance Abuse

To identify family characteristics that may lead to substance abuse, several researchers have asked alcoholic and other patients to describe their families of origin. Alcoholic patients tend to depict their family of origin as highly controlling and oriented toward achievement and as lacking in independence, expressiveness, and interest in intellectual and social pursuits. In contrast, patients describe their conjugal families as somewhat more expressive and independent and as somewhat less rigidly structured. Compared to black alcoholics, white alcoholics saw both their past and present families as more disturbed, that is, as less cohesive and organized and less oriented toward intellectual and religious activities (Patterson et al., 1981).

Other groups of substance abusers characterize their families of origin similarly. Compared to controls who did not abuse drugs, Penk and his colleagues (1979) found that men addicted to heroin typically came from families that value high achievement and inhibit the open expression of feelings. The researchers posited that substance abuse may be associated with setting unrealistic goals in the absence of appropriate role modeling and self-discipline. Substance abusers may develop problems because of their failure to achieve the high goals expected of them. Contrary to the findings for alcoholics, heroin abusers tended to recreate the social climate of their families of origin in their conjugal families.

Studies such as these may help to identify family characteristics associated with the development and maintenance of substance abuse. In this respect, cross-generational processes can shape the formation of conjugal family environments. The interaction patterns and values people learn in their families of origin may foreshadow those of their conjugal families. It is also important to recognize that retrospective ratings of one's family of origin are characterized by memories of parental control and dominance. Such ratings may reflect "natural" generational differences rather than a "real" variation in the functioning of one's present and past families (Carpenter, 1984).

Family Environment and Depression

A related line of research has identified associations between the family environment and depression. Wetzel (1978) found that women are vulnerable to depression if their tendency toward independence or dependence is not supported by the family environment. Women who were independent but not in autonomous families tended to be depressed, as did dependent women in autonomous families. Roehl and Okun (1984) noted that family support may reduce the risk of depression among women under high stress. In their study of married women who had children living at home, lack of family cohesion was related to more life stressors and higher depressed mood. As the level of family cohesion rose, increases in the number of life events were less strongly associated with depression. Similarly, we found an association between lack of family support and an increase in depression and physical symptoms in the subsequent 12 months (Holahan & Moos, 1987b).

Comparable findings have been obtained in studies of seriously depressed patients and their spouses. We compared more than 400 depressed patients with an equal number of demographically matched nondepressed adults. At intake to treatment, the depressed men and women and their spouses reported less family cohesion and expressiveness, less independence and organization, and less interest in recreational and religious pursuits. Lack of family support was associated with more severe depression among the depressed patients and with heightened depressed mood among their spouses (Billings, Cronkite, & Moos, 1983; Mitchell, Cronkite, & Moos, 1983). Bromet, Ed, and May (1984) identified more symptoms among depressed patients who were in less cohesive and expressive families that were lower in religious emphasis and organization and higher in conflict. These aspects of family environments are also related to poorer individual functioning in other groups of psychiatric patients (Spiegel & Wissler, 1983).

Family Environment and Life Stressors

Family climate is also related to how well people cope with illness and other family-related stressors. In general, high family cohesion and social connectedness, as reflected by an emphasis on cultural and recreational pursuits, are associated with better adjustment among adults and children who have a chronic illness and among their family members. Together with moderate organization and structure, these family characteristics can help to maintain control over problem members and to manage their psychiatric disturbance, to dampen the impact of relocation and temporary family separation, and to confront an array of other stressful life conditions (Moos & Moos, 1986).

In general, well-organized families characterized by moderate or high cohesion and expressiveness and low conflict are able to adapt successfully to varied changes and demands. Structured families may find it easier to deal with diverse stressors and maintain established routines; adequate rapport and openness help families to communicate and resolve problems effectively. High family conflict and lack of structure, often a response to stressors, are related to poor adjustment. Moreover, relatively disengaged families, as indexed by high independence in the context of lack of cohesion, may be more likely to be influenced by stressors exogenous to the family and to transmit their effects from one family member to another (Thomson & Vaux, 1986). As we shall see, these aspects of family environments have important consequences for individual and family adaptation among alcoholic patients.

CHARACTERISTICS OF WORK SETTINGS

The Work Environment Scale

The Work Environment Scale (WES) is a 90-item scale composed of 10 subscales that measure three domains of the social climates of work settings (see Table 6.2). Involvement, peer cohesion, and supervisor support

LIFE STRESSORS, SOCIAL RESOURCES, AND COPING RESPONSES

Table 6.2 Work Environment Scale dimensions

RELATIONSHIP DOMAIN
1. Involvement   The extent to which employees are concerned about and committed to their jobs
2. Peer cohesion   The extent to which employees are friendly and supportive of one another
3. Supervisor support   How much management supports employees and encourages employees to support one another

PERSONAL GROWTH DOMAIN
4. Autonomy   The extent to which employees are encouraged to be self-sufficient and make their own decisions
5. Task orientation   The emphasis on good planning, efficiency, and getting the job done
6. Work pressure   The degree to which the press of work and time urgency dominate the job milieu

SYSTEM MAINTENANCE AND CHANGE DOMAIN
7. Clarity   How much employees know what to expect in their daily routine and how explicitly rules and policies are communicated
8. Control   The extent to which management uses rules and pressures to keep employees under control
9. Innovation   The emphasis on variety, change, and new approaches
10. Physical comfort   The extent to which the physical surroundings contribute to a pleasant work environment

---

assess the relationship domain, that is, the quality of personal relationships at work. Autonomy, task orientation, and work pressure assess the goals toward which the setting is oriented (personal growth or goal orientation domain). Clarity, control, innovation, and physical comfort measure the amount of structure and openness to change in the workplace (system maintenance and change domain).

The procedures used to develop the WES were similar to those followed with the FES. We employed interview and observational methods to gain a naturalistic understanding of work settings and to generate a pool of items to tap the three domains. For example, an emphasis on peer cohesion is conveyed by the following kinds of items: "People go out of their way to help a new employee feel comfortable" and "People take a personal interest in each other." An orientation toward autonomy is inferred from these items: "Employees have a great deal of freedom to do as they like" and "Employees are encouraged to make their own decisions." An emphasis on clarity is captured by items such as: "Activities are well planned" and "The details of assigned jobs are generally explained to employees."

To ensure that the WES would be broadly applicable, information was obtained from work groups composed of employees in a diverse set of occupations and socioeconomic statuses. Normative data are available for more than 1,400 employees in a representative set of general work groups and more than 1,600 employees in varied health care settings. The internal consistencies of the 10 WES subscales range from .69 to .86 and their 1-month test-retest reliabilities range from .69 to .83. The intercorrelations among the subscales are moderate, indicating that they reflect distinct but somewhat related aspects of work climate (Moos, 1986c).

The WES taps four facets of work group climate that are associated with employee strain and lack of mental and physical well-being: high job demands, supervisor control, lack of clarity, and insufficient opportunity to participate in decision making (Moos, 1986b). Employees who are engaged in their work and form positive bonds with their peers and managers seem to experience fewer work stressors and to react less negatively to them. These social resources in the work setting are tapped by the three WES relationship dimensions: involvement, peer cohesion, and supervisor support.

Alcoholic Patients' Work Environments

As we illustrated with the FES, patients' appraisals of the quality of work environments can be profiled and compared to each other.

Cohesive Task-Oriented Work Settings

The first examples depict two cohesive and task-oriented work settings; one highlights innovation and physical comfort whereas the other does not. Figure 6.4 contrasts the WES profile for Mr. S, whose family environment we described earlier, with that obtained for Mr. M, a 53-year-old married Caucasian man who had been treated in the milieu-oriented program.

Mr. S had worked steadily for over 5 years as a warehouse clerk. He saw his job as involving and co-workers as friendly and supportive. He reported an emphasis on autonomy and task orientation but also experienced high work demands. This basically positive work setting probably facilitated Mr. S's recovery, since job involvement and autonomy provide a supportive context within which some work demands are acceptable. Prior to treatment in the hospital-based program, Mr. S reported that he occasionally drank at work with his fellow employees. This behavior stopped after treatment, implying that cohesion among work associates who drink need not lead to relapse. Mr. S also enjoyed a stable, supportive family environment (see Figure 6.2) that probably helped him to counteract any social pressure at work to resume drinking.

Mr. M had worked as a research engineer for one company for several years. Prior to his admission to the milieu-oriented program he had taken a job as a salesman in which he worked with fellow employees who regularly went on drinking binges. Although Mr. M did not consume alcohol on the job, he did develop a pattern of frequent drinking. After treatment, he obtained a new job as an engineer for a defense industry contractor.

Mr. M experienced his posttreatment work setting very positively. He was committed to his job and thought that relationships with co-workers

LIFE STRESSORS, SOCIAL RESOURCES, AND COPING RESPONSES

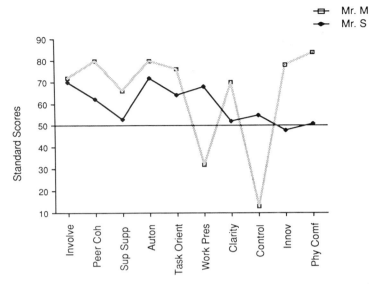

Figure 6.4 WES profiles for two alcoholic patients in cohesive and task-oriented work settings.

and supervisors were congenial. Mr. M saw his job as oriented toward independence and task performance but, unlike Mr. S, he reported work demands and supervisor control as well below average. Rules and policies were clear and innovation was valued. At this time, Mr. M was abstaining from alcohol and felt comfortable about his work, his family, and his life overall. Mr. M still held this job 18 months later, but then saw the workplace much less favorably, especially in terms of the relationship dimensions, task orientation, and clarity. Combined with the development of high blood pressure and bronchitis and sharply increased family conflict, these changes may have contributed to Mr. M's renewed heavy drinking.

Highly Demanding Work Settings

The WES profiles shown in Figure 6.5 illustrate two highly demanding work settings. The first profile was obtained from Mr. D, a 44-year-old, stably married, Caucasian man who had been treated in the Salvation Army program. After his release, he began a new job as a printer and graphic arts technician. Six months posttreatment, Mr. D saw the quality of job relationships as well above average but noted little emphasis on independence or task orientation. This lack of focus on planning and efficiency undoubtedly contributed to the high work demands. Although employees knew what to expect in their daily routine, Mr. D reported a lack of innovation; he also appraised the physical conditions at work as quite unpleasant.

The issue in this type of setting is whether the positive relationships among people on the job can offset the lack of autonomy and high work

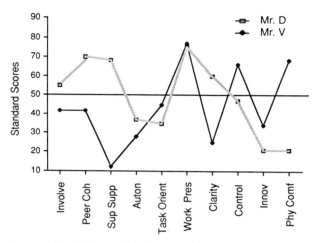

Figure 6.5 WES profiles for two alcoholic patients in highly demanding work settings.

demands. Unfortunately, a later WES profile indicated that Mr. D saw the work setting as much lower on all three relationship dimensions as well as on autonomy and clarity. In addition, he had resumed moderately heavy drinking and developed heart disease. The fact that Mr. D's wife reported an increase in family cohesion at this time (Mr. D did not agree) again points to the potential adaptive value of drinking in some family systems.

The final example is of Mr. V, a 44-year-old, stably married, Caucasian man with two children. Prior to treatment, he had consumed alcohol frequently on weekdays and occasionally at work. After his release from the milieu-oriented program, he began working as a structural engineer. As shown in Figure 6.5, his initial report on the work setting was quite negative. He experienced high work demands, saw supervisors as controlling and unsympathetic, and reported little job clarity, autonomy, or task orientation. Despite these problems, Mr. V stayed in this job for the ensuing 18 months, during which a pattern of supportive interactions among coworkers began to develop. This helped to promote improved relationships with supervisors and led to more autonomy and a substantial drop in work demands. Combined with his well-organized, achievement-oriented family setting, these improvements may have helped to maintain Mr. V's long-term abstinence from alcohol.

The foregoing examples illustrate the complexity of work settings and the need to consider their multiple dimensions in conjunction with one another as well as with a patient's family environment. Moderate job involvement and autonomy and a supportive family helped Mr. S manage the demands of his job and co-workers' social pressure to resume drinking. In contrast, the strain of personal illness and family conflict seemed to outweigh the positive resources that existed initially in Mr. M's work milieu. The cases of Mr. D and Mr. V highlight the importance of changes in work settings and their interplay with patients' families in influencing the process of recovery and relapse.

Work Climate and Well-Being

The WES has been used widely in studies of work settings. To illustrate some important applications, we provide a brief overview of three relevant areas (for more details, see Moos, 1986b, 1986c).

Job Morale and Performance

One line of research has identified characteristics of work settings that contribute to job morale and performance. As expected, considerate supervisors who specify clear goals and encourage participation in decision making tend to promote good employee morale and feelings of personal accomplishment, as do well-organized work settings that have flexible policies. Cohesive and independent work settings that also are well organized and provide meaningful and challenging tasks tend to produce high work performance.

In contrast, job ambiguity and group conflict are likely to spawn emotional exhaustion and alienation, as are situational constraints and highly structured tasks and leaders. Strain is most likely to occur when job demands are high and the employee has little discretion in deciding how to meet them. When employees are allowed to make decisions about their work, high job demands can be stimulating and can promote active problem solving and innovation. For example, Rosenthal and his colleagues (1983) found that the influence of high work demands depended on the personal and structural context in which they occurred. They were associated with personal accomplishment in a clear, involved, and task-oriented setting but with emotional exhaustion and alienation in a setting that lacked these qualities. These variations in work climate may affect the satisfaction and performance of staff in alcoholism treatment programs (see Chapter 11).

Work Climate and Depression

As mentioned earlier, we studied a large group of depressed psychiatric patients and demographically matched nondepressed controls. The depressed patients reported significantly more work stressors and less work support (Billings, Cronkite, & Moos, 1983). In addition, work stressors were related to more severe depression and physical symptoms among men patients and to lack of self-confidence among both men and women patients. These findings held more strongly among nonchronic than among chronic patients; work stressors and resources may be more salient for patients who do not experience recurrent depressive episodes (Billings & Moos, 1984a, 1984b).

We have also examined these issues in a representative community sample of employed women and men. Men who reported less involvement and cohesion at work were more likely to experience depression and psychosomatic symptoms even after the influence of family support was considered. When initial levels of dysfunction and stressful life changes were controlled in a predictive analysis, a decline in work support over a 12-month interval was related to an increase in psychological dysfunction among both women and men (Holahan & Moos, 1981). Comparable associations between work climate and psychological distress have been identified among patients in treatment for medical disorders (Feuerstein, Sult, & Houle, 1985).

Work and Family Settings

To understand fully the impact of work settings, we need to examine their connections to other aspects of an individual's life context, especially to family settings. In pursuing this issue, we have identified some associations among work stressors, work and family support, and individual adaptation. In our study of community adults, we found that high work stressors were associated with fewer work resources, less self-confidence, and more physical and emotional symptoms. Men who experienced more work stressors also reported less family support; high stressors in a married woman's job were associated with her husband's report of less positive family relationships and more physical symptoms. In contrast, family cohesion helped to dampen the negative impact of work stressors. By reducing the energy available to manage conflict and maintain a cohesive family, stress in the workplace can adversely affect spouse and family functioning (Billings & Moos, 1982b, 1982c).

Family cohesion can have an unintended influence on work adjustment. For example, Kobasa and Puccetti (1983) examined the connections among stressful life events, personal hardiness, and family and work support. The influence of family support varied according to the level of hardiness of the individual. Men who were low in hardiness and had cohesive families reported more illness, especially when they experienced more job-related stressors. While trying to protect a vulnerable man from stress, "supportive" family members may alienate him from his job and thus contribute to his illness. In general, these studies highlight the value of including information about stressors and social resources in the family and workplace in studies of alcohol abusers.

APPRAISAL AND COPING RESPONSES

Most life stressors do not foreshadow increased alcohol consumption or a decline in functioning. Aside from personal and social resources, the most important variables intervening between stressors and adaptation are cognitive appraisal and coping responses. Because no one can avoid all stressors, recovering alcohol abusers necessarily confront situations that can induce relapse; their appraisal and coping patterns help to determine whether stressors undermine the recovery process. Stressors may increase or reduce alcohol consumption, depending on how individuals appraise and manage them and their consequences.

Some theorists believe that stressors can either trigger or deter drinking, depending on their contingent relationship to drinking behavior (Abrams, 1983). For example, stressors that occur because of resumed drinking may provide a strong deterrent against drinking. However, both positive and negative consequences can flow from drinking in most high-risk situations. This raises the question of why people decide to attend more to one set of consequences than to another. The concepts of cognitive appraisal and coping responses try to answer this question by emphasizing people's active *selection* among specific consequences to which they attend and their *choice* among alternative coping responses in light of their appraisal of the consequences. Appraisal and coping responses influence the stressors to which a person is exposed, his or her reaction to the differential reinforcements they offer, and how stressors affect the process of remission or relapse.

There is growing interest in the role of coping processes in problem drinking and substance abuse. Perri (1985) identified coping strategies used by people who succeeded in self-management of a drinking problem. Abstainers and nonproblem drinkers used a greater variety of coping methods; in particular, active problem-solving responses such as stimulus control (spending less time with heavy-drinking friends, removing alcoholic beverages from their home), changing their daily routine, developing alternative pursuits (such as new hobbies and physical exercise), and searching for advice and support. Self-reinforcement for avoiding relapse was an especially valuable coping strategy.

Three Domains of Coping Responses

Considering the complexity and diversity of life stressors and of individuals' attempts to deal with them, it is not surprising that efforts to conceptualize coping responses are at an early stage. One approach has viewed coping as a cluster of cognitive processes that protect a person from external and intrapsychic threat. This line of inquiry encompasses research on ego defense mechanisms and trait definitions of coping. More recent ideas have broadened the concept of coping to cover problem-solving responses that aim to deal actively with external stressors as well as cognitive and behavioral responses that serve to manage the emotion aroused by a problem (Moos & Billings, 1982b).

Coping responses can be classified into three domains according to their focus. Appraisal-focused coping aims to define the meaning of a situation and includes cognitive strategies such as logical analysis and redefining a stressor in more positive terms. Problem-focused coping seeks to modify or eliminate the source of stress, to deal with the tangible consequences of a problem, or to change oneself and create a more satisfying situation. Emotion-focused coping aims to manage the emotions aroused by stressors and maintain affective equilibrium. These three domains include the major types of coping responses used to manage a variety of life stressors (Moos & Schaefer, 1986).

Some investigators have gathered information on how people typically deal with generalized and relatively enduring stressors, such as marital and economic strain. In contrast, we chose to examine the cognitive and behavioral methods people use in response to specific recent events. In this respect, we see coping responses as somewhat situation-specific ways of managing stressful conditions. This view is consistent with evidence that coping responses vary as much or more in line with situational as personal factors (Dohrenwend & Martin, 1979; Folkman & Lazarus, 1980). We divided active attempts to resolve the stressful event into cognitive and behavioral methods, while separately clustering methods that aim to avoid the problem or to reduce the emotional tension associated with it. Active cognitive responses are appraisal-focused strategies, while active behavioral responses are problem-focused strategies and avoidance responses are emotion-focused strategies.

Active cognitive coping includes six responses that aim to manage one's appraisal of the stressfulness of an event, such as "tried to step back from the situation and be more objective," "considered several alternatives for handling the problem," and "tried to see the positive side of the situation."

Active behavioral coping includes six responses that aim to deal directly with the problem and its effects, such as "tried to find out more about the situation," "talked with spouse or other relative about the problem," and "took some positive action."

Avoidance coping covers five responses that aim to avoid actively confronting the problem, such as "kept my feelings to myself" and "prepared for the worst," or to reduce indirectly emotional tension by behavior such as eating or smoking more. Alcohol consumption often is an avoidance-coping response, but we did not include it so as not to confound our measures of coping and of treatment outcome.

Use and Efficacy of Coping Skills

We used these three indices of coping methods to examine the nature of the coping process among a representative sample of normal adults. We found some variations in coping among different kinds of events. Active behavioral responses were used more often in confronting an illness than in adapting to a death or a sudden loss of income. This probably reflects the differential demands of these stressors as well as the relative ineffectiveness of problem-focused approaches in the latter two situations.

We also identified gender differences in the use and efficacy of these coping responses. Women were more likely to use avoidance coping, which was associated with somewhat more impairment of functioning among women than men. However, women's reliance on avoidance coping was affected more strongly by the stressful circumstances they experienced than by their prior functioning. Reliance on avoidance coping among men was associated more closely with their prior adaptation than with their experience of recent life stressors. Thus, avoidance coping may be more situationally determined among women but reflect poor functioning among men (Cronkite & Moos, 1984).

Although the outcome of specific coping responses varies in different situations, we can draw some general conclusions about their relative efficacy. A propensity to rely on active cognitive coping, such as making optimistic comparisons and setting high expectations, is associated with less occupational distress. These cognitive coping skills also help to lessen emotional distress in the areas of marriage and parenting. Direct problem-solving action also is generally helpful in managing acute stressors, although it may not lessen chronic marital or occupational strains (Menaghen & Mervis, 1984). Moreover, a higher ratio of problem-focused to emotion-focused coping is associated with better adaptation (Mitchell, Cronkite, & Moos, 1983). In contrast, avoidance coping tends to reflect a less effective way of managing stressors; it is linked to poorer adaptation (Holahan & Moos, 1987b).

Family and Work Contexts of Coping

The characteristics of family and work settings affect the way in which people cope with stressful circumstances; this influence of the family context may be stronger for women than for men. Supportive and structured families seem to promote active cognitive and active behavioral coping and make avoidance coping less likely. For example, in one community group we found that people in cohesive, well-organized families oriented toward achievement and intellectual and religious pursuits were more likely to use problem-focused coping responses. Family independence was also associated with the use of such coping responses, but active coping was less likely among members of conflict-oriented and controlling families (Billings & Moos, 1982a). High family support may lessen the need to rely on avoidance coping, especially among women.

We replicated these findings in a second community group and in our group of depressed patients. High family support was associated with greater reliance on active cognitive and active behavioral coping and less reliance on avoidance coping in both groups. More important, when initial coping propensities were controlled, family support was related to a decline in avoidance coping in both groups and to an increase in active cognitive and behavioral coping among the patients (Holahan & Moos, 1987a). An increase in family support foreshadowed a rise in problem-solving coping among depressed women and a decline in emotional discharge coping among depressed men (Fondacaro & Moos, 1987).

Kohn and Schooler (1983) have noted that occupational experiences can affect a person's value system and coping strategies. In essence, occupational conditions conducive to self-direction in one's work—such as high autonomy, innovation, and supervisor support—are associated with valuing self-direction and the use of active coping strategies. People's jobs affect their perceptions and values by confronting them with demands that must be met; coping strategies used to handle problems at work then are generalized to manage other situations.

As expected from Kohn and Schooler's (1983) observations, we identified some associations between occupational settings and coping responses. In general, people in cohesive, innovative, and independence-oriented work settings were more likely to use active cognitive and active behavioral coping. Increases in work support were related to greater reliance on affective regulation among women and to more information and support seeking among men (Fondacaro & Moos, 1987).

When faced with difficult work environments, people draw on a wider range of coping strategies. Accordingly, Parkes (1986) found that student nurses used more coping responses in situations of high work demand and low work support. In the absence of support from their supervisors, student nurses tried to cope directly with work problems, but only when they were not already overloaded. In contrast, when the work load was high, support and supervision tended to constrain students' direct coping activities.

These findings imply that characteristics of individuals' job and family situations can influence remission and relapse through their impact on the use and efficacy of different coping strategies. In general, cohesive, well-organized, and independence-oriented work and family settings are associated with more reliance on problem-solving coping. However, highly demanding jobs also can promote active coping.

Although our discussion has focused primarily on work and family settings as contexts for coping, we recognize that patterns of mutual influence are likely to form as coping strategies and life contexts affect each other. In the next chapters we examine the associations between these life stressor, social resource, and coping factors, and alcoholic patients' treatment outcome.

7
Context, Coping, and Treatment Outcome

We have provided a rationale for examining the influence of life stressors, social resources, and coping responses on the development and course of alcohol abuse. We constructed measures to assess these domains and have described their clinical and research applications. We turn now to an analysis of how these three domains influence the process of recovery and relapse in alcoholism. The first step is to extend the conceptual paradigm presented in Chapter 4 to encompass context and coping and how they are shaped by pretreatment and treatment factors. Next, we describe the 2-year and 10-year outcome of a subset of married patients in our sample. We then consider the associations between an array of life stressors, social resources, and coping responses and short- and long-term treatment outcome. Finally, we examine how well the overall conceptual paradigm of patient, treatment, life context, and coping factors helps us to predict several outcome criteria.

EXPANDING THE PARADIGM: CONTEXT AND COPING FACTORS

Guided by the foregoing ideas, we expanded our conceptual paradigm to include life context and coping determinants of treatment outcome. The paradigm in Figure 7.1 shows connections among six sets of factors associated with the process of remission and relapse of alcoholic patients: patient demographic characteristics, patient functioning at intake, treatment factors (the treatment program, experiences, and environment), life stressors, social resources, and coping responses. We have seen (Chapter 4) that patient characteristics at intake (Panels I and II) affect the treatment (Panel III) a patient receives and that these factors affect treatment

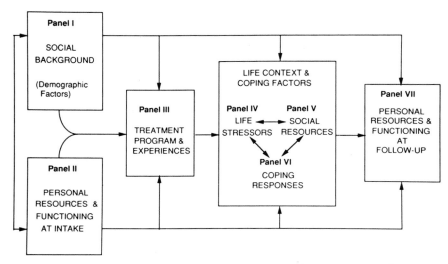

Figure 7.1 A model of the influence of treatment and extratreatment factors on treatment outcome.

outcome. The next two sets of factors describe the patient's life context (Panels IV and V). Coping responses (Panel VI), the final set, are characteristics of the individual that are initiated by and directed toward the environment. Accordingly, they may be viewed as proximal outcomes of person-environment transactions. In addition to indicating that each set of factors can influence outcome, the model highlights the dynamic nature of the links among the sets.

Patient and Treatment Factors

As reported in Chapters 3 and 4, we found relationships among social background, intake functioning, and treatment outcome. Specifically, married and better-educated patients tended to have less severe drinking problems and to function better at intake. In turn, patients with higher demographic status and less severe intake symptoms were more likely to enter the private programs. Patients in these programs and patients who became more actively involved in treatment experienced better alcohol-related, physical, and social functioning 6 months after treatment.

Life Stressors and Coping Resources

After discharge from a residential program, recovery is affected by the patient's life context, which can provide a supportive milieu for continued improvement, cushion the impact of stressors, or trigger relapse. As shown in Figure 7.1, we believe that stressful life conditions and social resources affect outcome. These contextual factors elicit coping responses that may contribute to relapse or prevent it. For instance, a cohesive family may foster good treatment outcome by promoting reliance on effective coping responses, such as taking direct action to confront modifiable stressors.

Life context and coping factors can alter one another, mediate the influence of patient and treatment characteristics on outcome, and affect outcome directly. Patients with more positive demographic characteristics and less severe symptoms may show better outcome because they return to less stressful settings and enjoy richer social resources. In addition, treatment can help patients learn coping skills that will improve the quality of their adaptation after treatment. Life stressors are less likely to foreshadow renewed alcohol abuse when patients use active cognitive or behavioral coping skills to manage them.

To examine the role of life stressors, social resources, and coping responses and their associations with patient, treatment, and outcome indices, we conducted follow-ups at 6 months, 2 years, and 10 years after treatment on a sample of patients who returned to their families following treatment. After describing the short-term and long-term treatment outcome of these patients, we use the conceptual model as a guide in pursuing three main questions: (1) How do patient demographic characteristics and functioning at intake influence short-term and long-term treatment outcome among this family subsample? (2) How are life stressors, social resources, and coping responses concurrently and predictively related to treatment outcome? (3) Compared to patient intake and treatment factors, how well can context and coping indices account for outcome?

PATIENTS IN FAMILY SETTINGS

Upon completing the initial follow-up, 6 to 8 months after release from treatment, the 157 patients who returned to family settings were asked if they and their families would participate in an extended study. Altogether, 124 patients and their families, or 79% of those eligible, agreed to participate. A group of 113 of these 124 patients (96% of the 118 persons still living) were followed 18 months later. Eight years later, we were able to follow 82 of the 93 patients who were still alive (20 had died).

At intake to treatment, the 113 patients followed both at 6 months and 2 years tended to be middle aged (74% were 40 years or older), white (88%), and educated beyond high school (68%), although only 19% were college graduates. There were 88 men and 25 women. Of the patients who indicated an occupation, most (56%) were employed in occupations of moderate prestige. During the month before entry into the program, most patients (75%) reported drinking daily, with a mean alcohol consumption of more than 13 ounces of ethanol from all beverages on a typical drinking day. Almost half (43%) of these patients had been hospitalized for alcoholism in the past 3 years.

This family sample is a distinctive subset of the larger group of patients. Compared to the nonfamily alcoholics, these patients had less severe drinking problems at intake, were more stable in their residences and jobs, were more highly educated, included more women, and usually were treated in one of the private programs. All but seven were married. Six months after treatment, the family patients consumed less alcohol, were more likely to be abstinent and to use outpatient services, and were less likely to be rehospitalized for alcoholism than the nonfamily patients.

Patient functioning for the family sample was assessed at intake with six indices: (1) *alcohol consumption* during the month prior to admission; (2) *abstinence* in the previous month; (3) *physical symptoms;* (4) *depression;* (5) *social functioning;* and (6) *occupational functioning.* The six indices of treatment outcome correspond to these measures of intake functioning (see Finney, Moos, & Mewborn, 1980).

HOMOGENEITY AND STABILITY OF TREATMENT OUTCOME

Relatively little is known about the interrelationships among multiple outcome indices used to tap alcoholism treatment effectiveness. In our study, we focused on the relationships of two drinking indices—alcohol consumption and 1-month abstinence—with indices of functioning in four other areas—physical, psychological (depressive symptoms), social, and occupational. Studies with two or more follow-ups of treated individuals provide valuable data on these relationships and on the long-term stability of various measures of outcome.

Cross-Sectional and Longitudinal Relationships among Outcome Indices

In Chapter 3, we saw that improvement in drinking behavior from intake to the 6-month follow-up was associated with improvement on other outcome criteria. Using the sample of treated alcoholics living with their families, we conducted similar cross-sectional and longitudinal analyses of the relationships among outcome criteria at the 6-month, 2-year, and 10-year follow-ups. For the most part, better functioning in each area was associated with more positive outcome in all other areas.

In cross-sectional analyses of the family sample, lower alcohol consumption was related to better functioning on three of the four nondrinking outcome criteria (all except employment) at the 6-month follow-up (average $r = .29$), to depression at the 2-year follow-up ($r = .36$), and to physical symptoms ($r = .24$) at the 10-year follow-up. Abstinence was associated with better outcome in all nondrinking areas except social functioning at 6 months (average $r = .24$), with physical symptoms ($r = .25$) and depression ($r = -.47$) at 2 years, and with physical symptoms ($r = .20$) at 10 years.

The cross-sectional associations indicate concurrent relationships between drinking and functioning in other life areas—especially physical symptoms and depression. We also wanted to know whether improvement in drinking status over time was related to improvement on nondrinking outcome criteria. Accordingly, we examined concomitant changes in outcome criteria across three intervals: (1) from intake to 6 months after the index treatment episode, (2) from 6 months to 2 years after treatment, and (3) from 2 years to 10 years after treatment. We calculated partial correlations between outcome criteria at time 2 of each interval, controlling for three background characteristics at intake (sex, age, and education) and for functioning on the two appropriate outcome measures at time 1 in each interval.

The results of these "change" analyses paralleled the cross-sectional correlations for the most part, although the magnitudes of the relationships were somewhat lower, especially over the 8-year interval between the last two follow-ups. Reduction in alcohol consumption correlated .25, on average, with improvement in the four nondrinking criteria for the intake to the 6-month interval, .16 for the 6-month to the 2-year interval, and .16 for the 2-year to the 10-year interval. A shift to abstinence by the month prior to follow-up was associated with improvement in the nondrinking domains for all three intervals (average correlations of .21, .25, and .16, respectively).

Thus, both cross-sectional and longitudinal analyses show some interdependence among outcome criteria. In general, there was more overlap among indices of drinking (alcohol consumption and abstinence), physical symptoms, and depression (average cross-sectional correlations of .33, .30, and .23 at 6 months, 2 years, and 10 years) than among drinking indices and social and occupational functioning (average correlations of .19, .12, and .08, respectively, for the three follow-ups). This pattern supports the conclusion that a reduction in drinking tends to be associated with improvement in intrapersonal domains but is less closely tied to better social and occupational functioning (see also Fink et al., 1985; cf. Babor et al., 1988).

Stability of Treatment Outcome

We examined both group and individual stability of the treatment outcome indices across the three follow-ups. Group-level stability helps to determine the average effectiveness of a treatment program for all patients or for particular groups of patients. Several studies have found that 6-month outcome on drinking indices tends to be stable at the group level (e.g., see Armor, Polich, & Stambul, 1978), whereas other research has found group-level stability only after 1 year or 18 months (Van Dijk & Van Dijk-Koffeman, 1973). However, group-level stability does not preclude individual change over time as long as the improvement shown by some patients is balanced by the decline of others.

Outcome at 6 Months and 2 Years

In general, patients as a group were doing somewhat less well at the 2-year than the 6-month follow-up (see the top half of Table 7.1). The 1-month abstinence rate declined from 68% at 6 months after treatment to 40% at 2 years. Alcohol consumption, physical symptoms, and depression increased and social functioning declined.

We also identified considerable fluctuation in individual adaptation. The correlations of 6-month with 2-year outcome indices range from .31 (social functioning) to .71 (occupational functioning), indicating that 10% to 50% of the variance in outcome 2 years after treatment is predictable from variation in outcome at 6 months. These associations are somewhat higher than those we identified in the overall sample between intake functioning and the 6-month outcome criteria (Chapter 3).

Outcome at 10 Years

A varied pattern of stability and change occurred between the 2-year and 10-year follow-ups (see the bottom half of Table 7.1). Patients who survived and were successfully followed showed improvement in drinking behavior (alcohol consumption and 1-month abstinence), no change in depression or physical symptoms, and somewhat fewer social activities and reduced employment. These last two changes are likely to be associated with aging.

The correlations between the 2- and 10-year outcome criteria are weaker than those between the 6-month and 2-year criteria, as is expected with a longer interval. The lower correlation for occupational functioning is partly due to an age effect, with older persons retiring, as well as a trend for women to enter or reenter the work force. Among the 82 patients successfully followed 10 years posttreatment, 10% were retired at the 2-year follow-up versus 24% at the 10-year follow-up. For the 19 women patients reassessed 10 years after treatment, 21% were employed part- or full-time at the 2-year follow-up versus 47% at the 10-year follow-up.

For alcohol consumption, a relatively modest 21% of the variation in 2-year levels was associated with drinking volume at the 6-month follow-

Table 7.1 Means, standard deviations, and correlations for outcome measures 6 months, 2 years, and 10 years after treatment

Outcome criteria	6 months ($N = 113$)		2 years ($N = 113$)			Correlation across the follow-ups
	Mean	Standard deviation	Mean	Standard deviation	t	
Alcohol consumption (oz. of ethanol)	2.25	5.71	4.56	7.62	−3.43***	.46***
1-month abstinence (proportion yes)	.68	.47	.40	.49	5.73***	.40***
Physical symptoms (no. yes of 6)	1.20	1.54	1.78	1.56	−4.13***	.54***
Depression (no. yes of 6)	2.29	2.09	2.88	2.31	−2.83**	.51***
Social functioning (no. yes of 5 activities)	2.07	1.35	1.78	1.29	1.99*	.31**
Occupational functioning (proportion employed)	.65	.48	.67	.47	<1	.71***

Outcome criteria	2 years ($N = 82$)		10 years ($N = 82$)			Correlation across the follow-ups
	Mean	Standard deviation	Mean	Standard deviation	t	
Alcohol consumption (oz. of ethanol)	3.84	6.16	2.54	5.62	1.49	.11
1-month abstinence (proportion yes)	.41	.50	.66	.48	4.13***	.40***
Physical symptoms (no. yes of 6)	1.57	1.47	1.71	1.70	<1	.37**
Depression (no. yes of 6)	2.22	2.01	2.20	1.91	<1	.47***
Social functioning (no. yes of 5 activities)	1.84	1.22	1.52	1.11	1.95†	.21†
Occupational functioning (proportion employed)	.72	.45	.61	.49	1.75†	.28*

†$p < .10$. *$p < .05$. **$p < .01$. ***$p < .001$.

up, but only 1% of the variation in drinking at the 10-year follow-up was associated with alcohol consumption 8 years earlier. These findings indicate that some alcoholic patients may alternate among heavy drinking, nonproblem drinking, and even abstinence across the three follow-ups. In the next section, we examine some life context and coping factors that may be responsible for such fluctuations in individual drinking behavior over time.

LIFE STRESSORS, COPING RESOURCES, AND TREATMENT OUTCOME

Only a few studies have examined patients' life contexts after alcoholism treatment in relation to outcome, and most of these studies have focused only on stressful life events or the family environment. However, another family member's dysfunction can also be a source of problems for patients attempting to recover. For example, a spouse's alcohol consumption, depressed mood, and chronic physical symptoms probably add to a recovering patient's burden, as do ongoing health problems of children in the family.

Although aspects of the work environment have rarely been related to prognosis, studies suggest the work climate affects outcome. Mayer and Meyerson (1970) found that better relationships with co-workers were associated with reduced drinking among stably employed treated alcoholics. In addition, Ward, Bendel, and Lange (1982) noted that patients who reported higher pretreatment work satisfaction were less depressed and more satisfied with life at follow-up. Alcohol abusers and their wives also emphasize the importance of the work setting in maintaining sobriety (Wiseman, 1981). However, high levels of drinking among co-workers can lead to increased alcohol consumption, especially in conjunction with high work demands and a stifling or meaningless job (see Chapter 5 and Whitehead & Simpkins, 1983).

To assess life stressors, social resources, coping responses, and treatment outcome, we used three sets of indices. These indices are drawn from the Health and Daily Living Form (Moos, Cronkite, Billings, & Finney, 1984) and the Family Environment Scale (Moos & Moos, 1986). We also used the Work Environment Scale (Moos, 1986c) to assess stressors and resources at work.

1. *Life stressors* were assessed by the following indices. (*a*) *Negative life events* is composed of 10 events that may have occurred in the last year, such as divorce, decline in income, and death of a close friend. *Spouse dysfunction* is tapped by indices of spouse (*b*) alcohol consumption, (*c*) depression, and (*d*) physical symptoms that are comparable to those used for the patients. (*e*) *Children's health problems,* assessed only at the 2-year follow-up, is a set of 13 items cov-

ering conditions such as asthma, frequent headaches, anxiety, and serious physical or mental disorder.
2. *Family environment* was assessed by six subscales drawn from the FES and an index of *family arguments,* which reflects the number of areas in which family members report disagreements. The index covers 16 areas, such as friends, relatives, politics, money, religion, and sex.
3. *Coping responses* were measured at the 2- and 10-year follow-ups by asking the patient to consider a stressful event and describe how it was handled in terms of the indices of active cognitive, active behavioral, and avoidance coping responses described in Chapter 6. We controlled for the fact that more severe life stressors tend to elicit more coping by constructing indices to reflect the proportion of each type of coping used by the patient.

In Table 7.2 we present cross-sectional correlations for these three sets of context and coping factors with outcome 2 years after treatment; we conducted similar cross-sectional analyses on the 10-year follow-up data. We obtained the partial correlations from hierarchical regressions in which three background characteristics (sex, age, and education) and the appropriate intake symptom were entered first, followed by the indices in each set of predictors. The multiple correlations for the background and intake symptom regressions in the first row of the table provide a baseline against which to gauge the effectiveness of each set of factors in accounting for additional outcome variance. The partial correlations reflect the residual variation accounted for by individual context and coping factors, that is, variation that is independent of background characteristics and intake symptoms. The partial correlations for social and occupational functioning are not shown; virtually none of the latter were statistically significant. We will note the few important findings regarding social functioning.

We also obtained comparable partial and multiple correlations from hierarchical regressions using life context factors assessed at the 6-month follow-up to predict 2-year outcome and regressions using life context and coping factors at the 2-year follow-up to predict 10-year outcome. The findings for three of the outcome criteria are shown in Table 7.3. Overall, the predictive relationships are similar to those obtained in the cross-sectional analyses, although the magnitude of the associations is somewhat lower, especially for the 8-year interval between the last two follow-ups.

Life Stressors and Treatment Outcome

Concurrent Relationships at the 2-Year Follow-Up

Stressful life events, spouse dysfunction, and children's health problems were related to poorer 2-year treatment outcome, especially physical

Table 7.2 Cross-sectional partial and multiple correlations between context and coping indices and two-year treatment outcome (N = 113)

	Outcome indices			
Posttreatment set or variable	Alcohol consumption	Abstinence	Physical symptoms	Depression
BACKGROUND AND INTAKE (R)	.31*	.15	.34*	.45***
LIFE STRESSORS (R)	.45	.36	.56***	.65***
Negative events	.03	−.27**	.37***	.40***
Spouse drinking	.21*	−.17	.25**	.27**
Spouse depression	.28**	−.20*	.27**	.34***
Spouse symptoms	.19*	−.12	.26**	.19*
Children's health problems	.20*	−.08	−.01	.16*
FAMILY ENVIRONMENT (R)	.47*	.34	.52**	.67***
Cohesion	−.28**	.21*	−.31**	−.47***
Expressiveness	−.01	.12	−.28**	−.32***
Conflict	.05	−.08	.26**	.25**
Active recreational	−.21*	.17*	−.12	−.26**
Moral-religious	−.15	−.03	.04	−.04
Organization	−.20*	.10	−.16	−.28***
Family arguments	.12	−.02	.28**	.30***
COPING RESPONSES (R)	.44**	.39**	.47**	.66***
Active-cognitive (%)	−.28**	.29**	−.17*	−.38***
Active-behavioral (%)	.01	.05	−.17*	−.13
Avoidance (%)	.27**	−.34***	.34***	.52***
Overall regression (R)	.49**	.43**	.59***	.71***

*$p < .05$. **$p < .01$. ***$p < .001$.

symptoms and depression (Table 7.2). Patients who reported more negative events experienced more physical symptoms and depression and were less likely to be abstinent. Patients whose spouses drank more and reported more physical symptoms drank more themselves and experienced more physical symptoms and depression. In addition, patients whose spouses were more depressed did less well in all four areas, while patients whose children had more health problems consumed more alcohol and were more depressed. Overall, the set of life stressors added significant increments in the explained variance on physical symptoms (19%) and depression (22%) over that accounted for by patient background and intake functioning (11% and 20%, respectively).

Concurrent Relationships at the 10-Year Follow-Up

We obtained generally comparable findings at the 10-year follow-up. Patients who experienced more negative events tended to be more de-

Table 7.3 Longitudinal partial and multiple correlations between 6-month and 2-year context and coping indices and 2-year (N = 113) and 10-year (N = 82) treatment outcome

	6-month predictors of 2-year criteria			2-year predictors of 10-year criteria		
Posttreatment set or variable	Alcohol consumption	Physical symptoms	Depression	Alcohol consumption	Physical symptoms	Depression
BACKGROUND AND INTAKE (R)	.31*	.34*	.45***	.21	.25	.55***
LIFE STRESSORS (R)	.34	.40	.53*	.47*	.32	.64†
Negative events	.01	.22*	.22*	−.04	.13	.23†
Spouse drinking	.10	−.01	.18	.36**	−.08	−.11
Spouse depression	.05	.07	.19	.10	.11	.29*
Spouse symptoms	.10	.09	.23*	.30*	−.03	.19
Children's health problems	—	—	—	−.06	−.10	.00
FAMILY ENVIRONMENT (R)	.37	.44	.60**	.58***	.39	.65*
Cohesion	−.19	−.03	−.32**	−.37***	−.22†	−.35**
Expressiveness	−.11	−.20*	−.18	−.05	−.02	−.07
Conflict	.15	.01	.18	.13	.05	.13
Active recreational	−.09	−.20*	−.27**	.08	.03	.04
Moral-religious	−.09	−.04	−.07	−.23*	−.16	.01
Organization	−.11	−.07	−.22*	−.15	−.22†	−.30*
Family arguments	.07	.13	.31**	−.12	.05	.20†
COPING RESPONSES (R)	—	—	—	.41*	.35	.62*
Active-cognitive (%)	—	—	—	−.35**	−.24†	−.33**
Active-behavioral (%)	—	—	—	.22†	.04	.07
Avoidance (%)	—	—	—	.14	.19	.26*
Overall regression (R)	.36	.47**	.61***	.58***	.36	.67*

†$p < .10$. *$p < .05$. **$p < .01$. ***$p < .001$.

pressed. Spouse dysfunction was related to patient functioning, but not in as many areas as were found at the 2-year follow-up. Spouse drinking was more strongly associated with patient alcohol consumption (partial $r = .52$) and abstinence (partial $r = -.29$) than was the case at the 2-year follow-up, but spouse drinking was not related to any of the other outcome indices. Spouse depression was associated with poorer patient outcome in all four areas (partial rs ranged from $-.24$ to $.41$). Overall, the set of life stressors added significantly to the prediction of alcohol consumption, abstinence, and depression.

Predictive Relationships

As shown in Table 7.3, negative events assessed at the 6-month follow-up predicted more patient physical symptoms and depression at 2 years. However, as would be expected because of the long interval, negative events at 2 years did not predict any of the outcome criteria at 10 years, although there was a trend ($p < .10$) for persons who experienced more events to be more depressed at the later follow-up.

Two-year spouse drinking and spouse physical symptoms predicted higher patient alcohol consumption at 10 years, and 2-year spouse depression was positively associated with 10-year patient depression. The set of life stressors 2 years posttreatment accounts for an increment of 19% in explained variance on alcohol consumption at the 10-year follow-up over the 4% that can be explained by background characteristics and intake functioning. Overall, the spouse's adaptation plays an important role in a patient's recovery from alcoholism; similarly, the partner's drinking affects the spouse's functioning (Chapter 9).

Although prior studies have highlighted the association between the spouse's drinking and the partner's relapse, few researchers have considered other aspects of spouse functioning. A spouse's poor mood and physical complaints can be a chronic source of stress, lead to more family conflict, and sharpen the detrimental influence of the spouse, especially when the spouse drinks excessively. In addition, these personal characteristics are associated with spouses' avoidance coping styles such as withdrawal and acting out, which also predict poorer outcome (see Chapter 9). Conversely, a spouse who abstains from alcohol and manages to function well in other areas can heighten the patient's chance of recovery.

Family Environment and Treatment Outcome

Concurrent Relationships at the 2-Year Follow-Up

As expected, several aspects of family climate were related to outcome at the 2-year follow-up. As a set, information about the family climate added significantly to the prediction of two of the four outcome criteria

(Table 7.2) and to social functioning. More specifically, patients in more cohesive families were functioning better in all areas. Whereas family expressiveness was associated with fewer physical symptoms and less depression, family conflict and arguments were associated with poorer outcome in these two areas. A recreational orientation in the family was associated with less alcohol consumption and depression, a higher likelihood of abstaining, and (as expected) more social activities. Patients in well-organized families also reported less alcohol consumption and depression. The family environment factors account for a mean increment of 15% of explained variance in the four main outcome criteria over the 11% that, on average, is accounted for by patient background and intake functioning.

Concurrent Relationships at the 10-Year Follow-Up

Again, we obtained comparable findings at the 10-year follow-up. Patients in more cohesive and better organized families consumed less alcohol. These patients also reported fewer physical symptoms and less depression, as did patients in more expressive families. Finally, a stronger moral-religious climate in the family was associated with fewer physical symptoms. Information about the family climate added to the prediction of three of the four outcome criteria (all but abstinence).

Predictive Relationships

In general, many of these findings held when we related family climate at 6 months to treatment outcome at 2 years. The predictive associations were strongest for the outcome criteria of physical symptoms and depression (Table 7.3). As a set, the 6-month family environment variables accounted for 15% more of the variance in 2-year patient depression over the 20% explained by background characteristics and intake functioning.

The long-term predictive analyses showed that higher family cohesion and moral-religious emphasis at the 2-year follow-up were related to less alcohol consumption 8 years later. High cohesion and organization at 2 years predicted fewer physical symptoms and depression at 10 years. Earlier family arguments also predicted later depression ($p < .10$). As a whole, information about the family environment at 2 years predicted 10-year alcohol consumption and depression (increments of 29% and 15% in explained variance, respectively), after controlling for patient background and intake functioning factors. The long-term stability of certain aspects of family climate probably explains their ability to predict functioning over an 8-year interval.

The Importance of the Family

More than three decades ago Jackson (1954) asked, "What are the factors within families which facilitate a return to sobriety or hamper it?"

(p. 585). We can now formulate an answer to this question. In broad perspective, we found that cohesive, well-organized, and socially active families are associated with better treatment outcome. Although each of these family climate factors is important by itself, the combination of all three seems especially beneficial.

In a predictive study of men patients and their wives, Orford and his colleagues (1976) identified a strong association between high marital cohesion at the beginning of treatment and better treatment outcome 1 year later. A good prognosis was related to emotional closeness between the spouses, the husband's involvement in family tasks, and the wife's positive view of the future of the marriage and of her husband when he was sober. Overall, only 18% of high-cohesion couples showed poor treatment outcome as compared to 51% of low-cohesion couples. Similarly, Vannicelli, Gingerich, and Ryback (1983) found that lack of family involvement and high family strain and conflict at treatment intake predicted poorer treatment outcome. As we note in Chapter 12, marital treatment that focuses on improving these areas of family functioning can enhance treatment outcome.

Work Environments and Treatment Outcome

We used the WES to obtain information about the work settings of two groups of employed patients. One group of patients ($N = 55$) was not living in families at the 6-month follow-up; the other group ($N = 56$) was a subset of our married patients. We found little or no association between aspects of work settings and 6-month, 2-year, or 10-year treatment outcome among the married patients. Among the patients not living with their families, however, a more positive experience at work was related to better 6-month outcome on both drinking and nondrinking indices. High job involvement, co-worker cohesion, and supervisor support were especially closely related to better outcome. Work stressors, such as high job demands and lack of autonomy and clarity, were associated with poorer treatment outcome.

Parker and Brody (1982) describe three models of risk factors in the workplace associated with drinking. The social control model posits that a weak occupational structure tends to promote deviant behavior and problem drinking. The alienation or stress model points to workers' lack of control over the job and workplace conditions as a detrimental influence on their morale and health-related behavior. The social availability model asserts that problem drinking is due to participation in group activities with heavy-drinking co-workers. When they tested these ideas, Parker and Brody (1982) found some support for the stress model: high work demands and routinization were associated with perceived job stress, which was related to more alcohol consumption and drinking problems.

Our findings support these ideas; they also imply that social integration into the workplace (presumably with non-heavy-drinking co-workers) may protect some high-risk individuals from experiencing a relapse.

Why do workplace conditions influence single more than married patients? A cohesive family may act as a buffer to improve the chance that a patient will make a good adjustment. Patients with families may view job problems with more detachment because their families cushion the workplace's adverse impact. Moreover, during the posttreatment "reorganization" phase, when emotional energy is focused primarily on the family, stressful work conditions may be less salient for patients. Unmarried patients have fewer significant relationships to help relieve the tension produced by an unsatisfactory work situation. Accordingly, work stressors and resources are more likely to affect their treatment outcome. However, work stressors can contribute to relapse among married patients who have few family resources (see Chapter 8).

Coping Responses and Treatment Outcome

Concurrent Relationships at the 2-Year and 10-Year Follow-Ups

As expected, reliance on active cognitive coping was associated with better treatment outcome, particularly at the 2-year follow-up (see Table 8.2), whereas the use of avoidance coping was strongly associated with worse outcome at both the 2- and 10-year follow-ups. Active behavioral coping was related to fewer physical symptoms at the 2-year follow-up and to a greater likelihood of abstinence at the 10-year follow-up. Taken together, information about the three types of coping responses predicted all four of the outcome criteria at both the 2-year (Table 7.2) and 10-year follow-ups, accounting for average increments of 14% and 9%, respectively, in explained outcome variance.

Predictive Relationships

We did not assess coping responses at the 6-month follow-up. In longitudinal analyses of the 2-year and 10-year data, we found that active cognitive coping at 2 years predicted less alcohol consumption, physical symptoms, and depression at 10 years (Table 7.3). More avoidance coping at 2 years predicted more later depression. Thus, even though coping responses are somewhat situation specific, they seem to capture stable personal tendencies that are associated with long-term functioning.

Only a few studies have examined the connections between coping responses and the recovery process. Jones and Lanyon (1981) found that alcoholic patients' performance on an adaptive skills battery was strongly related to good treatment outcome. Litman and her colleagues (1979) identified several types of coping responses among alcoholic patients: cognitive control (stopping to examine my motives, remembering the mess I've gotten myself in through drinking), distraction/substitution (doing some work around the house), and stimulus control (keeping away from friends who drink). Compared to relapsed patients, successful patients were more likely to use cognitive control as a coping strategy and showed more flexible coping in high-risk situations. Sjoberg and Samsonowitz (1985) found that alcohol abusers who used a greater variety of coping techniques in their efforts to give up drinking were more successful (see also Chaney & Roszell, 1985).

Overall Influence of Life Context on Outcome

In an attempt to determine the overall influence of life context on outcome, we conducted multiple regressions of the outcome measures on the three background characteristics at intake, the appropriate intake index, and the five best contextual predictors (negative events, spouse depression, family arguments, family cohesion, and family recreational orientation).

Concurrent Relationships at the 2-Year Follow-Up

The multiple correlations from these regressions for the 2-year follow-up data are shown in the bottom row of Table 7.2. They are all significantly higher than the multiple correlations from regressions using only background characteristics and intake symptoms (see the first row of Table 7.2). In fact, the five contextual factors accounted for increments of 14% to 30% of the variance in treatment outcome (mean = 20%), compared with 2% to 20% accounted for by the background characteristics and intake functioning (mean = 11%).

Concurrent Relationships at the 10-Year Follow-Up

The multiple correlations obtained at the 10-year follow-up were similar in magnitude to those obtained at the 2-year follow-up. The overall multiple Rs for alcohol consumption, physical symptoms, and depression (Rs = .49, .52, and .70, respectively) were significantly higher than those obtained from regressions using only background characteristics and functioning at intake. The five contextual factors accounted for an increment of 20% of the variance in alcohol consumption, 21% in physical symptoms, and 18% in depression (mean = 19%), compared with 4% to 31% (mean = 14%) accounted for by the demographic characteristics and intake functioning.

Predictive Relationships

We also conducted summary regressions in which information about the five contextual predictors obtained at the 6-month follow-up was used to predict 2-year treatment outcome after controlling for the background and intake indices. The five predictors accounted for increments of 9% of the variance in physical symptoms and 17% in depression beyond the 11%

and 20%, respectively, accounted for by background and intake functioning. In short, the life context factors at 6 months accounted for almost half of the predictable variance in two of the four treatment outcome indices at 2 years.

Summary regressions using life context factors at the 2-year follow-up to predict 10-year follow-up functioning yielded significant increments in explained variance in alcohol consumption and depression (Table 7.3). The life context factors accounted for an additional 29% of the variance in 10-year alcohol consumption and 14% in 10-year depression over the 4% and 31%, respectively, explained by demographic characteristics and intake functioning. Thus, even over an 8-year interval, life context factors can predict the course of treated alcoholism in two important areas.

EXAMINING THE CONCEPTUAL MODEL

Our final step in analyzing the effects of life context and coping factors was to examine their interrelationships and influence within the full model shown in Figure 7.1. Specifically, we estimated the associations among social background, intake functioning, treatment (the program, the intensity of residential and aftercare treatment, and the treatment environment), the three sets of extratreatment factors (life stressors, social resources, and coping responses), and treatment outcome using data from the larger 2-year follow-up sample. We focused on the four more highly related outcome criteria: alcohol consumption, abstinence, physical symptoms, and depression.

Five patient variables are included. *Social background* is indexed by four characteristics that reflect personal resources in that they tend to be positively related to treatment outcome: sex, age, education, and marital status (only seven patients were not married or cohabiting). *Intake functioning* corresponds to the relevant outcome criterion.

Three aspects of treatment are included. *Treatment program* is assessed by four dummy variables scored "0" or "1," depending on whether the patient received treatment in the specified program (the five programs are represented by distinct patterns of "0's" and "1's" on the four variables). *Treatment experiences* are indexed by the sum of scores on 13 standardized items that reflect the range of treatment and aftercare intensity for each patient (see Chapter 4). Finally, *Treatment environment* is tapped by the sum of standardized scores on the 10 COPES dimensions (see Chapter 2).

Two life context factors and one coping variable also were analyzed. *Life stressors* are measured by the sum of four standardized items: negative life events, spouse drinking, spouse depression, and spouse physical symptoms. *Family resources* are measured by the sum of the respondent's standardized scores on family cohesion, expressiveness, recreational and religious orientation, organization, conflict (reversed), and family arguments (reversed). *Coping responses* are indexed by the number of active cognitive and active behavioral coping strategies divided by the total number of coping strategies relied on to manage a recent stressful event.

For each outcome criterion, we used the procedure outlined earlier (Chapter 4) to partition the explained variance for each outcome criterion into the unique variance attributable to each predictor and the variance shared among combinations of predictors (Cronkite & Moos, 1980).

Associations among Patient, Treatment, and Extratreatment Factors

There were only a few significant relationships among the patient, treatment, and extratreatment factors. We estimated these relationships by using the earlier sets of variables in the paradigm to predict subsequent ones in regression analyses. For example, we used social background, intake functioning, and treatment program to predict the intensity of treatment; we then used these four sets of factors to predict life stressors, and so on.

With data from the larger sample (Chapters 2 and 3), we saw that more advantaged and less impaired patients were more likely to receive treatment in one of the private programs. These relationships remained among the subset of family patients. In turn, patients in the milieu-oriented program received more intensive treatment, as did patients in the Salvation Army Center and the halfway house. Overall, patient and program variables explained about 57% of the variation in treatment experiences.

The treatment program was the only factor uniquely accounting for perceptions of the treatment environment (about 26% of the variance explained). Patients in the two private programs and in the halfway house reported particularly positive milieus. Background characteristics, patient intake functioning, and treatment experiences had no independent "effects" on perceptions of the treatment environment. These findings are consistent with the results reported in Chapter 4; they suggest that the COPES provides a relatively objective portrait of the social environments of alcoholism treatment programs.

The sets of patient and treatment variables did not predict life stressors or family resources. The latter finding is probably because the programs offered little if any family treatment. However, patients who experienced more stressful circumstances had less positive family environments at both the 6-month and 2-year follow-ups. Overall, the prior predictors in the model explained about 20% of the variance in family resources at the 2-year follow-up.

Finally, coping responses at the 2-year follow-up were predicted uniquely only by family resources (as noted earlier, the coping indices were constructed to be somewhat independent of life stressors). Patients who enjoyed more family resources were more likely to use active coping responses. The treatment variables independently explained about 7% of the variation in coping responses; however, this proportion was not statistically significant. Thus, treatment did not have a significant effect on posttreatment coping responses. This result is expected, given that none of the five programs emphasized coping skills training.

Overall, these findings indicate that social background and intake functioning are associated with the program in which patients received treatment, but that once patients are in a program their characteristics have little influence on the intensity of treatment they receive or on their perceptions of the treatment environment. Between- and within-program treatment factors had little if any influence on patients' posttreatment life contexts (life stressors and family resources) or on the types of coping responses patients used. However, stressful life circumstances were related to less positive family environments, and patients with more family resources were more likely to employ active coping responses.

Influence of Patient, Treatment, and Extratreatment Factors on Outcome

Our next step was to identify the influence of each of the predictor sets on 6-month and 2-year treatment outcome.

Six-Month Outcome

We first focused on how well the patient and treatment variables in the family patient subsample predicted the four main 6-month outcome criteria. In combination, the patient and treatment variables explained between 14% (alcohol consumption) and 34% (depression; average = 23%) of the variation in short-term outcome. The patient variables uniquely accounted for an average of 6% of the variance in the two drinking criteria (alcohol consumption and abstinence) and 21% of the variance in physical symptoms and depression. The three sets of treatment variables (program, treatment experiences, treatment environment) independently explained an average of about 6% of the 6-month outcome variance. Thus, the patient and treatment variables combined explained comparable proportions of the variance in outcome for the smaller family subsample as for the full sample of patients (see Chapter 4).

Next, we added life context factors (coping responses were not assessed) to see to what extent they explain additional variance in 6-month treatment outcome after patient background, intake functioning, and treatment factors are controlled. Life stressors and family resources accounted for significant increments in explained variance for alcohol consumption (6%), physical symptoms (9%), and depression (5%). Patients who reported fewer stressful circumstances and had more family resources experienced better outcome. Family resources were more strongly related to outcome than were life stressors. Overall, life context factors provide a moderate increment in our understanding of the short-term outcome of alcoholism treatment, raising the explained outcome variance an average of about 6% over that accounted for by patient and treatment factors only.

Two-Year Outcome

As expected given the greater time span, both patient intake and treatment factors had weaker relationships with 2-year than with 6-month treatment outcome. In analyses considering *only* these sets of factors, the patient social background and pretreatment functioning variables accounted for averages of 7% of the variance in the two drinking criteria and 16% of the variance in the two nondrinking criteria. The three treatment factors independently accounted for an average of 4% of the variance in the 2-year outcome criteria (none of the proportions of variance explained was statistically significant). Together with the results for the full sample (Chapter 4), these findings suggest that treatment has some positive short-run influence, but that these modest effects diminish over time. As shown in Figure 7.2, patient intake and treatment variables explained 11% to 24% of the total variation in 2-year treatment outcome (average of 17%).

We obtained a more complete picture of 2-year posttreatment functioning and of the independent effects of the different predictor sets by adding life stressors, social resources, and coping responses to the analyses (see Figure 7.2). Patients who encountered fewer stressful situations and had more family resources experienced better outcome. We found that life stressors and family resources uniquely explained significant increments of the variance in abstinence (6%), physical symptoms (16%), and depression (17%).

When we considered coping responses along with the two sets of life context factors, the total unique explained variance (see Figure 7.2) rose even further. The three factors accounted for an average increment of 15% of the variance in alcohol consumption and abstinence and an aver-

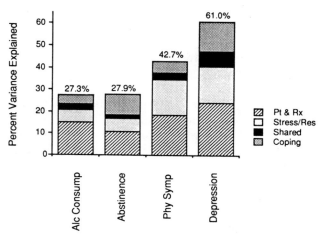

Figure 7.2 Percent variance explained in 2-year outcome by patient, treatment, life context, and coping factors.

age increment of 31% of the variance in physical symptoms and depression. Patients who used more active coping responses experienced better outcomes in these areas. Our overall model of patient, treatment, and life context predictor sets accounts for between 27% (alcohol consumption) and 61% (depression) of the variance in the four main outcome criteria. The overall model accounts for an average of 40% of the variation in patients' 2-year functioning on those four criteria. In short, considering life context and coping factors more than doubles the explained variance in 2-year outcome over that accounted for by patient pretreatment characteristics and treatment factors.

A UNIFIED MODEL OF REMISSION AND RELAPSE

We have examined some new aspects of treatment outcome, namely, the influence of life context and coping factors on the recovery process. The contribution of the life context factors to the four indices of treatment outcome confirms their importance in the recovery process. The inclusion of concurrent information about these factors added an average of more than 18% to the explained variance in 2-year and 10-year outcome for alcohol consumption, abstinence, physical symptoms, and depression. Information about life context factors at 2 years predicted more of the variance in these four criteria at 10 years (15% on average) than did patient demographic and functioning characteristics at treatment intake (12% on average). In fact, the life context factors accounted for almost as much of the variance in the four 2-year outcome criteria as did patient background, intake functioning, and treatment factors combined.

Personal coping responses also play a role in the process of remission and relapse. In cross-sectional analyses, the three coping variables contributed average increments of 14% and 9% in explained variance in the four 2-year and 10-year outcome variables, respectively, after patient background characteristics and intake functioning had been controlled. In predictive analyses, coping responses at 2 years accounted for significant increments in 10-year alcohol consumption (12%) and depression (8%). Finally, in analyses of the full conceptual model, coping responses explained, on average, an additional 8% of the variance in the four 2-year outcome criteria after the effects of patient, treatment, and life context factors had been taken into account.

More specifically, social resources and reliance on active coping skills promote remission, whereas stressful life conditions and avoidance coping responses increase the likelihood of relapse. These context and coping factors affect mood and health-related functioning as well as drinking outcomes. Similarly, Ward (1981) noted that patients' pretreatment satisfaction with their family roles and their spouse was predictive of less drinking behavior and better interpersonal attitudes at a 5-month follow-up. Thus, life context and coping factors are strongly associated with the process of remission and relapse among alcohol abusers (Brown, 1985; Marlatt & Gordon, 1985).

Some researchers have tried to specify mechanisms through which life context factors—particularly stressors—and coping responses affect drinking behavior. One main mediational model relies on a tension-reducing effect of alcohol to explain why an individual may drink more when confronted with a stressful situation. Vuchinich and Tucker (1988) offer a different model; they argue that stressful life events may lead to increased alcohol consumption by reducing available alternative reinforcers to alcohol or by providing more constraints on access to alternative reinforcers. For example, the sudden death of a spouse implies a reduction in the availability of reinforcers other than alcohol.

In regard to the impact of coping styles, Cooper et al. (1988) found that avoidance coping had an indirect effect on alcohol consumption. Individuals with a tendency to rely on avoidance coping to manage stressful situations were more likely to "drink to cope" or engage in "escapist" drinking. In turn, persons who drank to cope tended to consume greater quantities of alcohol—especially persons who held high positive expectations regarding the effects of alcohol.

Context and Coping in Other Addictive Disorders

There is growing evidence of commonalities in the recovery and relapse process for different addictive disorders. Brownell and his colleagues (1986) have described similarities such as the high rate of relapse after treatment, the fact that most persons try self-change strategies that can be quite effective, and the idea of three common stages of change: decision and commitment to change, initial change, and maintenance of change. More specifically, context and coping factors have been associated with each of these three stages in the process of recovery from heroin addiction, smoking, and obesity, as well as in alcohol abuse.

By fostering the ability to make difficult decisions and adhere to them, social resources may promote better treatment outcome in different addictive disorders (Janis, 1983). Accordingly, support from family and friends is associated with long-term success at smoking cessation and weight reduction (Brownell, 1984; Wilson, 1985). Coppotelli and Orleans (1985) identified aspects of partner facilitation such as problem solving, rewarding quitting, listening and understanding, and promoting coping and nonsmoking skills. Partner facilitation was the best predictor of maintenance of smoking cessation among newly abstinent married women smokers. In contrast, being married to someone who is a smoker may make it harder for a person to stop smoking (Lichtenstein, 1982).

The use of cognitive and behavioral coping skills has been associated with maintenance of smoking cessation. Shiffman (1985) found that the single best predictor of good outcome in a potential relapse crisis was reliance on one or more active coping responses. Cognitive and behavioral responses were equally effective in averting relapse; the combination of both types was better than either one alone. Cognitive coping was especially important in that it was used independently of situational stressors. Behavioral coping was more responsive to contextual factors such as alcohol consumption, which diminished its use, and depression, which lessened its effectiveness (Shiffman, 1984, 1986). More generally, long-term recovery may be enhanced by coping skills that reflect the belief that one can respond effectively in a given high-risk context. (For examples of the use of these ideas in relapse prevention programs, see Condiotti & Lichtenstein, 1981; Killen et al., 1984; Perri et al., 1984.)

Context and Coping in Depression

Context and coping factors also are related to remission and relapse in depression (Billings & Moos, 1985a, 1985b). We examined this issue in a 1-year follow-up of our group of seriously depressed treated patients. The measures were conceptually similar to those employed here; that is, we used indices of stressors and social resources from the Health and Daily Living Form (HDL), the FES, and the WES. Many of the findings are comparable to those for alcoholic patients.

Depressed patients showed substantial improvement after treatment; they reported less depression, fewer physical symptoms, and higher self-esteem. More important, patients who experienced more life stressors and fewer social resources after treatment showed poorer treatment outcome than expected based on their demographic characteristics and functioning at intake. There were especially strong associations between chronic stressors in the areas of health, housing, and family and poor treatment outcome. Lack of family support also predicted poorer outcome. Overall, the average level of stressors for the patients as a whole did not decline from intake to follow-up. Accordingly, the high rate of relapse among patients treated for unipolar depression may be due to the presence of ongoing stressors.

The characteristics of depressed patients' work climates were relatively stable between intake and follow-up. Remitted patients reported as much work support as nondepressed controls, but partially remitted and nonremitted patients reported less. Even after controlling for demographic factors and intake functioning, work stressors were associated with more depression and physical symptoms and less self-esteem and participation in family activities. Work support was linked to better functioning in each of these four areas (Billings & Moos, 1985b). These findings support the idea that experiences at work can affect treatment outcome.

Our findings on coping responses to stressful events highlight the role of coping as a stress-mediating factor that can affect treatment outcome. We found that, compared to their coping responses at intake, persons who had been treated for depression at follow-up reported more effort at controlling their feelings and less reliance on emotional discharge and avoidance. At follow-up, they also relied less on seeking information and advice, a coping response often overused by depressed persons who tend to ruminate and avoid acting decisively (Folkman & Lazarus, 1986). Patients who reported these changes experienced better treatment outcome. Thus, treatment may contribute to better outcome among depressed patients by promoting more effective coping responses. Overall, the strength of the connections between context and coping factors was comparable to what we observed in our study of alcoholic patients.

Life stressors and social resources also play a significant role in the posttreatment course of other psychiatric disorders. Spiegel and Wissler (1986) used information about the family environment obtained immediately after hospital discharge to predict subsequent adjustment and rehospitalization among psychiatric patients with varied diagnoses. Patients living in cohesive and expressive families were functioning better and were less likely to be rehospitalized at 3-month and 1-year follow-ups. Vaughn and her colleagues (1984) found that schizophrenic patients who returned to families characterized either by excessive criticism or emotional overinvolvement did worse than expected given the severity of their disorder (see also Leff & Vaughn, 1985).

The General Role of Context and Coping Factors

We raised three main questions at the outset of this chapter. Our findings show that (1) patients' social background and functioning at intake are moderately related to both short-term and long-term treatment outcome; (2) life stressors are associated with poorer treatment outcome, whereas both family resources and greater reliance on active coping responses are related to better outcome; and (3) life context and coping factors are associated as strongly or more strongly with treatment outcome as are patient intake and treatment factors. Some of these associations are quite robust over 18-month and 8-year intervals.

These sets of factors mutually influence each other. Accordingly, changes in stressful conditions and social resources can follow, as well as foreshadow, a patient's heavy drinking and depression. For example, we found that patients who were more depressed at intake were more likely to experience stressful life events subsequently. Moreover, the spouse both affects and is affected by the patient's adaptation. Context and coping factors can play a causal role in problem drinking; however, they also are an outgrowth of an individual's personal resources.

We have sketched a conceptual paradigm that can be used to examine the psychosocial processes involved in relapse and recovery in a variety of addictive disorders. The model also applies to depressed patients and their spouses (Moos, in press), persons with serious medical conditions (Moos, 1985a), and representative groups of healthy women and men (Cronkite & Moos, 1984). In this regard, we believe that some of the psychosocial variables and processes that are related to serious depression

CONTEXT, COPING, AND TREATMENT OUTCOME

and associated aspects of functioning such as self-esteem are comparable to those involved in alcoholism and other addictive behaviors. Because there are underlying commonalities in the formation and influence of life context and coping factors, the use of a general framework may help to integrate research on different psychiatric and behavioral disorders and thereby lead to a more comprehensive understanding of relapse and recovery processes.

8
The Process of Recovery and Relapse

We saw in the previous chapter that some alcoholic patients are able to quit drinking or reduce their alcohol consumption levels substantially 2 years after treatment. In addition, improvement in drinking behavior tends to be associated with improvement in some other areas of functioning. However, to evaluate the extent of remission and the full costs of continued alcohol abuse, we need a comparison group of demographically similar persons without drinking problems. In this chapter, we provide that comparison.

Although there is growing interest in the process of recovery from alcoholism, most prior studies have focused on the personal and social deficits of alcoholics and on how such deficits affect the onset and progression of alcohol abuse. This body of work examines the risk factors related to excessive alcohol use, but it has neglected the personal and social resources that enhance recovery. In fact, the development and cessation of alcohol abuse are part of a dynamic, long-term process that is influenced by multiple personal and psychosocial factors (Vaillant, 1983).

Some researchers have described stages involved in becoming an alcoholic and then linked these stages to the sequence of recovery. Mulford (1977) developed an Alcoholic Stages Index (ASI) that divides the process of becoming an alcoholic into four steps: initial troubles due to drinking, serious personal problems due to drinking, preoccupied drinking, and uncontrolled drinking. These stages were associated with different recovery patterns in two follow-ups. Individuals who had not been able to control their drinking were more likely to be abstinent at follow-up and less likely to maintain successful social drinking patterns than were earlier-stage drinkers.

De Soto and his colleagues (1985) traced the changes in cognitive and psychosocial correlates of abstinence following active alcoholism. Patients reported high levels of physical symptoms in the first few months of abstinence. Symptom levels decreased over time, but they only approached normal levels after 10 years or more of abstinence. Thus, full recovery may take some time; long-term follow-ups are needed to understand the conditions that facilitate recovery.

We examine the process of recovery from alcoholism here by addressing three issues: (1) Can remitted and recovered alcoholic patients function as well as demographically matched, normal-drinking community controls? (2) Do relapsed patients function more poorly than recovered patients or community controls in areas other than drinking? (3) Do patients who remit or recover from alcohol abuse benefit from an especially favorable life context that promotes good treatment outcome? Classifying patients as remitted or relapsed reflects the two global categories that are most often used in describing alcoholism treatment outcome. These categories summarize a patient's functioning on several drinking-related outcome dimensions and provide a way to compare patients who are doing well or poorly with community residents who do not have alcohol-related problems.

COMPARING ALCOHOLIC PATIENTS WITH COMMUNITY CONTROLS

We focus first on whether patients who are able to abstain or to moderate their drinking after treatment adapt as well as nonalcoholic community controls. As we have seen, patients who enter treatment for alcoholism typically function quite poorly and may lack personal and social resources. With treatment, many patients reduce or stop their drinking and improve their physical status, but they may or may not improve in areas less directly related to drinking, such as social and occupational functioning. Because studies of the outcome of treatment for alcoholism have focused primarily on comparisons between treated and minimally treated patients, we do not know how well remitted or recovered alcoholics function compared to matched community controls.

Alcohol abuse and its concomitant problems may be the primary factors that differentiate alcoholics from nonalcoholics. According to Vaillant (1983), there is little or no difference between these groups in predisposing personal factors or childhood stressors. Only two studies have explicitly compared long-term recovered alcoholics with nonalcoholic community controls. Kurtines, Ball, and Wood (1978) found no differences between controls and AA members who had been sober for an average of 9 years in their sense of well-being, self-acceptance, or concern about health, although the recovered alcoholics were more socially inhibited. Vaillant and Milofsky (1982) compared the functioning of 110 inner-city men who at some point between the ages of 21 and 47 met criteria for alcohol abuse with the functioning of 240 demographically similar, social drinking, community controls. Securely abstinent former abusers (abstinent 3 years or more; average = 10 years) exhibited almost the same level of psychosocial functioning and annual income as the social drinker controls. These findings imply that recovered patients should be able to attain normal adaptation in most areas if prolonged alcohol abuse has not produced residual deficits that resist change.

A second issue is the extent to which individuals who continue to abuse alcohol function more poorly than either remitted patients or matched community controls. Relapsed patients are likely to show some deficits in adaptation in nondrinking areas but, because such patients typically have not been compared with demographically similar recovered patients or matched community controls, we know little about the magnitude of the deficits. Moreover, some patients who cannot completely control their drinking nevertheless function quite well in other areas. The standard that remitted patients set is one that relapsed patients presumably could attain, while a comparison with normal-drinking community controls helps to estimate the full personal and social costs of continued alcohol abuse.

A third issue involves the role of life context and coping factors in treatment outcome. We have shown that social stressors and coping resources play an important role in treatment outcome (Chapter 7). We focus here on comparing the levels of stressors and resources among remitted and relapsed patients with those among matched normal controls. Alcohol consumption can help to alleviate the anxiety and tension caused by stressful life events, especially when the events signify personal failure and a loss of self-esteem (Hull, 1981). Thus, the maintenance of stable remission or recovery may require an especially supportive family context. In this respect, the wives of many sober recovering alcoholic men describe them as charming, considerate, thoughtful, and unusually attentive husbands and fathers (Wiseman, 1981). An avoidance of family conflict may help to promote the initial phases of recovery.

Families of active alcoholics are characterized by heightened conflict, marital disruption, disturbed communication, and role dysfunction (Jacob & Seilhamer, in press; Steinglass & Robertson, 1983; Zweben, 1986). Some investigators have speculated that the identified patient's alcohol abuse is not the major marital problem and that family functioning may continue to be marginal even when the alcoholic member recovers (Steinglass, 1981). One of our case examples (see Chapter 6) implied that problem drinking can serve an adaptive role and that family functioning can deteriorate when the alcohol-abusing spouse becomes abstinent. Here, we examine whether family functioning improves after the cessation of alcohol abuse and whether families of stably married recovering alcoholics function as well as those of matched normal controls.

The Value of Matched Community Controls

This is the first of three chapters that probe these issues by comparing a group of married alcoholic patients and their families with a group of matched community controls and their families. Here we compare community controls with remitted and relapsed alcoholic patients studied 2 years and 10 years after initiating residential treatment for alcoholism. Subsequently, we compare the patients' spouses and children with the controls' spouses and children (Chapters 9 and 10).

Our demographically matched community sample provides a realistic normative baseline for judging whether stably remitted or recovered patients are functioning adequately; it also identifies the personal and social costs experienced by patients who are unable to control their drinking. As Edwards and his colleagues (1979) noted, a normal community group can help to evaluate the impact of treatment, because the extent to which alcoholic patients function as well as their neighbors is one important measure of treatment effectiveness.

Some researchers rely on an implicit outcome standard of optimal functioning, which reflects an idealized goal rather than a practical standard that alcoholism treatment programs can reasonably hope to attain. In broad terms, using a standard of optimal functioning is analogous to assessing treatment implementation against individuals' preferences or ideals. Alternatively, the use of a community sample as a standard is analogous to using normative conditions in treatment programs as a baseline for comparing individual programs (Chapter 3). Moreover, information on community controls can reveal more about how normal individuals and their families function and how they differ from treated patients and their families (Jacobson, Follette, & Revenstorf, 1984; Kazdin & Wilson, 1978).

Alcoholic Patients

The patients were drawn from the larger group of 429 persons who were treated for alcoholism at one of the five residential facilities (Chapter 2). The samples used here were composed of 113 married patients who were followed 2 years after treatment and 83 of these patients who were followed 10 years after treatment. The 2-year sample is almost identical to the sample of 113 patients who completed 6-month and 2-year follow-ups (Chapter 7). However, the current sample includes seven married patients who were followed at 2 years but not at 6 months, and it excludes seven unmarried patients from the sample described in Chapter 7.

These 113 patients (88 men and 25 women) followed at 2 years had severe alcohol-related problems at the time of intake to treatment. Their mean alcohol consumption from all beverages on a typical drinking day was more than 13 ounces; 93% had been on binges and 72% had experienced delirium tremens in the past month. A total of 90% had physical symptoms, 85% had missed meals, and 80% had memory problems caused by drinking.

We identified two groups of patients on the basis of their drinking history during the 2 years after treatment. Patients in the stably remitted group ($N = 55$) met *each* of five criteria at *both* 6-month and 2-year follow-ups: (1) no rehospitalization for alcoholism and (2) no inability to work because of alcoholism in the follow-up period; (3) abstaining or consuming less than 5 ounces of 100% ethanol on a typical drinking day in the month prior to follow-up; (4) quantity-frequency (QF) index (average consumption of 100% ethanol per day) less than 3 ounces; and (5) no problems from drinking, with the possible exception of family arguments. The relapsed group was composed of 58 individuals who were rehospitalized for alcoholism or whose drinking was so severe that they could not be classified as remitted nonproblem drinkers.

Compared to spouses of relapsed patients, spouses of remitted patients were significantly less likely to report family arguments about alcohol. Moreover, only 1 of the 54 spouses of remitted patients reported having had to deal with an alcohol or drug problem in the family in the past year. These facts support the validity of the remitted/relapsed designations.

Matched Community Controls

In general, we tried to identify two demographically matched control families from the same census tract as each treated family. Census tract boundaries are designed to achieve some uniformity of population characteristics and living conditions. Accordingly, we assumed that control families selected from the same or an adjacent census tract would be relatively similar. We identified the census tract in which each treated patient resided at the 6-month follow-up. We then used census tract maps and reverse telephone directories to select community participants at random.

Of the 492 eligible families contacted in this manner, 132 (27%) declined to participate. A total of 294 (82%) of the remaining 360 families completed the survey and members of 93% of these families were followed about 15 months later. We did not include families in which drinking problems were reported or that included a family member who had been treated for alcoholism or who was a heavy drinker. The subgroup of 113 community participants used here was selected to match the patient sample on six sociodemographic factors: sex, age, ethnicity, religion, education, and family size. We were able to follow 101 of these 113 persons 8 years later.

The matching process was successful; there were no significant differences among the three groups, nor between any two of the groups, on any of the six matching variables. The patients and controls tended to be middle aged (average age between 45 and 50 years), white (about 85%), and educated beyond high school (about 65%). Most respondents were employed in occupations of moderate prestige. About half had children living at home. These groups were composed of stably married people; the average length of marriage was 22 years for the control group and 21 and 17 years for the remitted and relapsed patients, respectively.

Indices of Personal and Environmental Factors

The patients and community controls were given our three structured inventories: the HDL, the FES, and the WES. In brief, we compared the three groups on the following four sets of indices (see Moos, Finney, & Chan, 1981).

1. *Mood, health, and alcohol consumption* were measured by (*a*) *self-confidence* (the accuracy of six items as self-descriptors: aggressive, ambitious, confident, dominant, energetic, and outgoing); (*b*) *drinking patterns* as assessed by the quantity of alcohol consumed from wine, beer, and hard liquor; (*c*) indices of *current mood and health status* (depression, anxiety, physical symptoms, smoking, and symptoms caused by smoking); and (*d*) *use of health services* (medication use, visits to physicians, and instances of hospitalization).
2. *Occupational, social, and family functioning* was tapped by nine indices. *Occupational functioning* was indexed by part- or full-time employment, job changes, and annual family income. *Social functioning* was measured by (*a*) the frequency of informal social contacts and (*b*) family social activities as reflected by the spouses' reports of the number of joint family social activities during the past month. To assess performance of family roles, we asked the spouse to identify who usually performed each of 17 tasks, such as planning and cooking meals, cleaning the house, handling the bills, and making minor household repairs. *Role performance* was measured by the proportion of tasks performed (*a*) by the alcoholic or matched control, (*b*) by the spouse of the alcoholic or the spouse of the control, and (*c*) jointly by both husband and wife.
3. *Life stressors* and *social resources* were tapped by the selected subscales of the FES and WES described earlier. We also included the patients' report of *family arguments,* as measured by the proportion of applicable areas (areas such as "dating and curfews" were applicable only to families with children) in which there was conflict among family members. *Disagreement about the family environment* was assessed by husband-wife incongruence on the FES (see Chapter 6 and Moos & Moos, 1986). *Negative life events* was composed of 10 events that could have occurred in the last year, such as divorce, decline in income, and death of a close friend.

4. *Coping responses* were measured by the respondent's tendency to use active cognitive, active behavioral, and avoidance coping responses to manage a recent personal crisis or stressful event.

We conducted two preliminary analyses. To examine gender differences, we compared the women patients with a matched group of men patients. Because essentially no differences were found, data from the men and women were combined. Additional analyses showed that the controls who were matched to the remitted patients were very similar to those matched to the relapsed patients. Therefore, both remitted and relapsed patients were contrasted with the total control group. We compared the three groups with one-way analyses of variance (ANOVA) and the Student-Newman-Kuels Multiple Range Test. We obtained virtually identical results using analyses of covariance controlling for demographic factors and thus present the unadjusted means and F values from the ANOVAS here.

TWO-YEAR ADAPTATION AMONG STABLY REMITTED AND RELAPSED ALCOHOLICS

We examine the 2-year adaptation of stably remitted and relapsed patients and compare them with community controls in terms of the four broad domains of variables: (1) mood, health, and alcohol consumption; (2) occupational, social, and family functioning; (3) life stressors and social resources; and (4) coping responses.

Mood, Health, and Alcohol Consumption

Characteristics of Stably Remitted Alcoholics

Although the stably remitted patients were as self-confident as the controls, their mood and health were not as good as those of the controls (Table 8.1). Remitted patients reported more anxiety, consumed more medications (primarily vitamins and tranquilizers), and visited doctors more frequently; in addition, 20% had been hospitalized 3 days or more during the past year compared to 9% of the controls. Some remitted alcoholics may have had residual medical disorders that required continuing treatment. Alcoholic patients are more likely than nonalcoholics to report medical conditions, incur accidents, and use health care services (Roghmann et al., 1981).

Compared to the controls, the remitted patients were less likely to have had a drink in the last month. However, the remitted alcoholics who drank and the community controls who drank did not differ in frequency or quantity of alcohol consumption. This finding supports the idea that some stably remitted alcoholics can engage in normal patterns of social drinking (Miller, 1983). Although some of the 16 patients who were 2-year

Table 8.1 Comparisons between stably remitted and relapsed alcoholic patients and community controls on personal resources, patterns of alcohol consumption, and mood and health at the 2-year follow-up

Variable	Community controls ($N = 113$)	Stably remitted alcoholics ($N = 55$)	Relapsed alcoholics ($N = 58$)	F value
Self-confidence (0-24 scale)	15.09[b]	15.34[c]	12.41[b,c]	8.87***
Drank alcohol past month (% yes)	84.1[a]	23.6[a,c]	75.9[c]	44.03***
Quantity ethanol (oz.)	2.46[b]	2.27[c]	11.18[b,c]	43.93***
Mean daily ethanol (oz.)	0.74[b]	0.89[c]	5.09[b,c]	21.07***
Depression (no. yes of 7)	1.60[b]	1.67[c]	4.02[b,c]	33.49***
Anxiety (no. yes of 5)	0.82[a,b]	1.27[a,c]	2.10[b,c]	19.11***
Physical symptoms (no. yes of 12)	2.21[b]	2.29[c]	3.69[b,c]	9.56***
Medications (no. yes of 10)	1.35[a,b]	1.89[a]	2.10[b]	6.04**
Doctor visits (1-5 scale)	1.86[a,b]	2.45[a]	2.44[b]	8.39***
Hospitalized 3 days or more (% yes)	8.85[b]	20.00[c]	44.83[b,c]	17.16***

Note. Means that share a common superscript differ significantly ($p < .05$) by the Student-Newman-Keuls test.
**$p < .01$.   ***$p < .001$.

moderate drinkers eventually relapsed, an additional follow-up 4 years after treatment indicated that 7 of the 12 moderate drinkers we were able to recontact still met our criteria of remission (Finney & Moos, 1981).

Consistent with prior studies, the remitted patients were more likely than the controls to smoke, smoke more heavily, and report physical symptoms due to smoking (Istavan & Matarazzo, 1984). However, the remitted alcoholics did not increase their smoking as they cut down on their drinking. Although high levels of alcohol and cigarette use often occur together, these addictions can be independent of one another once they are established. Accordingly, staff in abstinence-oriented alcoholism programs need not be concerned that they are trading a decline in one addictive behavior for a rise in another. In fact, in-program exposure to smoking cessation techniques can teach some alcoholic patients specific procedures that may help them stop drinking excessively (Burling & Ziff, 1986).

Characteristics of Relapsed Alcoholics

Relapsed patients were functioning much worse in mood and health-related areas than either remitted patients or community controls. Even after matching the three groups on demographic factors, relapsed alcoholics reported more depression, anxiety, physical symptoms, and medication use; they also showed less self-confidence.

The current drinkers among the relapsed group differed from those among the remitted patients and the community controls in that they consumed a much greater quantity of alcohol and drank hard liquor somewhat more often. In fact, 14 of the relapsed patients reported consuming more than 12 ounces of ethanol per drinking day during the month before the second follow-up. About 25% of the relapsed alcoholics were making a renewed effort to control their drinking at the 2-year follow-up. Some of these patients were participating in additional inpatient or outpatient treatment.

In general, the quantity of alcohol consumption is more closely related to relapse and other aspects of dysfunction than is the frequency of consumption (Jacob, 1986; Jacob, Dunn, & Leonard, 1983). The consumption of large amounts of alcohol in drinking binges signifies a loss of control and may be the main factor contributing to the relatively poor adaptation of the relapsed patients. Although our findings are not decisive on this point, we believe that the functional deficits of the relapsed alcoholics are primarily consequences of their alcohol abuse. The relapsed patients' educational and occupational backgrounds are comparable to those of the remitted patients. Accordingly, if they were able to control their excessive alcohol use, many of the relapsed patients might be able to function as well as the remitted patients.

Occupational, Social, and Family Functioning

Stably Remitted Patients

The stably remitted patients were comparable to the controls in their occupational functioning (Table 8.2). The remitted patients and their families did not have as many social contacts in the prior month as did the community controls, but the differences are relatively small (Table 8.2). About 75% of these patients tried to abstain from drinking and may have reduced their participation in social pursuits to avoid the temptation to drink. Alcohol is freely available during many social activities; accordingly, alcoholic patients who are trying to abstain are likely to appraise leisure pursuits less positively than normal drinkers and to participate less actively in them (Smolensky et al., 1980; Tuchfeld, Lipton, & Lile, 1983). However, participation in family-oriented social activities is positively related to treatment outcome (Chapter 7), probably because it reflects and enhances family cohesion and tends to occur in a nondrinking social context.

The remitted alcoholics performed about the same proportion of household tasks as did the community controls. Remitted alcoholics performed more household tasks together with their spouses; accordingly, the spouses of remitted patients performed slightly fewer tasks than did the spouses of controls.

Relapsed Patients

Relapsed patients had a much lower level of occupational functioning and family income than did the remitted patients or the controls. Only 38% of the relapsed patients were employed full-time compared to about 60% of the remitted patients and controls; 44% had changed jobs during the past

Table 8.2 Comparisons between stably remitted and relapsed alcoholic patients and community controls on occupational, social, and family functioning at the 2-year follow-up

Variable	Community controls ($N = 113$)	Stably remitted alcoholics ($N = 55$)	Relapsed alcoholics ($N = 58$)	F value
OCCUPATIONAL FUNCTIONING				
Employed full time (% yes)	59.3[b]	60.0[c]	37.9[b,c]	4.15*
Employed part time (% yes)	23.0[b]	12.7	8.6[b]	3.32*
Changed jobs in last year (% yes)	23.3[b]	12.2[c]	43.6[b,c]	9.66**
Annual family income (in thousands of dollars)	18.3[b]	17.2[c]	14.0[b,c]	8.66***
SOCIAL AND FAMILY FUNCTIONING				
Informal social contacts (no. in last month)	11.6[a,b]	9.1[a]	9.2[b]	5.13**
Family activities (no. yes of 12)	3.24	2.98	2.71	1.37
Tasks performed by patient (%)	37.0[b]	39.0[c]	29.7[b,c]	3.99*
Tasks performed by spouse (%)	46.2	40.5[c]	49.7[c]	3.04*
Tasks performed jointly (%)	10.6[a]	17.0[a]	15.0	3.26*

Note. Means that share a common superscript differ significantly ($p < .05$) by the Student-Newman-Keuls test.
*$p < .05$.   **$p < .01$.   ***$p < .001$.

year compared to 23% of the control group. The relapsed patients and their families had fewer social contacts in the last month than the controls. Moreover, the alcoholic member in the relapsed families participated in fewer household tasks, while the spouse performed a larger share of them.

Life Stressors, Social Resources, and Coping Responses

Family Environment

The family environments of remitted alcoholics were as cohesive, expressive, and well organized and as free of conflict as the families of community controls (Table 8.3). Together with the fact that remitted alcoholics reported fewer family arguments, these findings are consistent with the idea that families of remitted alcoholics avoid conflict and tension for fear of triggering renewed drinking.

Compared to the controls, the relapsed alcoholics experienced less family cohesion and recreational orientation and more disagreement about their family climate. The families of the 14 currently heavy-drinking relapsed patients experienced even more conflict, less expressiveness and organization, and participated in fewer social activities. Even after considering demographic factors that might account for such differences, family functioning is poorer among relapsed alcoholics than among remitted patients or community controls.

Table 8.3 Comparisons between stably remitted and relapsed alcoholic patients and community controls on family and work environments, life events, and coping responses at the 2-year follow-up

Variable	Community controls ($N = 113$)	Stably remitted alcoholics ($N = 55$)	Relapsed alcoholics ($N = 58$)	F value
FAMILY ENVIRONMENT				
Cohesion	7.24[b]	7.52[c]	6.40[b,c]	5.88**
Expressiveness	5.76	5.94	5.18	2.44
Conflict	2.42	2.19	3.07	2.48
Active-recreational	5.07[a,b]	4.31[a]	4.07[b]	4.55**
Moral-religious	5.52	5.26	5.15	<1
Organization	5.89	6.28	5.31	2.44
Family arguments (% yes of 16)	26.4	18.1	26.4	3.14*
Husband-wife incongruence	17.50[b]	15.90[c]	23.50[b,c]	3.34*
WORK ENVIRONMENT†				
Involvement	5.80	6.42	5.69	<1
Peer cohesion	5.83	6.61	6.46	1.97
Task orientation	5.55	5.66	5.77	<1
Work pressure	4.78	3.92[c]	5.89[c]	4.17*
Clarity	5.76	5.18	4.77	2.07
Physical comfort	5.24[b]	5.84[c]	3.81[b,c]	4.63**
LIFE EVENTS AND COPING RESPONSES				
Negative life events	.85[b]	1.07[c]	1.71[b,c]	9.08***
Active cognitive (%)	45.47[b]	48.65[c]	40.33[b,c]	5.04**
Active behavioral (%)	42.25	40.45	40.68	<1
Avoidance (%)	12.28[b]	10.90[c]	18.99[b,c]	8.10***

†The numbers of cases are 82, 38, and 26 for the three groups.

Note. Means that share a common superscript differ significantly by the Student-Newman-Keuls test ($p < .05$).

*$p < .05$.   **$p < .01$.   ***$p < .001$.

These findings corroborate prior research (Jacob & Seilhamer, 1987; Wiseman, 1981). They indicate that families with an alcoholic member experience considerable strain, which diminishes when the alcohol abuser controls his or her drinking. The magnitude of the group differences we identified are moderate, perhaps because the relapsed alcoholics and their spouses had been married for some time and had developed ways of adapting to fluctuations in the severity of the patient's alcohol abuse. In addition, only a few of the alcoholic partners were drinking as abusively at the 2-year follow-up as when they entered treatment.

Work Environment

There were two differences between the work milieus of relapsed and remitted alcoholics. The relapsed patients reported higher demands and more difficult physical conditions at work. As noted earlier, only 38% of the relapsed patients were employed full time and 44% had changed jobs in the last year. These findings show that the relapsed patients experienced a substantial level of work-related stressors, some of which may have been generated by their excessive drinking. In contrast, remitted patients managed to obtain and hold more meaningful and less demanding jobs in settings that they appraised as more physically comfortable.

The characteristics of the work environment may be especially important for married patients in more permissive and socially active families. In this respect, we identified seven moderate drinkers at the 6-month follow-up, only one of whom remained a moderate drinker at the 2-year follow-up. Compared to abstainers' work settings at the 6-month follow-up, the work settings of the moderate drinkers were much more aversive: higher in work demands and supervisor control and lower in involvement, co-worker cohesion, and supervisor support. The families of the moderate drinkers were quite cohesive and socially oriented, but the moderate drinkers' spouses were more likely to drink themselves. In addition, moral-religious emphasis and family control were quite low. The unsatisfying work conditions may have combined with these family influences to contribute to the high rate of relapse (Finney & Moos, 1981).

Physical stressors in the workplace have been implicated as a risk factor in other disorders. Link, Dohrenwend, and Skodol (1986) studied the occupational careers of schizophrenic patients. Compared to community controls and to depressed persons, the first full-time occupations of the schizophrenic patient more often exposed them to work conditions characteristic of some blue-collar jobs, such as hazards, heat, noise, humidity, fumes, and cold. Accordingly, occupational stressors may play a role in the etiology and course of some psychiatric disorders.

Life Events and Coping Responses

Stably remitted patients were more likely to experience positive life events than either relapsed patients or community controls. In contrast, relapsed patients reported more negative and fewer positive events than members of the other two groups did. Some of the stressful events involved moving, separation, changing jobs, and experiencing a sudden loss of income; many of these probably were due to the relapsed patients' continuing alcohol abuse.

The remitted alcoholics and the community controls did not differ on the three coping indices. However, relapsed alcoholics were more likely to rely on avoidance coping responses and less likely to use active cognitive coping responses than either the remitted patients or the controls. In general, cognitive coping seems to increase the likelihood of stable remission, while avoidance coping is related to continuing dysfunction and relapse after treatment.

Overall, these findings show that some stably remitted alcoholics and their partners can attain normal personal and family functioning. Our 2-

year follow-up results do not support the assertion that families of remitted patients attain only marginal levels of adaptation or that family functioning deteriorates because previously suppressed problems emerge after the patient achieves abstinence or nonproblem drinking.

LONG-TERM ADAPTATION OF PATIENTS AND CONTROLS

Alcoholism is often described as a chronic condition characterized by frequent relapses. Nevertheless, some afflicted individuals are able to maintain long periods of sobriety. We focused on the long-term course of alcoholism among the treated members of our family sample by following them 10 years after their index treatment episode. We also followed the matched community controls to provide a baseline for evaluating the long-term functioning of the remitted and relapsed patients.

As expected on the basis of prior research, significantly more patients (19, or 16.8%) than community controls (2, or 1.8%) died between the 2- and 10-year follow-ups. Thus, the patients were more than nine times as likely to die as matched controls; this difference is higher than that found in prior studies (Mackenzie et al., 1986). The higher patient-control mortality ratio may be attributable partially to chance, given our relatively small patient and control samples. Had just three fewer patients lived and three more controls died, the ratio of patient-to-control deaths would have been 3.2—a ratio within the range of previous findings.

However, it is also possible that the use of minimally adjusted (usually only for age, sex, and race) general population data has resulted in underestimates of the risk of premature death among alcoholic patients in at least some previous studies. General population mortality data are upwardly biased (for comparison purposes) by deaths among alcoholic persons, and they do not take into account marital and socioeconomic status. Married and white-collar adults, especially men, have a lower mortality rate (Kotler & Wingard, 1989). Our control sample, like the patient sample, was composed largely of married, middle-class individuals. Thus, one would expect to find a lower mortality rate among these controls, which may have resulted in the higher observed/expected ratio for our patient sample. In this regard, Edwards et al. (1978) found higher observed/expected mortality ratios among alcoholic persons of high and moderate socioeconomic status than among those of lower socioeconomic status.

We obtained death certificates for 18 of the 19 patients who died. Among the listed causes of death were cirrhosis of the liver (2 patients), cancer (2 patients), suicide (3 patients), hemorrhages (2 patients), alcoholic cardiomyopathy (1 patient), and heart disease or attack (8 patients); heart disease is the most common cause of death among older alcoholics (Vaillant, 1983). Information provided by 16 spouses indicated that 12 of the patients had been drinking heavily prior to the illness or injury that resulted in their death. Of these 12 patients, 10 had been classified as relapsed at the 2-year follow-up, and only 2 as remitted.

Ten-Year Remission and Relapse Rates

Of the 94 surviving patients, we successfully followed 83 (88%); thus, with knowledge of 19 deaths, we have data on the fate of 102 (90%) of the 113 patients. We obtained long-term follow-up data from 101 (91%) of the 111 surviving controls; thus, we know something of the fate of 93% of the original group of 113 controls. Five of the community controls were consuming over 5 ounces of ethanol on drinking days according to our liberal consumption measure. We excluded these 5 individuals from further analyses, leaving 96 community controls to compare with the remitted and relapsed patients.

Stably remitted patients had to meet each of the same five criteria used at the 2-year follow-up: (1) no rehospitalization for alcoholism and (2) no inability to work because of alcoholism in the past 2 years, (3) abstaining or consuming less than 5 ounces of ethanol per drinking day in the past month, (4) abstaining or consuming less than 3 ounces of ethanol per day in the past month, and (5) no problems associated with drinking (except for family arguments) in the past year. Patients who met these criteria but who indicated some heavy drinking on occasional drinking binges in the past 2 years were considered relapsed. According to these criteria, 47 of the 83 patients (57%) we followed were in remission and 36 (43%) were relapsed at the 10-year follow-up.

Again, the validity of these designations is supported by the fact that spouses of remitted alcoholics were much less likely to report family arguments about alcohol than were spouses of relapsed alcoholics. Moreover, none of the spouses of remitted patients reported experiencing an alcohol or drug problem in the family in the past year.

How do our remission and relapse rates compare to other long-term follow-up studies of treated alcoholics? In a 16-year follow-up, McCabe (1986) found that 17 of 31 surviving former patients (55%) had a favorable outcome status for the prior year. However, the death rate (44%) for McCabe's initial cohort was substantially higher than ours, as might be expected with a longer follow-up period. O'Connor and Daly (1985) found that 82% of 40 traced survivors had been abstinent for 1 year or longer or were self-described social drinkers. The follow-up interval again was longer than ours (20 years), and the proportion of deceased patients (57%) was substantially higher.

In a study similar to our own, Edwards and his colleagues (1983) tried to trace 99 married patients after an average of 11 years subsequent to the initiation of treatment. On average, these patients had been 41 years old at the time of the index treatment episode. A total of 68 (69%) of the former patients were reinterviewed; 18 (18%) had died, and 13 (13%) were lost to follow-up. Among those who survived and were followed, 40% had a good outcome (19 abstinent at least 1 year and 8 social drinkers), 47% exhibited uncontrolled drinking, and 13% had an equivocal outcome. With the exception of a lower unequivocal remission rate, these findings are quite consistent with ours.

Patient Status at the 2- and 10-Year Follow-Ups

Table 8.4 presents the status of the 113 patients at the 2- and 10-year follow-ups. Contrary to prior findings (Barr et al., 1984; Smith et al., 1983), there was no relationship between 2-year remission-relapse status and mortality. Of the 55 patients in remission at the 2-year follow-up, 8 (15%) died, whereas 11 of the 58 patients (19%) initially classified as relapsed died. Table 8.4 also shows that we were less successful in following the relapsed than the remitted patients (14% versus 5% attrition rates).

Among the patients we followed, we identified a fairly high level of stability in both the 2-year remitted and relapsed statuses. Of the initially remitted patients, 77% (34/44) had the same status 8 years later; a somewhat lower proportion (67%) of the 2-year relapsed patients were classified as relapsed at the 10-year follow-up.

Comparing Long-Term Remitted and Relapsed Patients to Community Controls

At the 10-year follow-up, the long-term remitted patients were much less likely than the community controls to have consumed alcohol in the past month (19% versus 89%—see Table 8.5). The remitted patients who drank consumed less ethanol per drinking day than did the controls, but this difference was not statistically significant. In fact, we found no significant differences between the long-term remitted patients and the community controls on any of the mood and health variables, except that remitted patients were more likely to smoke. We had found only a few differences in these areas at the 2-year follow-up. Thus, patients who achieve long-term remission seem to be functioning normally.

The 36 relapsed patients showed a very different picture in terms of their alcohol consumption, mood, and health. Compared to the community controls, they were less likely to have consumed alcohol in the past month (some were making another attempt at recovery), but those who

Table 8.4 Two-year and 10-year statuses for the patient sample ($N = 113$)

2-Year follow-up status	10-Year follow-up status				
	Remission	Relapse	Not followed	Died	Total
Remission	34	10	3	88	55
Relapse	13	26	8	11	58
Total	47	36	11	19	113

Table 8.5 Comparisons among long-term remitted and relapsed alcoholic patients and community controls at the 10-year follow-up

Variable	Community controls ($N = 96$)	Stably remitted alcoholics ($N = 47$)	Relapsed alcoholics ($N = 36$)	F value
MOOD, HEALTH, AND ALCOHOL CONSUMPTION				
Drank alcohol past month (% yes)	88.54[a,b]	19.15[a,c]	52.78[b,c]	53.08***
Quantity ethanol (oz.)	2.20[b]	2.05[c]	8.03[b,c]	35.04***
Mean daily ethanol (oz.)	.71[b]	1.02[c]	3.46[b,c]	21.37***
Depression (no. yes of 7)	1.63[b]	1.76[c]	3.64[b,c]	13.48***
Anxiety (no. yes of 5)	.56[b]	.70[c]	1.94[b,c]	18.19***
Physical symptoms (no. yes of 12)	2.24[b]	9.96[c]	4.25[b,c]	13.76***
Medications (no. yes of 10)	1.53[b]	1.79	2.33[b]	4.20*
Hospitalized 3 days or more (% yes)	8.33[b]	17.02[c]	33.33[b,c]	6.60**
ANNUAL FAMILY INCOME ($ thousands)	32.95[b]	28.30[c]	25.91[b,c]	5.44**
FAMILY ENVIRONMENT				
Cohesion	7.37[b]	7.76[c]	6.52[b,c]	3.37*
Expressiveness	5.91	6.14	5.21	2.15
Conflict	2.03	1.95	2.14	<1
Active-recreational	4.80	4.36	3.83	2.03
Moral-religious	5.54	5.55	5.21	<1
Organization	6.22[b]	6.71[c]	4.69[b,c]	7.71***
Family arguments (% yes of 16)	15.66	16.22	17.19	<1
LIFE EVENTS AND COPING RESPONSES				
Negative life events	.56[b]	.64	.97[b]	3.58*
Active cognitive (%)	45.86	49.44	45.63	<1
Active behavioral (%)	41.25	36.23	37.44	1.18
Avoidance (%)	13.41	14.33	16.93	<1

Note. Means that share a common superscript differ significantly ($p < .05$) by the Student-Newman-Keuls test.
*$p < .05$.   **$p < .01$.   ***$p < .001$.

drank consumed much more ethanol on drinking days and per day than did either the controls or the remitted patients. Moreover, the relapsed patients reported more depressed mood and anxiety, more physical symptoms, used more medications, and were more likely to have been hospitalized for 3 days or more in the past year. The relapsed patients were also more likely to smoke and to have more smoking-related symptoms than the community controls.

The relapsed patients also had lower family incomes than either the community controls or the remitted patients. In addition, relapsed patients reported less family cohesion and organization and more negative life events in the past year. However, there were no significant differences among the three groups on any other occupational, social, family functioning, family environment, work environment, or coping variable.

Thus, for the survivors, the long-term costs of alcoholism are more narrowly confined to personal and family functioning than they were at the 2-year follow-up.

Overall, our data suggest that the average 10-year course of treated alcoholism among initially married patients who survive is one of modest improvement. Patients who were remitted at the 10-year follow-up were functioning better and enjoyed more positive life contexts than did the remitters at the 2-year follow-up. Relapsed patients showed more dysfunction in mood and health than remitted patients at each follow-up; however, relapsed patients at the 10-year follow-up were functioning somewhat better than were the relapsed patients at the 2-year follow-up. Part of this modest improvement may reflect the death of some patients who were functioning more poorly. However, as shown in Chapter 7 (Table 7.1), it also reflects a process of "maturing out" of alcoholism for some of the surviving patients, as discussed by Drew (1968).

TOWARD A THEORY OF RECOVERY AND RELAPSE

Although the average trajectory among the survivors is modestly positive, the 10-year paths of individual patients varied considerably. Our findings support the idea that life context and coping factors in the early posttreatment stages play a role in determining the long-term path an individual patient will follow. They also highlight substantial differences between remitted and relapsed alcoholics in areas such as income and hospitalization. Compared to the remitted patients, the relapsed patients at 2 years posttreatment had about 25% less family income and were more than twice as likely to be hospitalized for 3 days or more in the past year. Differences remained between the two groups on these variables at 10 years, although they were not quite as large. These findings indicate that substantial benefits may accrue when individuals are able to curtail their alcohol abuse.

Remission among Alcoholic Patients

At the 2-year follow-up, the stably remitted alcoholics experienced no more life stressors than the community controls and were somewhat more likely to experience positive events. Moreover, compared to relapsed patients, they had a more extensive social support network, reported more family cohesion and organization and less conflict, and experienced more physical comfort and less pressure at work. The remitted patients apparently tried to obtain help from physicians and persons in the community who are likely to respond supportively to an alcoholic who is making a concerted effort at recovery. These successfully treated alcoholics and their spouses managed to create relatively benign circumstances that may have contributed to long-term recovery. In fact, 77% of the successfully followed patients who were remitted at 2 years had the same status 10 years later.

Many of the relapsed alcoholics, however, were trapped in a vicious cycle in which stressful life conditions, which may have been caused in part by their alcohol abuse, contributed to its continuation. These conditions established a pattern in which the stressors were amplified and more heavy drinking ensued. This process was fostered by the high conflict and lack of cohesion and structure among families of the relapsed patients, by their recurrent lack of employment and frequent job changes and, for those who were employed, by high job demands and difficult physical conditions at work. The combination of more life stressors, lack of adequate social resources, and reliance on less effective coping seems to have made it hard for the relapsed patients to break their destructive drinking patterns. Only 13 of 39 patients followed 8 years later had gone into remission.

The relapsed patients' lack of personal resources and self-esteem at the 2-year follow-up undoubtedly contributed to their continued problems. Persons with low self-confidence are more likely to blame themselves for life stressors. Relapsed patients who are highly self-conscious and who experience life events indicative of personal failure may be especially prone to resort to alcohol to help them avoid the negative implications of such events (Hull, 1981). Hull, Young, and Jouriles (1986) found that 7 of 10 (70%) alcoholic patients with high self-consciousness who experienced life events that signified personal failure had relapsed at a 3-month follow-up. This was true of only 1 of 7 (14%) highly self-conscious patients who experienced positive self-relevant life events. The quality of life events was not associated with 3-month relapse rates among patients with low levels of self-consciousness.

Our findings are also consistent with other recent studies. Rosenberg (1983) noted that alcoholic patients who did not relapse experienced fewer negative and more positive life events, were less compliant in high-risk situations, and enjoyed more social support from family and friends. Large and dense social networks composed of close friends who are not heavy drinkers tend to discourage heavy drinking and help motivate alcoholics to enter and continue treatment (Strug & Hyman, 1981). In a 20-year follow-up of treated men alcoholics, Nordstrom and Berglund (1986) noted that more than 70% of recovered patients attributed their recovery to changes in social circumstances, social pressure to stop drinking, and negative social consequences of alcohol abuse. More generally, positive changes in a person's family and work milieu are associated with natural recovery and the maintenance of remission after treatment (Ogborne, Sobell, & Sobell, 1985).

The process of remission does not necessarily proceed smoothly. In an incisive paper, Wiseman (1980) pointed out that alcoholic men typically feel tense, irritable, and depressed and are more sensitive to physical aches and pains during moderate-term sobriety. Many recovering alcoholics describe this as a difficult period. Their wives may ventilate pent-up anger about their husband's past irresponsible and aggressive behavior. With longer-term sobriety, some men become model husbands and fathers, but a minority are lethargic and withdrawn and tend to create a somber home atmosphere. In either case, wives are tense and fearful of stimulating renewed drinking outbursts. None of the alcoholics or wives of alcoholics Wiseman studied felt that their lives fully returned to normal.

Vaillant (1983) has also noted that abstinence rarely brings instant relief and can be painful over the short term. Recovering alcoholics often experience difficult problems as they try to resume occupational and family responsibilities. Thus, even though recovering alcoholics seem to function well, they may continue to experience some personal and social strains.

Remission among Other Groups of Substance Abusers

Comparable psychosocial factors have been identified in recovery from heroin dependence. Krueger (1981) found that heroin abusers who relapsed while on a methadone maintenance program experienced more stressful life events relative to a control group and to their own prerelapse event levels. Like alcohol, heroin may help some addicts to regulate and dampen experiences of failure and depression. Wille (1983) studied 40 former heroin abusers who were no longer using opiates. One subgroup of remitters relied primarily on self-help and personal motivation that was triggered in part by community social supports and positive life events. A second subgroup of remitters initially needed external pressure or social control and then experienced positive life changes that facilitated their recovery. Just as with alcohol abuse, treatment for drug dependence must build on curative psychosocial factors and be grounded in a theory about the natural processes that promote recovery. Such processes include forming new personal relationships and investments in constructive activities and eventually developing a new social identity and perspective on life (Biernacki, 1986).

Environmental support has also been related to smoking cessation and maintenance. Mermelstein and his co-workers (1986) examined the role of partner support for quitting smoking and of general social resources in the maintenance of gains for treatment for smoking cessation and in relapse. Two groups of smokers participated in a smoking cessation program and were followed over a 12-month period. Partner support and general support were related to the cessation of smoking and to short-term (up to 3 months) abstinence. Supportive confidant relationships were associated with cessation in a sample that included a large proportion of single people. Supportive relationships influenced short-term but not long-term maintenance, perhaps because ex-smokers no longer sought support or partners and confidants got tired of providing it. As expected, the presence of smokers in the person's social network was predictive of long-term relapse.

Overall, common personal and environmental factors are involved in remission and relapse in different addictive disorders (Brownell et al., 1986). The most important personal factors are positive and sustained motivation, self-efficacy, and a varied repertoire of cognitive and behavioral coping skills. Critical environmental factors include life stressors, such as interpersonal conflict and social pressure to continue an addictive behavior, and social resources from family members and friends. Although common factors promote remission among different groups of substance abusers, it is likely that more pervasive environmental changes are needed to maintain recovery from heroin and alcohol abuse than to maintain smoking cessation (Biernacki, 1986; Marlatt & Gordon, 1985).

Remission among Patients with Unipolar Depression

Psychosocial studies of depression have concentrated mainly on the onset and treatment phases of the disorder. We studied the posttreatment phase of unipolar depression by examining the personal and social characteristics of remitted, partially remitted, and nonremitted depressed patients (Billings & Moos, 1985b). The sample was based on 12-month follow-ups of our groups of over 400 patients and a similar number of demographically comparable nondepressed community controls.

As expected, patients whose depression remitted also improved in other aspects of their adjustment as well as in personal resources such as self-esteem, and in their coping responses to posttreatment stressors. In contrast, nonremitted patients continued to experience deficits in these domains.

More specifically, remitted patients' mood and physical functioning was comparable to that of the normal controls, except that remitted patients still reported more physical symptoms, used more psychotropic medication, and were more likely to smoke. Remitted patients were comparable to controls with respect to most life stressors, but they experienced more stressful events and illness among their children. In addition, remitted patients reported a less extensive network of friends, fewer close relationships, and less interpersonal and family support. Such less supportive social contexts may make a relapse more likely, especially when these patients rely more heavily on avoidance coping strategies. Together with other studies of psychiatric treatment (Edwards et al., 1979; Spiegel & Wissler, 1983), however, the findings imply that some remitted patients function quite well and are able to establish near-normal social contexts.

Recovery and the Hope for a Normal Life

We conclude that some successfully treated alcoholic patients can establish normal lives and resume essentially normal patterns of functioning once they stop their excessive drinking. Many people who experience a significant life crisis or physical illness never feel quite the same again. Similarly, some stably remitted alcoholics and their spouses may not experience their lives as completely normal. However, our long-term follow-up shows that these patients typically are not seriously disturbed persons who create malignant social and family environments irrespective of their alcohol abuse.

Vaillant (1983) obtained similar findings in groups of treated and untreated alcohol abusers. In a treated clinic sample of 100 patients followed annually for 8 years, freedom from alcohol abuse was associated with improved social adjustment. In the study mentioned earlier of inner-city men, generally untreated alcoholics who were able to maintain abstinence were less likely to die and more likely to enjoy their life than were chronic alcoholics. Moreover, their current psychiatric functioning and their marital, parental, and occupational adaptation were comparable to that of men for whom alcohol was never a problem. In contrast, chronic alcoholics were four times as likely to remain unemployed and four times as likely to die. Likewise, the findings of Kurtines et al. (1978) suggest that long-term remitted alcoholics can attain essentially normal levels of self-acceptance and a sense of well-being.

There is a vast difference between progressive alcohol abusers and stably remitted individuals who previously were severely symptomatic. Overall, stably remitted alcoholics are similar to people in the general population and different from active alcoholics or individuals with psychiatric disorders. The fact that adaptation among recovering alcoholics can return to normal is an unexpected positive outcome. It provides the hope that the personal and social problems fostering alcoholism need not lead to permanent residual deficits, that the stigma of alcoholism can be overcome, and that after treatment some stably married alcoholics can attain essentially normal lives.

III

ALCOHOLISM AND THE FAMILY

9
Spouses of Alcoholic Partners

The functioning and life circumstances of spouses of alcoholics are of interest because the spouse can affect the partner's recovery and because spouses may be burdened by the problems of their alcoholic partners. As we saw in Chapter 7, outcome was poorer for alcoholic partners whose spouses consumed more alcohol and experienced more depression and physical symptoms. In this chapter we focus on how the alcoholic partner and other contextual factors affect the spouse. Although spouses of alcoholics experience their own problems, in part as a reaction to the partner's heavy drinking and other dysfunction, the long-term outlook for the spouse of a recovered alcoholic may be quite positive. The spouse may benefit from the partner's renewed interest in social activities and increased energy to share in household tasks. Moreover, the recovering alcoholic's initially inward focus may be replaced with renewed attention and interest in the spouse and family.

How does a partner's illness influence his or her spouse? What factors mitigate the stress of a partner's dysfunction and enable a spouse to continue to function effectively? There is growing interest in these issues in a number of disorders, including alcoholism and drug abuse, depression and schizophrenia, and varied medical conditions (Beardslee et al., 1983; Emery, Weintraub, & Neale, 1982; Leff & Vaughn, 1985; Orford & Harwin, 1982). Investigators have sought to learn how spouses of impaired persons differ from normal controls, how they alleviate or contribute to the problems their mates experience, and how they can learn to cope with their partner's impairment.

We address these issues by examining personal and social factors that affect adaptation among spouses of remitted and relapsed alcoholic patients. We compare these two groups of spouses with spouses of matched community controls. We then formulate a general perspective on spouse functioning that considers the alcoholic family member's problem drinking and dysfunction, other life stressors, and the social resources and coping responses that help to manage such stressors.

PERSPECTIVES ON SPOUSES OF ALCOHOLICS

Three perspectives have dominated an extensive search for unique characteristics of the spouses of alcoholic patients. One set of studies has tried to identify personal traits that increase the likelihood that individuals will select alcoholic or prealcoholic mates and then nurture their partners' tendency toward alcohol abuse. A second line of research has focused on the stressors associated with being married to an alcoholic partner and how they contribute to distress and dysfunction among spouses. A third group of studies has identified ways in which spouses cope with their alcoholic partners and establish satisfactory life-styles even though they are enmeshed in disturbed marriages.

The first approach assumes that alcoholics' spouses suffer from long-standing personal deficits, whereas the second contends that they are essentially normal people who experience severe intermittent strain. The third approach posits that many spouses can cope with the stressors that confront them and lead reasonably normal lives (for reviews, see Jacob 1986; Kaufman & Pattison, 1982; Orford & Harwin, 1982; Paolino & McCrady, 1977). These ideas can be integrated within a stress and coping framework that considers the influence of personal and contextual factors on spouse functioning. In this respect, it is important to distinguish between long-standing personal characteristics that may antedate a partner's alcohol abuse and proximal personal factors that influence how a spouse manages current life stressors.

The Personality Perspective

Research on the spouses of alcoholics began with a series of clinical descriptions of the wives of heavy-drinking men. These women were depicted as demanding, dependent, masochistic, self-righteous, sadistic, psychopathic, and so on. Although only a few studies focused on the husbands of women alcoholics, these men were characterized as introverted, unsociable, emotionally distant, self-righteous, sadistic, and defensive. These studies were cross sectional, but the findings were construed to imply that a spouse's dysfunction contributes to his or her partner's abusive drinking.

In a related line of research, some investigators noted instances of depression, psychological or psychosomatic illness, and problem drinking among wives of alcoholics who became abstinent. Such findings were interpreted in terms of a decompensation hypothesis. The spouse's personality was thought to create a need for an alcoholic partner; accordingly, the spouse's functioning should deteriorate when this need is no longer met after the partner stops drinking. However, empirical evidence does not support the disturbed personality or decompensation hypotheses; in general, spouses of current or recovered alcoholics are not characterized by neurotic or disturbed personality traits (for reviews, see Nace, 1982; Paolino & McCrady, 1977).

The Stress Perspective

The stress hypothesis has been examined by comparing spouses whose mates were heavy drinkers but who currently are abstinent with spouses of currently heavy-drinking alcoholics. Women whose husbands are abstinent typically report less mood and personality disturbance and fewer psychosomatic symptoms than women whose husbands are still actively drinking. Spouses of alcoholics in treatment report a decline in anxiety and depression as their partner's drinking problem improves. These findings support the stress hypothesis, because wives of abstinent alcoholics, who should experience fewer stressors, are less impaired than wives of active alcoholics. In contrast, women family members of active alcoholics make more visits to physicians and have more distinct diagnoses and a higher prevalence of trauma and stress-related disorders than do women in nonalcoholic families (Roberts & Brent, 1982). Moreover, Zweben (1986) found that the degree of stress or hardship experienced by the spouse mediated virtually all of the association between the partner's alcohol use and marital dysfunction.

An alcoholic patient's return to sobriety does not necessarily alleviate stress-related disturbances in other family members. As we saw earlier, the cessation of alcohol abuse may or may not be associated with improvement in other areas of personal and social functioning. Residual dysfunction of the alcoholic partner, such as depression and social withdrawal, can create continuing strain for the spouse. Some wives see their husbands as emotionally distant, angry, and suspicious when the husbands are trying to achieve long-term sobriety (Wiseman, 1981), indicating that alcohol abuse may not be the primary personal or marital problem. Therefore, a finding that spouses of remitted alcoholics do not function as well as spouses of nonalcoholics may be consistent with the stress perspective.

The Coping Perspective

Whereas the personality perspective focuses primarily on the deficits of spouses of alcoholics, the coping perspective emphasizes spouses' personal resources and coping skills. Wiseman (1980) described a developmental progression in the coping responses that wives use to "treat" their husbands' problem drinking. Wives initially believe their husbands' drinking is voluntary, and they rely on logical arguments to persuade their husbands to drink less. When this strategy fails, a wife may intensify her efforts and try to convince her husband that drinking will ruin his health or cause him to lose his job. Disappointed wives then step up their efforts and nag their husbands. Next, wives may resort to pleading and threatening to leave, but their husbands often respond to such pressure with anger and disdain.

When these approaches fail, wives try to manipulate the environment so their husbands will have less opportunity or desire to drink. One strategy is for a wife to pretend her husband does not have a drinking problem. Another strategy is to assume control of the situation. In this stage, women manage demanding tasks and try to be "better" wives in the hope that this will free their husbands of burdens and cause them to drink less. Wives also choose nondrinking companions for their husbands, limit the money available to them, and keep their husbands busy so they will have less time to drink. Such coping strategies may be effective in some situations, but they did not work for the women Wiseman (1980) studied. Many of these women gave up their attempts at home treatment and sought professional help.

Orford and his colleagues (1975) identified ten styles of wives' coping behavior, some of which were associated with a good prognosis for the alcoholic partner. Active behavioral coping responses that imply some bond between the partners, such as the wife's pleading, were related to improvement in the husband's drinking behavior. In contrast, some wives create an independent existence for themselves while remaining married. These women increase their work and hobby skills, gain job promotions, schedule their time to avoid contact with their husbands, and make their own friends and social plans. Thus, wives of alcoholics modify their coping strategies in response to changes in their husband's drinking behavior. In turn, the coping patterns adopted by spouses may affect the course of their partners' recovery and their own adaptation (see also Gorman & Rooney, 1979).

SPOUSES OF REMITTED AND RELAPSED ALCOHOLICS

We focused on these ideas by comparing the spouses of our remitted and relapsed patients with the matched spouses of our community controls. As noted before, patients and their spouses were studied 2 years and 10 years after treatment; the patients provided independent information about their drinking patterns and levels of functioning. We first examine whether spouses of remitted patients can attain normal lives and normal levels of functioning. We then compare adaptation among spouses of relapsed alcoholics with that among matched spouses of controls and of remitted alcoholics.

Consistent with the idea that the strain of being married to an alcoholic partner leads to personal and psychosocial problems, we expected spouses of relapsed patients to function more poorly than spouses of remitted patients. Because such strain should be most evident when the partner is drinking heavily, we distinguish between spouses of heavy-drinking relapsed patients and those of relapsed patients who are making a renewed effort to control their alcohol abuse.

Selecting Matched Groups of Spouses

In Chapter 8, we described a group of 113 married alcoholic patients. We obtained information from 105 of the spouses (84 wives and 21 husbands) of these 113 patients at the 6-month and 2-year follow-ups. Of the respondents, 54 were spouses of remitted alcoholics and 51 were spouses of relapsed alcoholics. The sample of 105 community control spouses was selected to match the spouses of the alcoholic patients on six demographic factors (sex, age, ethnicity, religion, education, and family size). The groups did not differ on these variables or in the occupational status of those spouses who were working or seeking work. In brief, the spouses tended to be in their late forties (mean age = 48), Caucasian (over 80%), Protestant (about 50%), and educated beyond high school (over 50%). As noted before, all three groups of spouses were stably married when we began to study them.

The spouses completed our three structured inventories: the HDL, the FES, and the WES. We measured four sets of variables, which correspond to those we used with the patients (Chapter 8). These variables tapped mood, health, and alcohol consumption (13 indices); family and social functioning (5 indices); life stressors and social resources, especially in the individual's family and work settings (13 indices); and three types of coping responses (see Moos, Finney, & Gamble, 1982).

We conducted two preliminary analyses. To examine gender differences, we compared the husbands of women patients with a demographically matched group of wives of men patients. Because we found essentially no differences, data on the husbands and wives of patients were combined in subsequent analyses. Additional analyses identified no differences between control spouses who were matched to spouses of remitted patients and those matched to spouses of relapsed patients. Accordingly, spouses of remitted and relapsed patients were contrasted with the total control group. The three groups were compared using one-way ANOVAs and the Student-Newman-Keuls Multiple Range Test. We obtained virtually identical results using analyses of covariance controlling for demographic factors and thus present the unadjusted means and F values from the ANOVAs here.

Two-Year Posttreatment Adaptation among the Spouse Groups

Alcohol Consumption and Social Psychological Functioning

The proportion of spouses who were current drinkers was about the same among the community control and the relapsed alcoholic spouse groups; it was somewhat lower among spouses of remitted patients (Table 9.1). Among spouses who drank, spouses of relapsed patients consumed more

Table 9.1 Comparisons among stably remitted and relapsed alcoholics' spouses and control spouses on alcohol consumption and social and psychological functioning—2-year follow-up

Variable	Spouses of community controls ($N = 105$)	Spouses of remitted alcoholics ($N = 54$)	Spouses of relapsed alcoholics ($N = 51$)	F value
Drank alcohol past month (% yes)	90.4[a]	63.0[a,c]	78.4[c]	9.19***
Quantity ethanol (oz.)	2.05[b]	1.93[c]	3.39[b,c]	4.18*
Mean daily ethanol (oz.)	.49[b]	.73	1.53[b]	4.11*
Depression (no. yes of 7)	2.52[a]	1.81[a,c]	2.76[c]	3.21*
Anxiety (no. yes of 5)	1.05	1.06	1.20	<1
Physical symptoms (no. yes of 12)	3.11	2.46	2.92	1.30
Medications (no. yes of 10)	1.87	2.02	1.86	<1
Informal social contacts (no. in last month)	13.06[a,b]	9.61[a]	9.43[b]	11.11***
Negative life events (no. yes of 10)	.90[b]	.76[c]	1.29[b,c]	3.29*
Family environment				
Cohesion	7.37[b]	7.60[c]	6.60[b,c]	4.31**
Active-recreational	5.21[a,b]	4.23[a]	3.87[b]	6.67**
Organization	5.86	6.23	5.49	1.31
Family arguments (% yes of 16)	27.1[a]	15.5[a,c]	25.2[c]	6.53**

Note. Means that share a common superscript differ significantly ($p < .05$) by the Student-Newman-Keuls test.
*$p < .05$.   **$p < .01$.   ***$p < .001$.

alcohol than the other two groups of spouses, but their average daily ethanol intake was within normal limits.

There was only one significant difference in mood and health. Spouses of remitted alcoholics were less depressed than spouses of controls or of relapsed alcoholics.

Spouses of both groups of alcoholics reported fewer informal social contacts than did spouses of community controls, but the three groups did not differ in participation in structured family activities or religious pursuits or in the proportion who were currently employed (about 60%) or had changed jobs (about 15% to 20%) in the past year. In agreement with their partner's reports (Chapter 8), spouses of relapsed alcoholics reported less family income than spouses in the other two groups.

Life Events, Social Resources, and Coping Responses

The spouses also agreed closely with their partner's reports of life events and social resources (Chapter 8). The spouses of relapsed patients experienced more negative events than the other two groups did. The spouses of relapsed alcoholics also reported less family cohesion than those in the other two groups; the spouses of remitted and relapsed patients reported less family recreational orientation than the spouses of community controls. The spouses of remitted patients reported fewer family arguments. The three groups were similar in social networks and perceived work environments and in their use of coping responses.

Spouses of Heavy-Drinking Relapsed Patients

All the patients in the relapsed group either had been rehospitalized for alcoholism or had been drinking abusively sometime during the initial 2-year posttreatment interval. However, at the 2-year follow-up, some relapsed patients were trying to reduce their alcohol consumption, whereas others were drinking as heavily as when they entered treatment.

To examine whether spouses experience more strain when their alcoholic partners are drinking abusively, we compared the spouses ($N = 14$) of relapsed patients whose partners were consuming more than 12 ounces of ethanol per drinking day with the spouses of controls. The differences between these two groups were more extreme than those just reported. The spouses of currently heavy-drinking partners were more depressed and anxious, engaged in fewer social activities, and reported more stressful life events than the spouses of controls. They complained of more physical symptoms and medical conditions (64% reported one or more) and were much more likely to have visited doctors and to have changed jobs in the past year (57%). They also reported more reliance on avoidance coping and saw their families as characterized by more conflict and less cohesion, organization, and recreational orientation.

Long-Term Adaptation among the Spouse Groups

Overall, 19 of the 83 surviving patients we followed at 10 years had gotten divorced some time after the 2-year follow-up. This 23% divorce rate is comparable to the 28% rate Berglund and Tunving (1985) observed in a 20-year follow-up of treated alcoholics and the 19% rate McCabe (1986) identified among patients 16 years after treatment.

There was a clear relationship between the alcoholic partner's 2-year follow-up functioning and the fate of the spousal relationship over the next 8 years. Whereas 91% of the initially remitted patients who were followed still had the same spouse, that was true for only 56% of the initially relapsed patients. In 2 cases (5%) the spouse died, but in the other 15 cases (39%) a divorce occurred. The community controls had a 9% divorce rate. Thus, the initially remitted patients and the community controls had comparable divorce rates (9%), but the initially relapsed patients were more than four times as likely (39%) to experience a breakup of the relationship by the 10-year follow-up.

Of the 83 patients we were able to follow at 10 years, 62 were married to the same spouse, who was originally contacted 6 months after the patient received treatment. We obtained long-term follow-up data from these spouses (1 spouse had not participated in the 2-year follow-up). Our analyses focus on these 62 spouses as compared to 85 spouses of the controls who were also studied initially. We obtained information on the same set of variables at the 10-year as at the 2-year follow-up.

At 10 years posttreatment, there were no differences among the three spouse groups on the alcohol consumption variables (Table 9.2). The

Table 9.2 Comparisons among stably remitted and relapsed alcoholics' spouses and control spouses on alcohol consumption and social and psychological functioning—10-year follow-up

Variable	Spouses of community controls ($N = 85$)	Spouses of remitted alcoholics ($N = 37$)	Spouses of relapsed alcoholics ($N = 24$)	F value
Drank alcohol past month (% yes)	74.0	78.0	58.0	1.59
Quantity ethanol (oz.)	2.08	2.60	3.53	2.54*
Mean daily ethanol (oz.)	.49[a]	1.04[a]	1.08	3.09**
Depression (no. yes of 7)	2.13[b]	1.81[c]	3.42[b,c]	5.44***
Anxiety (no. yes of 5)	.67[b]	.92	1.45[b]	3.77**
Physical symptoms (no. yes of 12)	3.16	2.68	3.00	<1
Medications (no. yes of 10)	2.07	2.08	2.04	<1
Informal social contacts (no. in last month)	15.11	14.33	14.63	<1
Negative life events (no. yes of 10)	.74	.43	.92	2.38*
Family environment				
Cohesion	7.17	7.70	6.71	1.75
Active-recreational	4.65[c]	4.43	3.38[c]	3.05*
Organization	6.05	6.78	5.75	2.12
Family arguments (% yes of 16)	17.6	14.2	19.0	<1

Note. Means that share a common superscript differ significantly ($p < .05$) by the Student-Newman-Keuls test.
*$p < .10$.   **$p < .05$.   ***$p < .01$.

spouses of remitted patients shifted from being less likely to drink alcoholic beverages than spouses of controls at the 2-year follow-up to being equally likely to drink at the 10-year follow-up. This shift reflects both an increase in the proportion of remitted patient spouses' drinking and a decline in drinking among the spouses of controls. Among persons who drank, the spouses of both remitted and relapsed patients drank somewhat more than the spouses of controls.

In other areas of functioning, the spouses of remitted patients were somewhat (but not significantly) less depressed than the spouses of the controls, whereas the spouses of the relapsed patients were more depressed than the spouses of both remitted patients and controls and more anxious than the spouses of the controls. We did not find this difference in anxiety level at the 2-year follow-up. Also in contrast to the 2-year follow-up, there were no differences among the three groups in informal social contacts at the 10-year follow-up. However, spouses of relapsed patients reported marginally more negative life events than did either the remitted patient or control spouses.

The family environments of relapsed patients' spouses again were characterized as less recreationally oriented than those of the control families. They were also somewhat less cohesive and well organized, but these differences were not significant. The proportions of spouses who changed jobs at least once did not differ, but the spouses of relapsed patients changed jobs significantly more often in the previous year than did the remitted patient or control spouses. There were no group differences on any of the work environment or coping variables.

Implications for Personality and Stress Perspectives

At the 2-year follow-up, we identified only a few differences between the spouses of remitted alcoholics and those of community controls. The spouses of the remitted patients were less likely to have consumed alcohol during the past month and reported fewer social contacts and recreational pursuits. Otherwise, these spouses achieved comparable levels of occupational functioning, reported comparable social resources in their family and work settings, and coped with ongoing stressors in similar ways. They reported less depression and did not experience any more stressful events, anxiety, or physical symptoms than did the control spouses. There were even fewer differences between these two groups at the 10-year follow-up. Thus, spouses of remitted alcoholics function as well as demographically comparable spouses of nonalcoholic community members.

We found no support for the idea that spouses of alcoholics are likely to suffer from underlying deficits in personal functioning or coping resources. Nor was there support for the idea that they experience new problems due to their partner's successful control of alcohol abuse. Although spouses of remitted alcoholics experience some anxiety and physical symptoms, these problems are comparable to those of spouses of community controls.

Our findings are most consistent with the stress and coping perspectives. At the 2-year follow-up, spouses of relapsed patients consumed more alcohol, experienced more stressful events, participated in fewer social activities, and enjoyed less family cohesion and recreation. Most of these spouses had been married for some time and had made accommodations to their partner's alcohol abuse. A less stably married group of spouses might show more pronounced impairment. However, spouses whose alcoholic partners were drinking heavily at the 2-year follow-up experienced much more dysfunction than spouses of controls or of remitted patients. These spouses may exacerbate their problems by relying more heavily on avoidance coping responses to manage stressors when their partner is drinking abusively.

Compared to spouses of initially (2-year) remitted patients, spouses of 2-year relapsed patients were four times as likely to dissolve the marital relationship in the next 8 years (39% versus 9%). We examined the characteristics and functioning of the spouses of the relapsed patients at the 2-year follow-up to see if we could identify factors predictive of divorce. Given the small sample sizes, we found few statistically significant differences. In general, spouses who eventually divorced their alcoholic partners were functioning as well as or better than the spouses whose marriages remained intact.

Some of the deficits associated with having a relapsed partner were still evident at the 10-year follow-up. Spouses of relapsed patients reported more depression and more life events than did either the remitted patient or control spouses, more anxiety than the remitted patient spouses, and a less active family recreational orientation than the control spouses. However, these problems were in fewer areas than was the case for spouses of relapsed patients at the 2-year follow-up. One reason these spouses may have shown less distress is because their relapsed partners were less severely impaired at the 10-year follow-up than were the relapsed patients at the 2-year follow-up (see Chapter 8). Also, these spouses had more time to develop effective adaptations to their partners' impairment.

We conclude that spouses of alcoholics are basically normal individuals trying to cope with disturbed marriages and dysfunctional partners. These spouses experience cyclical crises and severe strain created by their life with an alcoholic partner, but these consequences diminish when the partner makes a concerted effort to control his or her abusive drinking. Such findings are consistent with evidence that alcoholic husbands who maintain sobriety for 2 years or longer tend to participate more actively and to express less anger in interaction with their spouse than husbands whose sobriety is more short term (Roberts et al., 1985). Marital adaptation seems to improve and normalize as alcoholic patients recover.

A STRESS AND COPING MODEL OF SPOUSE FUNCTIONING

Research on spouses of alcoholics has progressed independently of work on spouses of partners with other types of problems or of normal marital partners. Some of the stressors and coping processes involved in being married to an alcoholic person may be similar to those of being married to a physically ill, depressed, physically abusive, or unemployed person. There also may be special factors in alcohol abuse, such as its insidious onset and the typical assumption that a person should be able to control it. To examine these issues, spouses of alcoholics need to be studied in light of a stress and coping framework that is applicable to other groups of spouses as well.

We pursue these points by formulating a conceptual paradigm that tries to integrate the personality, stress, and coping perspectives. The paradigm shown in Figure 9.1 depicts the connections among six sets of variables presumed to affect current spouse adaptation: spouse social background, spouse initial personal resources and functioning, impairment of the alcoholic partner, life stressors, social resources, and spouse coping responses. The model recognizes that spouse functioning is affected by stressors associated with both the severity of the alcoholic partner's drinking problem and other aspects of the partner's dysfunction (Finney et al., 1983). The paradigm also incorporates extrafamily stressors, such as some negative life events. In addition, it reflects the fact that a spouse's social resources and coping responses can alter the effects of stressors as well as directly influence spouse functioning.

SPOUSES OF ALCOHOLIC PARTNERS

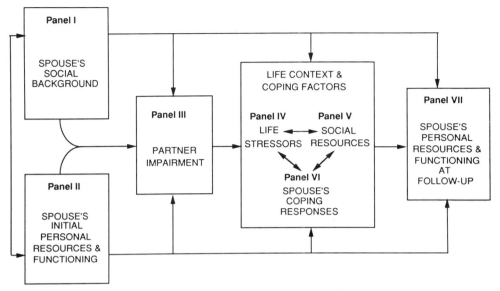

Figure 9.1 A stress and coping model of the determinants of spouse functioning.

Two spouses exposed to the same level of social stressors and resources may differ in functioning because their personal characteristics differ. Conversely, spouses with comparable initial personal resources may be affected differently by exposure to varied levels of stressors and support. Accordingly, the model specifies both personal and contextual determinants of spouse adaptation. The first two domains (Panels I and II) reflect personal characteristics, whereas the next three (Panels III, IV, and V) reflect contextual factors; the next domain (Panel VI) reflects coping responses, which are proximal outcomes of person-environment transactions.

Indices of Personal and Environmental Factors

Using our three structured inventories, we assessed the predictor and criterion variables. In brief, *spouse social background* was indexed by the spouse's age, sex, and education. *Spouse initial functioning* was measured at the 6-month follow-up by indices of alcohol consumption, depression, physical symptoms, and medication use.

The other five sets of variables were measured at both the 2-year and 10-year follow-ups. *Partner impairment* was tapped by six indices: alcohol consumption, drinking problems, anxiety, depression, physical symptoms, and occupational functioning. *Life stressors* were measured by the number of negative events experienced in the past year and by a 13-item index of children's health problems (2-year follow-up only). *Family resources* were measured by six of the FES dimensions: cohesion, expressiveness, lack of conflict, moral-religious emphasis, active-recreational orientation, and organization. *Spouse coping* was tapped by the indices of active cognitive, active behavioral, and avoidance coping responses. The four *spouse functioning* criteria correspond to the four initial indicators of spouse functioning.

Cross-Sectional Predictors of Spouse Functioning at 2 Years

We focus first on regression analyses to examine the concurrent relationships between the individual predictors and sets of predictors and the four indices of spouse functioning at the 2-year follow-up. These analyses examine the influence of specific factors, such as family cohesion and conflict, on spouse functioning; they also focus on entire sets of predictors, such as all six family climate factors.

Table 9.3 shows the partial and multiple correlations for the 2-year criteria from stepwise regressions in which the three background variables (age, sex, and education) and initial spouse functioning were entered first, followed by the measures in each of the predictor sets. The multiple Rs for the demographic and initial functioning indices in the first row of the table provide a baseline against which to gauge the effectiveness of each predictor *set* in accounting for additional criterion variance. The partial correlations indicate the extent to which the individual indices account for variation in functioning that is independent of demographic factors and initial spouse functioning.

As expected, the spouses of alcoholics were affected by their partners' problems. Spouses whose partners consumed more alcohol reported more depression and physical symptoms. The partner's reports of more problems in areas other than drinking, such as depression and physical symptoms, also were positively related to the spouse's alcohol consumption, depressed mood, and physical symptoms. Thus, the amount of alcohol consumed is only one among several aspects of the alcoholic partner's functioning that may be associated with the spouse's mood and health.

Negative life events were associated with increased alcohol consumption among the spouses, whereas children's health problems were related to more physical symptoms and medication use. The influence of negative events on spouse alcohol consumption extends our earlier finding indicating that the spouses were quite labile in their drinking habits (Chapter 7). As a set, the two life stressor variables add significantly to the explanation of all the spouse functioning indices except depression.

Spouses in families that were lacking in cohesion reported more physical symptoms, while those in families that were high on conflict experienced more depression and physical symptoms. As might be expected, spouses who were in less expressive families were more depressed. Moral-religious emphasis was positively related to physical symptoms, probably because health problems often stimulate a search for a deeper explanation for sudden life stressors (Moos, 1984). Finally, spouses who reported more family arguments were more depressed and had more physical symptoms; they also indicated using more medications.

A spouse's reliance on avoidance coping is related to poorer treatment

Table 9.3 Partial and multiple correlations between predictor measures and functioning criteria for spouses of alcoholics ($N = 105$)—2-year follow-up

	Alcohol consumption	Depression	Physical symptoms	Medication
BACKGROUND AND INITIAL FUNCTIONING R	.23	.40**	.38**	.53***
PARTNER CHARACTERISTICS R	.35	.58***	.56**	.58
Alcohol consumption	.11	.30**	.29**	.19
Drinking problems	.13	.17	.07	.09
Anxiety	.13	.23*	.15*	.11
Depression	.25**	.32***	.15	.15
Physical symptoms	.16	.33***	.25*	.12
Occupational functioning	−.04	−.15	−.20*	−.18
LIFE STRESSORS R	.47***	.44	.48**	.57*
Negative events	.41***	.17	.10	.10
Children's health problems	.10	.14	.30**	.24*
FAMILY ENVIRONMENT R	.36	.53*	.55**	.60
Cohesion	−.03	−.14	−.21*	−.10
Expressiveness	.09	−.22*	−.10	−.19
Conflict	.09	.21*	.24**	.11
Moral-religious emphasis	.12	.17	.21*	.19
Active recreational orientation	.07	−.09	.14	.11
Organization	−.15	−.09	−.04	.01
Family arguments	.11	.20*	.34***	.23*
COPING R	.30	.52***	.44	.57
Active cognitive (%)	−.03	−.21*	−.09	−.04
Active behavioral (%)	−.11	−.04	−.08	−.14
Avoidance (%)	.18	.34***	.23*	.23*

Note. The probability levels for the Rs (except those for background and initial functioning) refer to the significance of the increment in R after adding variables beyond the original background and initial functioning characteristics.
*$p < .05$.   **$p < .01$.   ***$p < .001$.

outcome for the alcoholic partner (Gorman & Rooney, 1979; Orford et al., 1975). The present findings show that avoidance coping also is associated with poorer spouse functioning. Moreover, additional analyses showed that reliance on avoidance coping by both the alcoholic partner and the spouse was associated with less family cohesion and more family arguments. In contrast, active cognitive coping responses were associated with less depression.

In general, these sets of context and coping factors tended to improve the prediction of spouse functioning, especially spouse depression and physical symptoms. In fact, information about partner functioning explained more of the variance in these two criteria (17.6% and 16.9%, respectively) than did the spouse's demographic and initial functioning characteristics (16.0% and 14.4%, respectively). Thus, life context and coping factors affect the patients' spouses as strongly as they do the patients themselves.

Cross-Sectional Predictors of Spouse Functioning at 10 Years

We conducted similar cross-sectional analyses with the 10-year data from the 62 spouses who were still married to the successfully followed patients. Except for alcohol consumption, the overall association between the spouse functioning criteria and the spouses' demographic characteristics and initial functioning (at the 6-month follow-up) were comparable to those for the 2-year analyses (Table 9.4). The findings for medication use are not shown; the only significant predictor was reliance on avoidance coping.

Again, spouse functioning—especially spouse depression—was affected by the functioning of the alcoholic partner. Each of the components of alcoholic partner functioning, except occupational functioning, was associated with spouse depression, even after controlling for the spouse's initial level of depression and demographic characteristics. The alcoholic partner's drinking problems, depressed mood, and physical symptoms were also associated with spouse physical symptoms.

Although negative events in the past year did not add to the prediction of spouse functioning, the family environment was associated with alcohol consumption and depression. Spouses with more conflict-ridden families consumed more alcohol, and spouses whose families were less cohesive, less expressive, less recreationally oriented, less well organized, and less argumentative were more likely to be depressed and/or to report more physical symptoms. Finally, spouses who used fewer active behavioral coping methods were more depressed at the 10-year follow-up, while those who relied more on avoidance coping had more physical symptoms.

These results extend our earlier findings on the remitted and relapsed patients' spouses. The group comparisons show that spouses of relapsed patients were more depressed than spouses of stably remitted patients at the 10-year follow-up. Similarly, the partial and multiple correlation analyses indicate that current partner functioning has an impact on the spouse, especially on spouse depression. In fact, information about partner functioning predicted an increment of 32% of the variance in spouse depression over the 21% predicted by demographic factors and initial spouse functioning. Although the life stressor, family environment, and spouse coping variables showed few between-group differences at the 10-year follow-up, they nevertheless showed some correlations with spouse depression and the other spouse functioning indices. Overall, most of the relationships we identified between context and coping indices and spouse functioning at 10 years are comparable to those we obtained at the 2-year follow-up.

Longitudinal Predictors of Spouse Functioning

We wanted to learn to what extent spouse functioning at the 10-year follow-up could be predicted by spouse background characteristics and initial functioning, as well as by partner functioning, negative life events,

Table 9.4 Cross-sectional and longitudinal partial and multiple correlations between predictor measures and functioning criteria for spouses of alcoholics ($N = 61$)—2-year and 10-year follow-ups

	10-Year cross sectional			Longitudinal		
	Alcohol consumption	Depression	Physical symptoms	Alcohol consumption	Depression	Physical symptoms
BACKGROUND AND FUNCTIONING *R*	*.62****	*.46***	*.21*	*.62†****	*.46***	*.21*
PARTNER CHARACTERISTICS *R*	*.71*	*.73****	*.45*	*.64*	*.65***	*.39*
Alcohol consumption	.21	.44***	.20	.02	.36**	.02
Drinking problems	.24†	.40**	.30*	.10	.27*	.01
Anxiety	-.20	.49***	.20	.01	-.02	.13
Depression	-.08	.59***	.33**	.05	.10	.07
Physical symptoms	-.03	.34**	.34**	.02	.16	.28*
Occupational functioning	-.11	-.04	-.04	-.15	.07	.02
LIFE STRESSORS *R*	*.63*	*.48*	*.23*	*.63*	*.51*	*.29*
Negative life events	.10	.16	.08	-.04	-.04	-.12
Children's health problems	—	—	—	.14	.24†	.17
FAMILY ENVIRONMENT *R*	*.73**	*.73****	*.56**	*.73†*	*.62†*	*.53*
Cohesion	-.09	-.45***	-.13	-.11	-.39**	-.21
Expressiveness	-.11	-.26*	-.26†	-.23†	-.17	-.13
Conflict	.39**	.21	.23†	.25†	.25†	.10
Moral-religious emphasis	.11	.07	.24†	.32*	.18	.33*
Active recreational orientation	.20	-.24†	-.08	.28*	.03	.19
Organization	-.09	-.30*	-.08	.03	-.09	-.09
Family arguments	.15	.48***	.38**	.19	.36**	.21
COPING *R*	*.62*	*.55**	*.34*	*.64*	*.57**	*.26*
Active cognitive (%)	.00	.15	-.01	-.10	.17	.00
Active behavioral (%)	.03	-.30*	-.15	-.01	-.35**	-.09
Avoidance (%)	-.05	.17	.24†	.17	.24†	.14

Note. The probability levels for the *R*s refer to the significance of the increment in *R* after adding variables beyond the original background and initial functioning characteristics.

†$p < .10$.   *$p < .05$.   **$p < .01$.   ***$p < .001$.

family environment, and spouse coping at the 2-year follow-up. We identified some predictive relationships over this 8-year interval, but they were fewer and weaker than those we obtained in the cross-sectional analyses (Table 9.4).

Spouses whose partners were consuming more alcohol and had more drinking problems at the 2-year follow-up tended to be more depressed at 10 years. These findings reflect the relatively high stability (see Chapter 8) in the partner's relapse/remission status at the two follow-ups. If a spouse's children had been experiencing more health problems at the 2-year follow-up, he or she was likely to be more depressed at the 10-year follow-up.

Spouses whose family environments were more cohesive and who relied more on active behavioral coping and less on avoidance coping at 2 years were less depressed at the 10-year follow-up. Higher family conflict and less family expressiveness at 2 years were predictive of more spouse alcohol consumption and depression at 10 years. Consistent with the cross-sectional findings, there was a positive association between family moral-religious emphasis and spouse physical symptoms later on. Finally, more family arguments at 2 years was associated with more spouse depression at 10 years.

In addition, there were two longitudinal relationships that did not emerge in the cross-sectional analyses. Spouses whose families had a greater moral-religious and a greater recreational orientation at the 2-year follow-up tended to consume more alcohol at 10 years. The association between spouse drinking and recreational orientation reflects the fact that participation in social activities tends to increase alcohol consumption. The link between spouse drinking and moral-religious emphasis is probably because a religious orientation often occurs as a response to an increased incidence of stressful life circumstances.

The 2-year follow-up data showed that spouses who experienced more family conflict were more depressed and that children's health problems were associated with more spouse physical symptoms. These findings held up over the 8-year interval between the last two follow-ups. Consistent with our results on the patients (Chapter 8), earlier life events did not predict later spouse functioning. Coupled with the findings on the influence of the alcoholic partner's functioning, these results suggest that spouses are more profoundly affected by chronic family strain than by acute negative life events. Thus, to provide a comprehensive account of spouse functioning, one needs to look beyond the alcoholic mate's functioning—especially in global terms—and to examine other factors that can affect the spouse.

The Conceptual Model of Spouse Adaptation

The data just presented indicate the extent to which individual variables and various predictor sets are associated with spouse functioning. We also examined the overall stress and coping framework and analyzed the interrelationships among the *sets* of predictors and their associations with spouse functioning. Our analyses of these issues focus on the data from the larger sample of spouses who were followed 6 months and 2 years after their partners' index treatment episodes.

Associations among Predictors of Spouse Functioning

We focused first on the connections among the sets of predictors of spouse functioning. We calculated standardized regression coefficients to estimate the direct effects of each antecedent variable set on subsequent variable sets in the four models (one for each criterion) of spouse dysfunction. The sets of variables were described earlier; standardized composites were used to construct the overall partner impairment, life stressors, and family resources indices. Spouse coping was measured by the proportion of active cognitive and active behavioral coping responses.

We examined the relationships among the six sets of predictors for each of the four criteria of spouse functioning. In brief, the earlier sets of variables in the models were used to predict the subsequent ones. Thus, spouse social background (Panel I) and spouse initial functioning (Panel II) were used to predict partner impairment (Panel III), while these three sets of variables were used to predict life stressors (Panel IV), and so on (see Figure 9.1).

Spouse social background and initial functioning, both assessed at the 6-month follow-up, were not associated with partner impairment at the 2-year follow-up. As expected, however, spouses who functioned better initially (Panel II) experienced fewer subsequent life stressors (Panel III). More important, a high level of partner impairment (Panel III) was associated with spouses' reports of more life stressors (Panel IV) and fewer family resources (Panel V). An average of 21% of the variance in life stressors and 9% of the variance in family resources was accounted for by these predictor variables.

Finally, spouses who had a better social background and reported a more positive family environment tended to rely more heavily on active coping, that is, they were more likely to use active cognitive or active behavioral coping responses. These predictors accounted for an average of 20% of the variance in active coping.

Predictors of Spouse Functioning

We also examined the overall influence of the six sets of antecedent variables on spouse functioning. In general, the findings were comparable to those of the partial and multiple regression analyses shown in Table 9.3, although the influence of partner impairment on spouse adaptation was somewhat stronger whereas the effect of life stressors and family resources was somewhat weaker (Finney et al., 1983).

We calculated the variance explained by the six sets of antecedent factors in spouse functioning. Overall, the predictor sets accounted for 18% of the variance in spouse alcohol consumption, 34% in depression, 24% in physical symptoms, and 36% in medication use. Consistent with the regression analyses, the three sets of contextual factors accounted for a substantial proportion of incremental variance in depression and physical symptoms over that accounted for by the background and intake factors.

AN INTEGRATED PERSPECTIVE ON SPOUSES OF IMPAIRED PARTNERS

We have tried to integrate and extend prior research on spouses of alcoholic patients by formulating a conceptual paradigm that considers personal and contextual determinants of spouse functioning. The six sets of predictors account for 18% to 36% of the variance in spouse functioning (an average of 28%), which shows the overall value of the paradigm. These proportions of variance are substantially greater than the proportions (2% to 12%) accounted for by partner drinking alone.

The Stress and Coping Approach

Consistent with the stress and coping approach, the impairment of the alcoholic partner was strongly related to poorer spouse functioning. Our measures of partner impairment included both drinking and other components. To examine the relative impact of these two facets of partner dysfunction, we separated drinking from other aspects of partner impairment and assumed that drinking problems preceded problems in other areas. The partner's drinking did not have an independent influence on spouse functioning. In contrast, partner social and psychological impairment had a significant independent effect on spouse depression and physical symptoms. Moreover, partner drinking had a substantial impact on partner impairment in other areas.

The influence of the partner's drinking problems on spouse functioning is mediated by the partner's impairment in other areas. Information on partner drinking provides only a partial account of the impact of an alcoholic partner on his or her spouse. Accordingly, the symptoms of the nonalcoholic spouse may be linked more closely to the social and behavioral consequences of drinking than to the level of alcohol consumption itself. Likewise, spouses of some sober alcoholics may continue to experience strain caused by their partner's continuing psychosocial dysfunction (Wiseman, 1981).

Spouses' coping strategies predict their level of adaptation. Spouses who rely more on avoidance coping responses report poorer mood and health and use more medications than spouses who place less reliance on them. In fact, spouses who employed more avoidance coping responses experienced poorer mood and health even after the partner's level of alcohol consumption was considered. Spouses who used mainly active coping strategies when their partner was drinking heavily were functioning much better than those who used avoidance responses.

These findings support the stress and coping framework. Because individual characteristics affect the selection of active or approach rather than avoidance coping, there also is some support for the importance of personal factors. As we noted earlier, spouses who had a less favorable social background were more likely to rely on avoidance coping to manage stressors. Thus, some spouses of alcoholics may amplify the influence of stressful life conditions by employing ineffective methods of dealing with them. The consistency in spouse functioning over time also bolsters the idea that stable personal factors influence spouse adaptation.

Our model of the determinants of spouse functioning is one of many that could be formulated. In addition to other predictors, such as better indicators of personal resources, there may be alternative causal connections between pairs of predictors. Some predictors are likely to have a mutual influence on each other—especially the functioning of the mates in a married couple. More generally, although we see our model as applicable to both women and men, we believe that future studies should look separately at husbands and wives when possible.

Risk Factors and Contextual Influences

Researchers should consider several other issues in planning future studies of spouses of alcohol abusers. One issue is personal risk factors predictive of spouse dysfunction. Even though most prior research supports the idea that spouse dysfunction is linked primarily to current stressors, personal factors are likely to be important as well. Our findings imply that some spouses of alcoholics tend to rely more heavily on avoidance coping responses to manage current stressors. Similarly, O'Farrell and his co-workers (1981) found that wives of alcoholics who were shy as children were more likely than their more outgoing counterparts to endure their husband's verbal abuse of them and their children. These women probably experience low self-efficacy and tend to employ avoidance coping strategies.

The second issue is to find out whether alcoholics and their spouses are similar to each other in some personal characteristics. deBlois and Stewart (1983) identified assortative mating among alcoholics and their spouses, that is, rebellious and unconventional young women were more likely to marry men with these same traits who later became alcoholic. Phenotypic assortative mating occurs when people select spouses with traits similar to their own. To the extent that alcohol abusers have predisposing personality characteristics, evidence for this process is consistent with the personality perspective. However, spouse similarity also may be attributed to environmental factors such as common life conditions and the postmarital influence of the spouses on each other (Hall, Hesselbrock, & Stabenau, 1983; Merikangas, 1982). A comprehensive perspective on spouse functioning needs to consider personal as well as contextual factors.

A third issue concerns the potential adaptive consequences of heavy drinking in some families. Most families function better when the alcoholic member regains sobriety, especially if that person is a violence-prone binge drinker. Among steady in-home drinkers, however, higher alcohol consumption may be associated with more marital satisfaction and fewer symptoms among some spouses (Dunn et al., 1987; Jacob, Dunn, & Leonard, 1983). As Wiseman (1981) noted, some sober alcoholics are tense, irritable, and depressed and create a dreary home life. From a different perspective, a newly abstinent partner may upset a carefully crafted pattern of spouse and family adaptation to a "missing" husband or wife. In this respect, there are some striking parallels between coping with an alcoholic husband and coping when a husband is imprisoned or missing in action in a time of war (Moos, 1986a).

Finally, in order to understand spouse functioning better, researchers need to consider the stage in the family's life history and the family's cultural context. Steinglass (1980) described a developmental cycle in which families progress through recognizable stages, each associated with a specific set of tasks. Failure to manage the tasks at one stage may compromise family resources in dealing with subsequent stages. Accordingly, processes of adaptation may be different at different stages. Steinglass (1980) describes a late resolution phase and two distinct resolution patterns: the stable-wet and the stable-dry family. Compared with families in the stable-dry phase, families manifested much more rigid patterns of behavior in the stable-wet phase (Steinglass, 1981). Because families may conform to cultural expectations, these patterns of development and resolution need to be examined within a broad social context.

Formulating a General Paradigm of Spouse Functioning

We have taken an initial step in developing a general paradigm to understand adaptation among spouses of alcoholic partners. A multivariate model can help to integrate research in this area with studies of spouses of partners who have other types of impairments, such as depression and physical illness, as well as with research on spouses of healthy partners.

Spouses of Depressed Partners

Spouses of depressed persons tend to experience their own problems. They are often psychiatrically impaired and they report more depression and physical symptoms, more illness, more stressful life circumstances, and less family support than comparable spouses of nondepressed persons (Merikangas, Bromet, & Spiker, 1983; Mitchell, Cronkite, & Moos, 1983). Just as with spouses of alcoholic partners, spouses of depressed persons in treatment report more distress than spouses of former patients who are not currently in a depressive episode (Coyne et al., 1987). However, spouses of depressed patients may experience some remaining burdens even though the partner is no longer in a depressed episode.

We examined these issues by comparing the functioning and life circumstances of our depressed patients at the patient's treatment intake and again after 1 year. Spouses of patients whose symptoms later remitted were functioning almost as well at intake as spouses of healthy controls, although they reported more physical symptoms and were somewhat more depressed. Compared with the control spouses, however, the spouses of to-remit patients initially reported poorer relationships with their partners, more family conflict, and less family cohesion and expressiveness. As expected, the initial functioning and life contexts of the spouses of patients who were not to remit were much worse than those of control spouses and somewhat worse than those of spouses of to-remit patients (Krantz & Moos, 1987).

The spouses of remitted patients did not improve markedly during the following year even though their partner's depression subsided. In fact, the spouses' levels of functioning were not related to changes in the depressive symptoms of their partners. However, when the partner's depression improved, there was some improvement in the spouse's life context: more family cohesion and social activities, a less negative home environment, and fewer work stressors. Notwithstanding these improvements, spouses of remitted patients still experienced more social and family problems than control spouses 1 year after the beginning of the index treatment episode.

Spouses of remitted depressed patients still face continuing problems. Some remitted patients experience intermittent depressed mood and other low-grade difficulties that continue to create strain for the spouse. In addition, well-established maladaptive interchanges between spouses are likely to continue, even after the depressive symptoms of one partner diminish. When Lutz, Appelt, and Cohen (1980) compared husbands of women alcoholic and depressed patients, they found no differences in the severity of associated difficulties between the two groups of husbands. However, the husbands of the depressed women were more likely to attribute their wives' disorder to stable factors that were beyond their control and, accordingly, to be more resigned to their ongoing family problems.

Overall, stably remitted alcoholics and their spouses seem to have fewer residual problems and to establish a more cohesive family context than do remitted depressed persons and their spouses. A person's depression may have a long-term residual effect on spouse and family functioning. However, we used a longer follow-up period and more stringent criteria in the study of alcoholic patients; this provided more opportunity for improvement among their spouses and family contexts.

Spouses of Healthy Partners

The stress and coping model can help to identify predictors of functioning among healthy husbands and wives and to understand how they influence each other. We used such a model to examine stress among normal-drinking community adults. We found that personal resources, such as self-esteem, and contextual factors, such as stressful life events and family social resources, were predictably associated with changes in depressed mood, physical symptoms, and alcohol consumption over a 1-year interval (Cronkite & Moos, 1984).

The symptoms and behavior of each spouse influenced the other spouse. For example, wives who had higher self-esteem seemed to influence their husbands to drink less; however, when a wife consumed more alcohol, her husband also drank more. On the other hand, men who consumed more alcohol seemed to exacerbate their wives' depressed mood.

Reliance on avoidance coping was associated with more depressed mood among men and more depressed mood and alcohol consumption among women. Avoidance coping also heightened the effects of a spouse's dysfunction. Having a wife who was more depressed or had more physical symptoms led to a greater increase in the husband's own depressed mood when he relied more heavily on avoidance coping. Similarly, having a husband who reported more depression or physical symptoms led to a greater increase in the wife's alcohol consumption when she relied more on avoidance coping. Healthy husbands and wives exert mutual effects on each other; such reciprocal influence processes also occur among problem drinkers and their spouses.

Spouses of Partners in Life Crises

The spouse functioning model also applies to spouses of partners in a variety of life crises. For example, Mitchell and Hodson (1986) used a similar model to identify the personal and contextual factors that influence social support, coping, and well-being among battered women. Women with more personal resources reported more social support and less avoidance coping, whereas women who had been exposed to more violence in their childhood reported less support and more avoidance coping. In turn, the mediating factors of social support and coping were predictably related to women's well-being (Mitchell & Hodson, 1983). Moreover, women whose husbands are imprisoned cope more effectively with this long-term stressor if they are better educated, enjoy higher social status, come from cohesive families with an egalitarian division of labor, and have more personal and family resources (Lowenstein, 1984). Because there are underlying commonalities in the impact of different crises and spouses' attempts to deal with them, a broad conceptual paradigm can lead to a deeper understanding of the adaptation of marital partners to a variety of stressful conditions.

10
Children of Alcoholic Parents

Problem drinking and alcoholism have a pervasive influence on the children in involved families. An estimated 6.5 to 15 million school-age youth in America are children of problem drinkers. More than 20 million adults in the United States were raised by problem-drinking parents (Deutsch, 1982; Russell, Henderson, & Blume, 1985). The prevalence of alcohol-related problems is more than twice as high among children of alcoholic parents than among children of normal-drinking parents.

To study the impact of parental alcoholism on children, Rydelius (1981) conducted a 20-year prospective follow-up comparing children of alcoholic fathers with children of normal-drinking controls. The daughters of alcoholic fathers adapted reasonably well, but the sons experienced more restlessness and hyperactivity, school problems, delinquency and alcohol abuse, and mental and physical illness. Nylander and Rydelius (1982) reported that such problems were equally prevalent among children of alcoholic fathers from high and low social status families. Similarly, Drake and Vaillant (1988) found that, as adolescents, sons of alcoholic fathers had more emotional problems and poorer physical health and were less competent in age-appropriate tasks such as academic performance relative to IQ, participation in extracurricular activities, and relationships with peers. By the time they were in their mid- to late forties, they were significantly more likely to receive a lifetime diagnosis of alcohol dependence than were sons of nonalcoholic fathers. Both genetic and environmental factors contribute to these familial associations (Cloninger, Bohman, & Sigvardsson, 1981; Gabrielli & Plomin, 1985).

Some of the health and behavior problems that children of heavy drinkers experience may foreshadow the later development of alcoholism. Such problems include impulsivity and rebellious behavior, hyperactivity, a more disturbed school career, and lack of verbal proficiency and academic achievement. Compared with children of moderate drinking or abstaining parents, these children also are more likely to experience physical and emotional problems such as insomnia, nightmares, depression, and low self-esteem and to visit physicians more frequently (for overviews, see Adler & Raphael, 1983; Deutsch, 1982; Knop et al., 1985). The insidious impact of parental alcohol abuse is clear, but little is known about how it is mediated or how it can be overcome.

Just as we saw with spouse functioning, the severity of a parent's alcohol abuse is only one among several factors associated with children's adaptation. Alcoholic parents may refrain from excessive drinking, but their other residual problems, such as depression and social dysfunction, can maintain stress-related problems among their children as well as their spouse. Conversely, a child may show good adaptation because his or her alcoholic parent has recovered or because of other compensating factors, such as a well-functioning nonalcoholic parent and a cohesive family climate. The literature focuses primarily on dysfunction among children of alcoholics; however, the majority of these children adapt normally and do not develop serious drinking problems or alcoholism (West & Prinz, 1987).

Constitutional factors and the early family environment can buffer the risks of parental alcoholism. In her cohort of children who were followed from birth to age 18, Werner (1986) identified aspects of the child and qualities of the caregiving environment that differentiated between offspring of alcoholics who did and those who did not develop serious problems. Although children of alcoholics were more likely to be delinquent and to have serious mental health problems overall, almost 60% were functioning quite well at age 18. Girls and the children of alcoholic fathers had fewer problems than boys and the children of alcoholic mothers. More important, the resilient children tended to be rated as "cuddly and affectionate" as infants and to receive more attention from their caretaker. They also experienced fewer stressful events in the first 2 years of life and developed better communication skills and a more positive self-concept.

Research on childhood risk factors has begun to examine the mechanisms by which parental illnesses or impairments adversely affect children. Factors such as disrupted communication and parenting abilities, parent-child conflict and rejection, and lack of family cohesion may be more important than the severity of parental psychiatric or behavioral disorder (Adler & Raphael, 1983; Drake & Vaillant, 1988; Reich et al., 1988; Roosa et al., 1988; West & Prinz, 1987). Other family stressors that may be associated with parental psychiatric problems also impact the child's functioning. Such stressors include parental divorce and job loss, marital conflict, poverty, relocation, and so on. In contrast, the health and adjustment of the other parent and his or her ability to maintain family rapport can be protective factors.

THE FAMILY CONTEXT OF CHILDREN'S ADAPTATION

These ideas led us to formulate a paradigm to depict the way in which family-related factors influence children's adaptation (Figure 10.1). We use the paradigm to understand adaptation among children of alcoholic and depressed parents, but we believe the ideas apply to other types of parental dysfunction as well. Most generally, family demographic factors, such as size and socioeconomic status, and the child's personal resources, such as self-esteem, can influence the child's adaptation.

More specifically, we expected that the severity of the impaired parent's dysfunction would have a major impact on the child's well-being. Thus, a child is likely to be more affected when the alcoholic parent is drinking more heavily. We thought that the alcoholic parent's impairment in areas other than drinking also would have a detrimental influence on the child, just as it had on the spouse. Because a child's observation and modeling of the parents' ineffective problem-solving behavior may make the child more vulnerable, we posited that a parent's tendency to rely on avoidance coping responses also would create problems for the child. In this respect, the child is affected both by the parent's general mood and health and by his or her daily behavior.

Because each parent's health and functioning affects the child, we emphasize the importance of the nonalcoholic as well as the alcoholic parent.

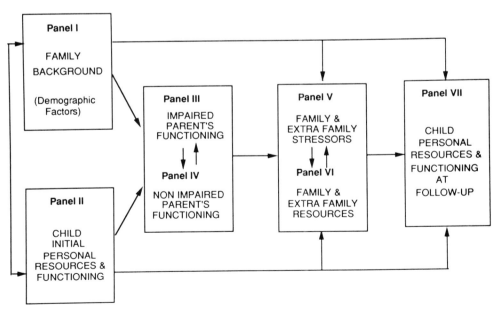

Figure 10.1 A model of the influence of parental and family functioning on children's adaptation.

Poor adaptation of the nonalcoholic parent is an added risk factor. Stressful life events, marital conflict, and family disorganization comprise another set of risk factors. In contrast, family resources such as cohesion, expressiveness, and interest in recreational and religious activities may be resistance resources. We try to capture these diverse influences on children by presenting a child's adaptation as affected by both parents and by life stressors and the family climate.

We use these ideas to address two related issues: (1) What are the effects of a parent's stable remission from alcoholism on his or her children and on the family environment? (2) To what extent is children's adaptation altered by family factors other than the alcoholic parent's drinking pattern and impairment in other areas, such as the level of functioning of the nonalcoholic parent and family stressors and resources?

Children in Alcoholic-Parent and Matched Control Families

We first compared children among the families of 2-year remitted ($N = 28$) and relapsed ($N = 23$) alcoholic patients with children among families ($N = 59$) of the matched community controls. As in the larger samples, the patient and control families were comparable in their demographic characteristics. Parents were primarily young and middle-aged adults (mean = 42 years). The majority of each group (about 80%) was Caucasian, and most (about 55%) had graduated from high school. There were no group differences in the number, age, or sex of children living at home (Table 10.1).

The adaptation of the children was determined from the mother's responses to questions about her children's health. This information was obtained at the 2-year follow-up. There were five items about *emotional problems:* depression, anxiety, nightmares, headaches, and indigestion. Another five items tapped common *physical problems:* allergies, anemia, asthma, frequent colds or coughs, and overweight or underweight. Mothers also were asked about the presence of a serious physical or mental disorder and about the use of alcoholic beverages, drugs or medication, and cigarettes among their children (Moos & Billings, 1982a; Moos et al., 1984).

Children's Health and Functioning

Compared to children of control families, children in families of relapsed alcoholics suffered from more depression and anxiety, experienced more indigestion and nightmares, and were more likely to have serious physical and mental problems (Table 10.1). As indexed by a composite measure of emotional problems (two or more of five), more than twice as much disturbance was reported among relapsed (52%) as among control (22%) families. In contrast, health and functioning among children in families of remitted alcoholics was comparable to that among control children.

These findings confirm prior reports on the negative impact of parental

Table 10.1 Comparison between children in families of remitted and relapsed alcoholic patients and families of community controls

Children's variables	Families of community controls ($N = 59$)	Families of remitted alcoholics ($N = 28$)	Families of relapsed alcoholics ($N = 23$)
Demographic characteristics			
Mean number of children	2.0	2.0	2.1
Mean age	11.3	14.0	10.8
Sex (% male)	48.8	50.0	52.0
Emotional problems (% 2 or more of five)	22.0	14.3	52.2***
Depression (% yes)	20.3	10.7*	43.5**
Anxiety (% yes)	20.3	25.0	43.5**
Nightmares (% yes)	3.4	7.1	17.4**
Indigestion (% yes)	8.5	3.6	21.7*
Headaches (% yes)	13.6	10.7	21.8
Physical problems (% 2 or more of 5)	8.5	10.7	21.7*
Serious mental or physical problems (% yes)	3.6	3.7	14.3*
Total health problems (% 4 or more of 12)	13.6	14.3	26.1
Smoke (% yes)	18.6	28.6	30.4
Use alcohol or drugs regularly (% yes)	15.3	14.3	17.4

Note. Two-tailed binomial comparisons of children from families of remitted and relapsed alcoholics with control family children.
$*p < .10$. $**p < .05$. $***p < .01$.

alcoholism on children; they also provide new information about how well children can adapt when their parents cease to abuse alcohol. The stress-related influence of parental alcoholism seems to diminish or disappear when the parent succeeds in controlling his or her alcohol abuse. This finding is consistent with our observation of normal mood and health among the spouses of these remitted alcoholics (Chapter 9). It strengthens the conclusion that alcoholic family systems need not continue to place undue strain on their members when the identified patient's alcohol abuse is in remission (Callan & Jackson, 1986). In contrast, continued parental alcohol abuse has a sharply detrimental influence on children.

Although the children of remitted alcoholics were functioning normally, they may be at increased risk over the long term. As noted earlier, the offspring of alcoholics are more likely to develop personality disorders and alcoholism that typically do not emerge until early adulthood or later. The academic difficulties and antisocial behavior seen among offspring of alcoholics may not appear until later during adolescence. Some children of alcoholics may remain symptom free until they encounter adult stressors that touch on areas of latent vulnerability. In any case, our findings imply that the remission of the alcoholic parent and other compensatory family factors reduce these long-term risks.

More work is needed to identify the ways in which parental drinking practices are transmitted to children. Wolin and his colleagues (1980) found that families in which alcohol problems were transmitted from parents to their offspring were more likely to misuse alcohol during ongoing family interaction and rituals, such as on vacations and holidays. The alcoholic parent in these families tended to drink heavily at home and to be intoxicated at family gatherings. However, some children who are raised by parents who drink heavily in the home may curtail their own drinking precisely because they wish to avoid the consequences their parents experienced. This reaction against the alcoholic parent may help to explain why many persons who have a family history of alcoholism are themselves normal drinkers or abstainers.

Family Stressors and Resources

We saw in Chapter 8 that the stably remitted alcoholic patients established basically normal family functioning, whereas the relapsed patients experienced more family stressors and fewer resources. These group differences were more extensive among families with children living at home than in the broader sample, which included families without children or whose children were no longer at home.

Continuing parental alcohol abuse creates stressful conditions among families with children living at home. Compared with families of controls (plotted at a standard score of 50 in Figure 10.2), families of relapsed alcoholics with children living at home were less cohesive and expressive and less likely to promote independence, achievement, intellectual and recreational pursuits, and a moral-religious orientation. In addition, these families were less well organized and the parents disagreed more about

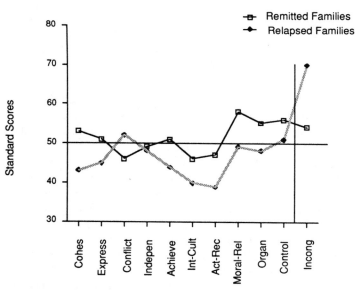

Figure 10.2 Family environments of remitted and relapsed alcoholic parents.

the family climate. The families of the remitted alcoholics did not differ significantly from those of the controls.

These aspects of the family environment are closely linked to adaptation among young children and adolescents. Baer and his colleagues (1987) found that lack of family cohesion and expressiveness and more family conflict were related to more alcohol use among junior high school students. More generally, children in cohesive and well-organized families tend to show better social and emotional adaptation, be more self-confident, and experience fewer behavioral and psychiatric problems. Children in families oriented toward independence and achievement are likely to be more assertive and self-sufficient, while those in active, stimulating families, as indexed by intellectual and recreational pursuits, tend to show better intellectual development and more adequate school adjustment. In general, children seem to benefit by a family emphasis on personal growth within the context of supportive parent-child relationships, clear rules, and well-defined limits (Moos & Moos, 1986).

More specifically, the family environment may increase the vulnerability to develop alcoholism in adulthood by shaping a child's temperament. Tarter, Alterman, and Edwards (1985) have suggested that the risk for alcoholism is increased by high emotionality, low attention span, and longer maintenance of arousal after stimulation. These temperament characteristics are more likely to develop among infants in families that are high in conflict and lack cohesion, expressiveness, and an emphasis on independence and intellectual and recreational pursuits (Plomin & DeFries, 1985). As we have noted, these qualities characterize the families of alcoholic parents, especially those with ongoing serious drinking problems. By fostering a family environment that promotes certain temperamental characteristics, parental alcoholism may increase a child's risk for alcohol abuse and other behavioral dysfunctions. Such an effect is likely to be mediated both genetically and environmentally (Plomin & DeFries, 1985).

Determinants of Functioning among Children of Alcoholic Parents

After comparing children of remitted and relapsed patients and community controls on individual variables, we examined the combined influence of parental and family functioning on children's adaptation. We followed the logic of the paradigm shown in Figure 10.1 and conducted partial and multiple correlation analyses in which we used three sets of variables to predict children's emotional and physical functioning. After controlling for group membership (alcoholic versus control) and size of family, these sets measured (1) the functioning of the alcoholic or matched control parent, (2) the functioning of the spouse of the alcoholic or matched control, and (3) family stressors and resources. Parent functioning was tapped by alcohol consumption, drinking problems (alcoholic parent only), anxiety, depression, physical symptoms, occupational functioning, and reliance on avoidance coping. The stressors were negative life events, family arguments, and parental disagreement about the family climate; the resources were family cohesion and organization.

Predicting Children's Functioning

As in earlier analyses (Chapters 7 and 9), the first set of variables (group membership and family size) provides a baseline against which to judge the incremental value of the subsequent sets. The multiple correlations for this set are shown in the first row of Table 10.2. Other demographic variables, such as parents' age and occupation and family income, are not

Table 10.2 Partial and multiple correlations between predictor measures and children's symptoms ($N = 110$)

	Child functioning criteria			
Predictor variables	Depression	Emotional problems	Physical problems	Total health problems
Group membership and size R	.07	.11	.20	.17
ALCOHOLIC OR CONTROL MATCH CHARACTERISTICS R	.46**	.51**	.34	.43*
Alcohol consumption	.25**	.28**	.15	.27**
Drinking problems	.29**	.38**	.17	.29**
Anxiety	.31**	.35**	−.04	.16
Depression	.31**	.41**	.12	.26**
Physical symptoms	.00	.25**	.05	.14
Occupational functioning	−.14	−.24*	.01	−.22*
Avoidance coping	.32**	.23*	.17*	.16
SPOUSE OR SPOUSE MATCH CHARACTERISTICS R	.35*	.47**	.34	.42**
Alcohol consumption	−.01	.17	.03	.02
Anxiety	.12	.11	.21**	.20*
Depression	.24*	.33**	.10	.28**
Physical symptoms	.17	.17	.20	.27**
Occupational functioning	.04	.08	.04	−.02
Avoidance coping	.29**	.35**	.15	.30**
FAMILY STRESSORS AND RESOURCES R	.37**	.39**	.27	.39*
Stressful life events	.23*	.26**	.10	.14
Family arguments	.23*	.26**	.03	.30**
Husband-wife incongruence	.24**	.20*	.15	−.19*
Cohesion	−.28**	−.27**	−.04	−.25**
Organization	−.14	−.20*	−.11	−.16

Note. The probability levels for the multiple Rs (except those for group membership and family size) refer to the significance of the increment in the Rs over those from regressions using only group membership and family size to predict the criteria.
*$p < .05$. **$p < .01$.

included because they were not related to the criteria. The partial correlations index how much additional variation in children's functioning is accounted for by the individual variables within each set.

In general, indices of parental and family dysfunction were related to children's depression and emotional problems but not to their physical problems. Aside from the expected influence of the alcoholic parent's alcohol consumption and drinking problems, the emotional dysfunction (especially depressed mood) of *both* parents and their reliance on avoidance coping were associated with more emotional problems among their children. The alcoholic parent's physical symptoms and occupational functioning were predictably related to the children's adaptation. Stressful life events and family conflict, spouse disagreement, and lack of family cohesion and organization also predicted children's emotional symptoms.

Information about the functioning of the alcoholic or matched control parent increased the explained variance in children's emotional problems by 16% over that obtained from knowledge of group membership and family size (increase in R from .11 to .51). The increment in explained variance due to information about the functioning of the nonalcoholic parent and to family stressors and resources was 13% and 8%, respectively.

Risk and Resistance Factors

We considered the extent to which parental drinking problems and depression, the nonalcoholic parent's reliance on avoidance coping, and lack of family support were independent risk factors associated with children's multiple health problems. We defined multiple health problems as present when one or more of the children in a family had three or more health problems. We identified the prevalence of multiple health problems among children exposed to four risk factors: parental drinking problems (one or more), parental depression (above the mean), an unsupportive family environment (below the mean on family cohesion), and the nonalcoholic or control match parent's reliance on avoidance coping (above the mean).

The proportion of families with multiproblem children increased with the number of risk factors. There were no multiproblem children in any of the families that had no risk factor. The prevalence of multiple problems rose to 28% among families with one risk factor and 46% among families with two or more risk factors (Figure 10.3).

While parental dysfunction and an unsupportive family place children's health at risk, low stress and high support may function as protective factors. The presence of these factors was associated with lower rates of multiple problems among children of alcoholic parents. Four of the 8 (50%) alcoholic-parent families with no resistance factors had children with multiple problems. This rate dropped to 15% among families in which neither parent was depressed, to 8% among those who also enjoyed high family cohesion, and to zero when the nonalcoholic parent also did not rely on avoidance coping (Figure 10.3). Thus, we were able to identify

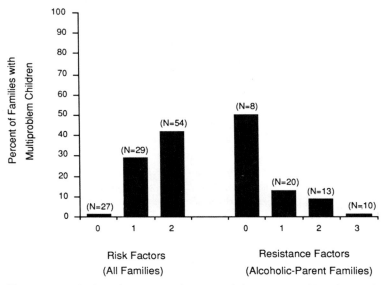

Figure 10.3 Risk and resistance factors and the percent of families with multiproblem children.

a group of alcoholic-parent families that had relatively healthy children, as shown by a comparatively low rate of multiple health problems. In addition, when two or more protective factors are present, the prevalence of multiproblem children among the controls is zero.

We have highlighted how a family-oriented conceptual paradigm can help to understand some of the determinants of child functioning. Clair and Genest (1987) found that a similar paradigm helped to understand adjustment among young adult children of alcoholic fathers. Compared to children of nonalcoholic parents, children of alcoholic fathers reported more conflict and less cohesion, organization, and intellectual orientation in their family of origin. In addition, they were more prone to depression and more likely to endorse emotion-focused coping strategies such as wishful thinking and avoidance coping. High family conflict and a lack of family cohesion, expressiveness, and independence were related to depression proneness and low self-esteem. Benson and Heller (1987) emphasized how family cohesion and support contribute to good adjustment among young adult daughters of alcoholic and problem-drinking fathers.

The conceptual framework can be used to integrate findings from studies of children with other risk factors such as parental divorce, depression, or chronic physical illness (Peters & Esses, 1985). Both general and disorder-specific factors that affect children may be identified. We need conceptually comparable studies of children exposed to different types of parental disorders. Such studies should examine the family stressors and resources that serve to accentuate or moderate the impact of one family member's dysfunction. We took a step in this direction by conducting a study of children of depressed parents.

THE FAMILY CONTEXT OF CHILDREN OF DEPRESSED PARENTS

Just as with alcohol abuse, parental depression is a significant risk factor for children. The offspring of depressed parents consistently have high rates of depression (Klein et al., 1988) and psychosocial dysfunction (Beardslee et al., 1983). In fact, children of a depressed parent show as much dysfunction as children of parents with other serious psychiatric disorders. For example, children of a depressed parent are as much at risk as children of a schizophrenic parent, as measured by impaired cognitive development, maternal ratings of child behavior, and teacher and peer judgments of competence and school adjustment (Cohler et al., 1983; Emery, Weintraub, & Neale, 1982).

Despite the risk of parental depression, however, most children of depressed parents function well. Their resiliency may stem from a remission in the parent's depression or from the depressed parent's adequate social and occupational functioning (Cohler et al., 1983). It may also be due to a positive family climate, a supportive relationship between the child and the disturbed parent, or other family resources such as a well-functioning, nondepressed parent. In their study of "superkids," those children who seem to be invulnerable to parental psychiatric disorders, Kauffman and her colleagues (1979) found cohesive yet independent relationships with the mother and positive social contact with an adult outside the family. The influence of serious parental psychopathology may be mitigated by beneficial family and extrafamily factors.

Children in Depressed-Parent and Matched Control Families

To examine these issues, we compared children in 133 families with a depressed parent with those in 135 demographically matched families with nondepressed parents. Depressed parents were selected from persons with a unipolar depressive episode entering psychiatric treatment. The measures were comparable to those we used in our work with alcoholic patients and their families. Children of depressed parents had much higher rates of psychological symptoms and behavioral problems. More specifically, 49% of the depressed parents had at least one child who experienced depressed mood and 44% had at least one child with anxiety problems, whereas this was true of only 32% and 19% of the control families. A total of 35% of the depressed parents had a child with academic problems compared to 17% of the control parents (Billings & Moos, 1983a).

Just as with alcoholic families, we found that parental dysfunction (in this case, depression), life stressors, and lack of family social resources were independent risk factors associated with an increased likelihood of a family having a child with multiple health problems. Only 3% of families with no risk factor had multiproblem children. The prevalence of multiple problems rose to 26% among families with a depressed parent, to 33% if the parent was acutely depressed, to 38% when such families were also experiencing many stressors, and to 41% when these three risk factors were combined with lack of family support. In contrast, the prevalence of multiproblem children was just 22% among families with few stressors and 11% among those with few stressors and high support. Stressors and an unsupportive family place children's health at risk, but low stress and high support act as protective factors in the presence of serious parental dysfunction.

Adolescent Children of Depressed Parents

Parental dysfunction and family stressors are thought to have an especially strong influence on adolescents. For instance, Weissman (1983) found that depressed mothers had serious problems communicating with their adolescent children and were unable to provide them with adequate affection and guidance. Accordingly, we compared adolescent children of a depressed parent with adolescent children of parents free from psychological or physical disability. In addition to the risk factors of parental disorder and stressful life events, we focused on the adaptive value of family support (Hirsch, Moos, & Reischl, 1985).

Compared to the normal group, adolescent children of a depressed parent reported lower self-esteem and more symptoms. We also found that stressful life events were strongly related to poorer adjustment among the adolescent children of depressed parents. Parental disability and stressful events had a joint influence on symptomatology. Adolescents in the depressed-parent group who experienced the most stressful events reported the highest symptom levels. In contrast, when adolescent children of a depressed parent experienced few life stressors, they reported symptom levels equivalent to those of the normal group. Moreover, a cohesive family environment was related to better adolescent adaptation.

Our study also included a group of adolescent children of a parent with rheumatoid arthritis. These adolescents had lower self-esteem than did adolescent children of normal parents. Together with our findings on children of alcoholic parents, the results imply that the principal risk factor for children is the presence of parental disability or distress rather than a specific parental diagnostic category.

Parental Remission and Children's Functioning

Earlier we saw that children's functioning returns to normal when parental alcohol abuse is in remission. Do children of remitted depressed parents also show normal levels of adjustment or improved functioning compared to when their depressed parent entered treatment? To address this issue, we compared three groups at a 1-year follow-up: (1) children of depressed parents whose symptoms remitted ($N = 23$), (2) children of depressed parents who continued to be depressed ($N = 34$), and (3) children of demographically matched nondepressed parents ($N = 95$) (Billings & Moos, 1986).

As expected, children of nonremitted parents showed much more dysfunction at follow-up than children of controls. We observed this finding for psychological symptoms such as depression, physical health problems, and behavioral difficulties such as school discipline problems. A high proportion (52%) of the nonremitted parent families had one or more children with multiple health problems. Surprisingly, children of remitted parents showed little improvement and continued to evidence more dysfunction than children of controls, even though the family contexts improved. Children whose depressed parents improved were still more likely to have multiple health problems than children of controls (27% versus 10%).

These findings indicate that children of remitted parents were doing better than those of nonremitted parents, but not as well as those of controls. Moreover, especially high levels of child dysfunction were reported among the nonremitted parent families. Nonremitted depressed parents had more severe symptoms at treatment intake and reported more family stressors and conflict and less cohesive and expressive family interactions. This pattern was relatively unchanged at follow-up. Consistent with the studies cited earlier, these results suggest that parental depression is a serious risk factor for children that persists into the early phase of recovery.

COMPARING CHILDREN OF ALCOHOLIC AND DEPRESSED PARENTS

Are children of an alcoholic parent as much at risk as children of parents with serious psychiatric disturbances such as depression? Do they experience as many family-related stressors and as conflicted family environments? Because unipolar depression tends to be a chronic recurrent condition, we expected children of depressed parents to be at greater risk than children of alcoholics. Some of the alcoholic parents were long-term steady drinkers stably married to well-functioning spouses who could protect their children from the effects of alcohol abuse. Moreover, children rarely feel responsible for their alcoholic parent's drinking behavior, but they typically do feel responsible and guilty for their depressed parent's sadness. In addition, depression is a cognitive as well as an affective disorder that often results in severe interpersonal dysfunction.

Two prior studies on this issue have obtained somewhat different results. El-Guebaly and his colleagues (1978) focused on offspring of psychiatric inpatients. Children of depressed fathers had somewhat more health problems than children of alcoholic fathers, but the differences were not statistically significant. Jacob and Leonard (1986) found that children of alcoholic and depressed fathers experienced more behavioral problems and social competence deficits than children of healthy control fathers. Most children were functioning in the normal range, but alcoholic fathers were somewhat more likely to have an impaired child than were depressed fathers. Compared to fathers of nonimpaired children, fathers of impaired children reported more alcohol-related problems and were more depressed. Together with other family and extrafamily stressors, these parental functioning factors are closely associated with the risk of child impairment in both alcoholic and depressed parent families.

We examined these issues by contrasting children in families of alcoholic and depressed parents. The two groups of families were roughly comparable demographically, although the parents in depressed families were somewhat younger (mean age of 38 compared to 42 years), had somewhat fewer children (average of 1.6 versus 2.0 per family), and were less likely to be stably married (about 30% were single parents).

Children's Functioning

Children tended to experience problems similar to those of their impaired parent. For example, mood and emotional disturbance was more common among children of depressed parents than among children of alcoholic parents, especially among the remitted parent groups. Specifically, 56% of families of remitted depressed parents had one or more children who themselves experienced depressed mood as compared to just 11% of families of remitted alcoholic parents. However, children in families of alcoholic parents were more likely to smoke cigarettes (29%) and use alcohol regularly (16%) than were children in families of depressed parents (15% and 6%, respectively). Rimmer (1982) found a higher rate of discipline problems among children of alcoholic parents than among children of depressed parents.

Family Stressors and Resources

In general, depressed parents and their spouses were functioning more poorly than their counterparts in alcoholic families. Depressed parents reported more physical symptoms than alcoholic parents; the spouses of depressed parents also reported more symptoms than the spouses of alcoholics. In addition, depressed parents had more serious medical conditions, used more medications, and had lower annual incomes even though they were as likely to be employed full time.

Although the family climates of the two groups of remitted parents were comparable to each other and to those of the normal controls, the families of nonremitted depressed parents were much more stressful for children than those of relapsed alcoholics. Specifically, the nonremitted depressed families experienced more conflict, were much less cohesive and well organized, and were less oriented toward independence and the open expression of feelings. In fact, families of nonremitted depressed parents were higher on conflict and lower on these other aspects of the family environment than our normative group of 500 distressed families (Moos & Moos, 1986).

Predictors of Children's Adaptation

We compared the two groups of families on the associations among parental functioning, the family environment, and children's adaptation. The findings point to common risk and resistance factors for children's health in alcoholic- and depressed-parent families. As expected, the focal parental dysfunction (alcohol abuse and depression) was the most salient risk factor. However, other aspects of the patient parent's dysfunction, especially depression among alcohol abusers and medical conditions among depressed parents, were also important, as was depressed mood among nonpatient spouses. In this respect, when parental alcoholism is associated with depression, children have a threefold greater risk of alcoholism than children of depressed parents or children of normal controls (Merikangas et al., 1985).

Parental reliance on avoidance coping, high family conflict, lack of family cohesion and organization, and less focus on expressiveness and recreational pursuits in the family were closely associated with children's dysfunction in both groups of families. Similarly, Stiffman, Jung, and Feldman (1986) found that mother-child discord and a high proportion of mentally ill family members who lived with a child were associated with more behavior problems among children of parents with a mental illness. The child's participation and competence in extrafamily activities, such as hobbies and sports, buffered these family stressors.

We identified similar risk and resistance factors among children of normal parents. Specifically, higher levels of depressed mood and physical symptoms and greater reliance on avoidance coping by both the mother and father were associated with poorer health among their children. High family conflict and lack of family cohesion and expressiveness were also closely related to children's dysfunction. Even though parental and family functioning is much better among normal families, the same risk and resistance factors are related to children's health problems (Holahan & Moos, 1987b). We also identified comparable predictors of adjustment among children with rheumatic disease and their siblings (Daniels et al., 1987).

Increased family and extrafamily stressors, lack of social resources, reliance on less effective coping strategies, and a diminished sense of parental self-confidence probably are the primary mechanisms by which parental disorders increase the risk of children's impairment. Conversely, a close relationship with one well-functioning parent and a benign family and extrafamily context may buffer the influence of parental alcoholism or depression. In the absence of other risk factors, these parental dysfunctions may be only minimally associated with children's health and psychological problems. Accordingly, when there is little or no marital discord in families with an affectively disturbed parent, the risk of school behavior problems is comparable to that among children of normal parents (Emery et al., 1982). In this respect, family climate is a more important predictor of children's adjustment than family structure, such as whether they live in a two-parent or single-parent family (Enos & Handal, 1986; Slater & Haber, 1984).

We have seen that the family climate can moderate the influence of parental dysfunction on children. Together with the strong connections between characteristics of the family and adaptation among children of alcoholic and depressed parents, these ideas led us to examine the factors involved in creating disturbed family environments.

A PARADIGM OF FAMILY FUNCTIONING

Families vary widely in the quality of interpersonal relationships, the emphasis on intellectual and social pursuits, and the level of organization and control. These aspects of family climate influence children. Such findings raise an intriguing question: Why do family social climates develop in such disparate ways; that is, what leads to an emphasis on cohesion, or recreational pursuits, or organization? The paradigm we formulated earlier (Figure 10.1) implies that the family environment is affected by family-related as well as extrafamily factors.

Family-related determinants of family climate include demographic factors, such as size and socioeconomic status, and aspects of parental functioning. Larger families tend to be less cohesive and more structured; the educational and social status of the adult partners is related to more family cultural and recreational pursuits. Parental dysfunction typically has a detrimental influence on the family, often by creating conflict and impaired relationships among family members. Overall, there is a reciprocal connection between child and parental functioning and the family climate (Mink & Nihira, 1986; Nihira, Mink, & Meyers, 1985). We saw earlier that family cohesion and recreational orientation can foster long-term recovery from alcohol abuse; here we focus on how parental functioning influences family adaptation.

Characteristics of parental work settings, an extrafamily factor, influence the family (Moos, 1986c). As we noted in Chapter 6, work stressors experienced by one spouse can alter the family climate and the other spouse's adaptation. In this respect, Piotrkowski (1979) has described how work overload and job role conflict can cause strain and create family tension. As work stressors increase, families often have fewer resources available to buffer them. Similarly, a person who fulfills both work and family roles may face interrole conflict and overload. This experience may lead to reduced involvement in the family and to a decline in the quality of family relationships.

We used indices of these sets of variables to develop a clearer understanding of the determinants of family climate. We used our alcoholic family sample to conduct hierarchical regression analyses in which family background characteristics (education of each spouse and number of children living at home), the alcohol-related functioning of the alcoholic parent (alcohol consumption, drinking problems), other aspects of both parents' functioning (depression, physical symptoms, and coping responses), life stressors, and high performance demands in parents' work were linked to four indices of family functioning: cohesion, expressiveness, conflict, and disagreement about the family environment (Moos & Moos, 1984).

Parental Functioning as a Predictor of Family Climate

As expected, family functioning was strongly affected by the adaptation of the alcoholic partner. Families in which the alcoholic member reported more alcohol consumption and drinking problems and complained of more depression and physical symptoms were less cohesive and expressive and had more family arguments and disagreement. Moreover, there were more family arguments when the alcoholic partner relied more on avoidance coping.

In general, there were comparable associations between the characteristics of patients' spouses and family climate. Thus, for example, families in which the spouse reported more depression and physical symptoms were less cohesive and higher in conflict.

These findings are consistent with results we presented in Chapter 7. They show that both alcohol consumption and other aspects of psychosocial functioning of the alcoholic partner influence family climate. Moreover, poorer functioning of the nonalcoholic spouse also is related to less adequate family adaptation. There may be a cumulative influence of the marital partners because, for example, families in which both spouses reported depression and physical symptoms had more arguments than those in which only one spouse gave such reports. In addition, a spouse's tendency to rely on avoidance coping predicted family arguments even after his or her partner's tendency toward avoidance coping was considered.

The relationships between parental and family functioning are reciprocal. Aspects of the family climate are associated with treatment outcome even after patients' demographic and intake functioning characteristics are considered (Chapter 7). This implies that a supportive family environment can have a positive influence on the adaptation of the alcoholic member. Conversely, the adequacy of a patient's adaptation can alter the quality of the family environment. Parental dysfunction may heighten family stress and interfere with children's health and development. However, conflicted family environments and poorly functioning children also may lead to parental alcohol abuse or depression. Future research can focus on the interplay between the behavior of each of the marital partners and the functioning of the family unit.

Life Events and Work Stressors as Predictors of Family Climate

Consistent with our earlier findings (Chapter 7), stressful life events were associated with more family arguments and less cohesion. Conversely, positive life events were linked to higher family cohesion. Some life events may be closely tied to parental functioning and thus tap an indirect way in which parents affect the family climate.

Performance demands in the alcoholic patient's and his or her spouse's job were indexed by the WES work pressure subscale. High work demands on the alcoholic family member were associated with less family cohesion. Similarly, high work demands experienced by the nonalcoholic spouse were related to less family expressiveness and more family arguments and incongruence. Work overload can influence the family by draining a parent of the energy necessary to promote family rapport or by creating tension and irritability that contribute to family conflict. From the social support perspective, however, a cohesive family can reduce the impact of work stressors. In this regard, we noted earlier (Chapter 7) that work stressors were related to poorer treatment outcome only among patients who were not living in family settings.

When Cooke and Rousseau (1984) examined these ideas, they found that high work demands were linked to family-work role conflict and overload, which were associated with more physical symptoms and lack of job and life satisfaction. The association between work demands, such as taking on extra duties and finishing job tasks by staying overtime, and perceived overload was progressively stronger among single persons, those who were married, and those who had children. However, once interrole conflict was controlled, family roles helped to buffer the influence of work stressors on physical strain. Family role expectations can promote strain among workers due to interrole conflict, but family cohesion also can provide the support to reduce it.

THE BROADER SOCIAL CONTEXT

We have found that parental disorder, stressful conditions, and the quality of family life influence children's health. To understand fully the determinants of family functioning and how they join with parental dysfunction to affect the children in a family, we need to consider the broader social context, including the interrelation between family and school and between work and family. We should also examine the influence of settings that can affect a person even though he or she does not take an active part in them, such as the influence of a parent's work setting on his or her children.

Specific aspects of work have been linked to an individual's values and patterns of problem solving in family and leisure settings. As described in Chapter 6, Kohn and Schooler (1983) believe that structural job conditions alter a person's way of dealing with the larger world. More complex jobs promote cognitive differentiation and the capacity for abstract thought, which contribute to an individual's active orientation, self-confidence, and well-being. People whose jobs require intellectual flexibility learn to exercise their cognitive skills in family and leisure activities as well as on the job. Accordingly, aspects of parents' work settings can influence family functioning and their children's adaptation. For instance, more cognitive complexity in a mother's job has been associated with her child's better school performance (Piotrkowski & Katz, 1982). Moreover, we found that an adolescent girl experienced considerable strain due to the impact on her family of stressors in her parents' work settings (Moos & Fuhr, 1982).

Some high-risk adolescents who become involved in school and develop a supportive peer social network may adapt successfully despite parental dysfunction and lack of family cohesion (Stiffman et al., 1986). For example, we found that satisfactory school involvement was associated with better adjustment among the adolescent children of depressed parents (Hirsch, Moos, & Reischl, 1985). When positive family and school influences reinforce each other, they can have an especially strong effect in promoting good adaptation among adolescents (Moos, 1987a).

Consistent with the idea that connections between different settings may promote well-being, Hirsch and Reischl (1985) noted that more contact between parents and peers was related to better adjustment among adolescent children of normal parents. Among adolescent children of depressed parents, however, more contact between parents and friends was associated with poorer adjustment and lower self-esteem. These adolescents also reported more strain in their relationship with their best friend than did adolescent children of healthy parents. Close contact between their impaired parent and their friends may distress some adolescents who fear embarrassment and rejection and who are forced to confront the parent's dysfunction.

Schneewind and his colleagues (1983) have carried this systems perspective one step further in their studies of adolescent personality development. They showed that a father's social context and job conditions can influence the quality of his family environment. For example, an impoverished social context and a father's experience of his job as monotonous and constraining were associated with a controlling and nonstimulating family climate. These conditions contributed to the father's and his son's authoritarianism and external control orientation. In contrast, an emotionally stimulating and well-organized family was related to children's orientation toward internal control. Thus, aspects of the broader social context influence parents' work settings. In turn, the work milieu can change their orientation to the world and alter the outlook of their children.

Future research on the impact and moderators of parental dysfunction should be guided by a conceptual framework that encompasses the interconnections among family, work, school, and peer influences (Moos, 1987a). Such research may identify general processes by which impaired parents—including alcoholic parents—influence their children and how these processes can be modified by beneficial factors in family and extrafamily contexts.

IV
PRACTICAL APPLICATIONS

11
Improving Treatment, Work, and Family Settings

We have identified some aspects of treatment and community settings that are associated with the process of recovery and relapse in alcohol abuse. Patients tend to do better in cohesive, well-organized treatment programs that are oriented toward a practical problem-solving approach. Patients who are in cohesive and well-organized families in which there is an emphasis on family social activities and relatively little conflict are more likely to maintain their remission. Clearly structured, supportive work settings seem to facilitate the recovery process among individuals who do not have the benefit of family support. These findings raise an important question: How can treatment and community settings be changed to promote their beneficial qualities? We address this issue here by describing how to monitor and improve treatment programs, work settings, and families. We emphasize the social climate, but the underlying logic and approach also apply to other aspects of these settings.

MONITORING PROGRAM DEVELOPMENT

In Chapter 2, we showed how an implementation assessment can obtain information about the way in which treatment is actually delivered. We identified three sources of information that may be used to develop implementation standards: normative conditions in other programs, specification of an ideal treatment, and theoretical analysis and expert judgment. The normative approach was illustrated by the COPES profiles of our five alcoholism programs (Figures 2.1 to 2.4). We also noted that the preferences of patients and staff could help to specify an "ideal" form of an intervention. We return to these issues here, because implementation assessment is the first step in monitoring a treatment program.

Maturation and Change in Psychiatric Programs

Information about the quality of the social environment can indicate how well psychiatric treatment programs are implemented. Mosher and his colleagues (Mosher & Menn, 1978; Wendt et al., 1983) established Soteria House, a community-based residential program for acute schizophrenic patients. They tried to develop a therapeutic community milieu that would differ from a comparison program in a large community mental health center. In fact, patients and staff appraised Soteria House as much more supportive and spontaneous and oriented toward autonomy, self-understanding, and the open expression of anger. The Soteria program was well below average in organization and structure. Patients and staff saw Soteria House as quite close to their preferred program. Thus, the Soteria House treatment climate was well implemented with respect to participants' preferences and, except for the system maintenance areas, to normative conditions in other programs.

Patients' and staff members' reports about the treatment milieu can help to monitor the impact of policy changes, new treatment components, or a shift to a fundamentally different program orientation. Accordingly, the Ward Atmosphere Scale (WAS) and the COPES have been used to track stability and change associated with patient and staff turnover, development of new administrative policies, formation of mutual support groups for nursing staff, alteration of physical features and program relocation, and the like (Moos, 1988a, 1988c).

Some researchers have monitored changes following the introduction of new treatment components or an entirely new orientation toward treatment. For example, Ng, Tam, and Luk (1982) found that the addition of nondirective community meetings in an inpatient psychiatric unit helped to promote a feeling of spontaneity and personal concern among patients. More generally, Verhaest (1983) followed the maturation of a therapeutic community by administering the WAS four times over a 6-year interval. The initial changes focused on improving personal relationships and promoting autonomy; they were followed by increases in involvement and the expression of anger and a decline in staff control. When staff set limits for disturbed patients, autonomy and anger decreased and perceptions of staff control increased. This emphasis on limit setting and structure eventually led to a further evolution of the therapeutic community emphasizing reality confrontation, sharing of decisions, and active exploration of personal problems.

Ryan, Bell, and Metcalf (1982) monitored the changes that occurred during a 4-year period when an insight-oriented program was modified to focus primarily on social rehabilitation and work-related training. Thirteen administrations of the COPES at 4-month intervals revealed several predictable changes in the quality of the treatment climate, including increases in autonomy, practical orientation, and staff support and a decline in staff control. These changes mirrored the conceptual shift in treatment

IMPROVING TREATMENT, WORK, AND FAMILY SETTINGS

orientation. Moreover, Bell and Ryan (1985) found that prevailing treatment practices were consistent with staff ideology in a rehabilitation program but not in programs with a biological or a psychoanalytic orientation. Such studies provide valuable information about the process of program development and the milestones involved in implementing an intended treatment ideology. We used this approach to monitor the impact of policy and other changes in the halfway house program.

Maturation and Change in the Halfway House Program
Initial Assessment of the Treatment Milieu

We have described how patients and staff initially saw the treatment environment at the halfway house (Figure 2.2). Both groups portrayed a program that was relatively well implemented as compared with normative data in the relationship and personal growth domains but somewhat lacking in system maintenance compared to normative conditions in other programs.

A more individualized method for generating an implementation standard is to identify an ideal form of the intervention. Form I (ideal) of the COPES allows patients and staff to specify their preferences about the treatment milieu. Figure 11.1 illustrates the changes residents and staff wanted in the halfway house program. The amount of change desired is obtained by subtracting the average score for the actual program from the average score for an ideal program for each subscale. The profile shows how much change is needed to match the preferences of residents and

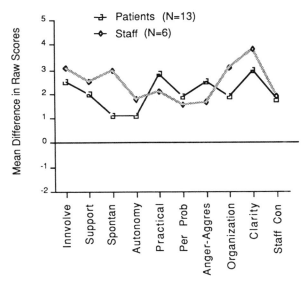

Figure 11.1 Real-ideal COPES discrepancies as seen by patients and staff in halfway house program—first assessment.

staff. The line marked zero in the center of the profile indicates no change is desired, or no discrepancy between the actual and preferred program. Positive scores indicate a desire for more emphasis, whereas negative scores point to a wish for less.

Residents and staff of the halfway house saw a need for more emphasis on all aspects of the program. Staff wanted more spontaneity than residents did, whereas residents preferred more open expression of anger. Overall, staff preferred a clear and orderly program characterized by supportive relationships and practical and personal problem orientation. They did not wish to be faced with the management problems that might ensue from placing priority on resident autonomy and the open display of anger. Thus, aspects of a program that are judged to be well implemented on the basis of normative data, such as involvement and spontaneity, may be found wanting when compared to patient and staff preferences.

Several developments took place in the subsequent 6 months. The original 16-person community was expanded to 27, and a more experienced director and new house manager were hired to stabilize the program. Transactional analysis became the major treatment modality, and the number of therapeutic activities increased. A new individualized recovery program allowed patients more freedom to plan activities suited to their needs. This led to an increase in the number of patients who accepted paid or volunteer work with community agencies or found regular part- or full-time employment.

The Interim Treatment Milieu

We readministered the COPES to residents and staff to identify the impact of these changes. Involvement and support diminished, reflecting the increase in program size and a corresponding decline in the quality of relationships among clients. House meetings were appraised as more businesslike, and the program became less intimate and more routine. The focus on practical orientation increased as more patients participated in vocational activities. Staff reported more autonomy and personal problem orientation, as expected from the new priority on individualized recovery and transactional analysis. Clarity and staff control were augmented by the more defined program structure and the leadership of the program director and house manager. Thus, the changes in the treatment milieu followed predictably from the changes in the program.

More developments took place in the subsequent 8 months. Staff gave the more experienced residents responsibility for leading group sessions and counseling new members. Changes in the admissions procedure enabled new patients to participate more actively. Community meetings were organized more clearly, and effective lines of communication were established to consider patients' ideas and grievances. In addition, the administrators became more actively involved in the day-to-day aspects of the program and added several new activities and therapy groups.

Longer-Term Program Development

The COPES was readministered to residents and staff about 8 months after the second assessment, or 15 months after the initial assessment. Involvement increased as patients participated more fully in the program by making decisions about how grievances should be resolved and by selecting new members. Support was enhanced by the counseling role of senior residents, improved communication among members, and increased responsiveness of the administrators (Figure 11.2).

The insight-oriented treatment groups and the focus on transactional analysis stimulated an increase in personal problem orientation. The strengthened priority on vocational activities led to a rise in practical orientation, and the increase in responsibility assumed by residents was reflected in a rise in autonomy. Organization increased as the new director stabilized the program structure. Staff and patients reported more clarity as they became familiar with the new routine.

The changes in the halfway house program reflect a dynamic and involved pattern of maturation. Initially, the program was a small, close-knit community with moderate emphasis on treatment goals and relatively little structure. The overall program moved toward the staff's preferred treatment milieu, that is, more clarity and organization and somewhat more emphasis on the relationship and treatment program dimensions. However, some aspects of the program still remained unsettled, as shown by the high level of anger and the discrepancy between staff and resident views of clarity and staff control.

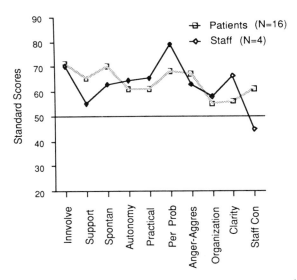

Figure 11.2 COPES form R profiles for patients and staff in halfway house program—third assessment.

Implementation Standards and Program Development

Standards for evaluating program implementation become more valuable as we accrue dependable information on the major types of psychiatric programs and their impacts. For example, we identified six types of treatment climates in cluster analyses of WAS and COPES data obtained on large samples of hospital-based and community-based programs. We labeled one of these six as a therapeutic community type, because of its high priority on personal relationships and treatment goals with moderate to low organization, clarity, and control (Moos, 1988a, 1988c). The Soteria House program described earlier is an example of a therapeutic community type of treatment milieu.

Subsequently, several investigators examined the goodness of fit between the WAS or COPES profiles of their treatment units and our therapeutic community type. Bell (1983) compared three Second Genesis programs for drug abusers to determine whether consistent treatment principles would produce comparable social environments. The three facilities had similarly shaped COPES profiles, but one consistently failed to measure up to the therapeutic community type. This program had the highest dropout rate, which may have been a consequence of inadequate treatment implementation (Bell, 1985).

Conversely, evidence of adequate implementation may point out that a particular treatment orientation is not effective for certain types of patients. Ryan and Bell (1983) studied a long-term, analytically oriented inpatient program that emphasized self-understanding and the open expression of anger but was poorly organized and lacking in support, autonomy, and practical orientation. The COPES profile was closely comparable to an insight-oriented program type we identified in our cluster analysis. Ryan and Bell (1983) found that schizophrenic patients in the program showed little overall improvement; they concluded that this finding was generalizable to comparable insight-oriented treatment climates.

Implementation analysis can clarify whether specific kinds of treatment climates can be developed in particular administrative contexts. Pullen (1982) evaluated the Street Ward Community, which is an acute admission unit that tries to function like a therapeutic community, even though patients stay an average of less than 3 weeks. Staff saw the atmosphere as high in autonomy, self-understanding, and the open expression of anger. Lindsay (1986) obtained similar findings in an evaluation of a psychiatric unit in a general hospital. Patients and staff saw the program as cohesive and expressive, oriented toward autonomy and self-understanding, and clear and well-organized. These results imply that a therapeutic community milieu can be established in short-stay admission programs and psychiatric units in general hospitals (but see Steiner, Haldipur, & Stack, 1982).

Implementation analysis is a valuable way to understand new forms of treatment programs better. For instance, Steiner (1982) showed that an

IMPROVING TREATMENT, WORK, AND FAMILY SETTINGS

active, well-organized treatment milieu can be developed in a joint psychiatric and medical inpatient program for adolescent patients. The combined emphasis on intensive psychiatric and pediatric treatment led to placing high priority on self-understanding and the expression of anger, as well as on clarity and staff control (Terry el al., 1984). These findings imply that the inclusion of medical approaches in alcoholism treatment need not have a detrimental influence on the program climate. Overall, such analyses can help to specify the staff resources needed to support and maintain a therapeutic community and other types of treatment programs, identify the consequences of variations in program organization, and monitor the process of program development.

ENRICHING TREATMENT ENVIRONMENTS

We have shown how information about the social environment can help to monitor the process of program development and maturation. Such information can be provided to program participants and used to stimulate program change and assess its impact. Several investigators have given feedback to treatment programs that were assessed with the WAS or COPES (Fairchild & Wright, 1984; Friedman, Jeger, & Slotnick, 1982); some have followed this procedure by planning modifications designed to improve the program. We have outlined a method by which information about a setting can be used to promote change. This method has been used to alter treatment, work, and family settings.

The Process of Feedback and Change

Our procedure consists of four steps: (1) program assessment, (2) feedback and discussion of the resulting information with special emphasis on real-ideal differences, (3) planning and implementing change, and (4) program reassessment. We use an ideal program standard as the basis for comparison.

Program Assessment

As discussed in Chapter 2, we administer the WAS or COPES to measure treatment quality. Form R and Form I provide data about the real and ideal social climates. Patients complete the WAS or COPES after they have been in treatment long enough to become familiar with the program.

Feedback and Discussion

First, we score responses to the environmental measure and identify discrepancies between the actual and preferred program. Next, we hold a meeting to present and discuss this information. Participants often express their ideas in light of the conceptual framework provided by the social climate scale dimensions. This framework helps to elicit ideas from persons who are hesitant to voice their opinions. In the feedback process, we pay special attention to similarities and differences in the reports and values of clients and staff, as exemplified by the data shown in Figure 11.1. When there is considerable disagreement, we provide item-by-item feedback to identify the reasons for it.

Planning and Implementing Change

After areas of shared concern are identified, we plan innovations to try to bring about the desired modifications. We often identify specific changes by considering three broad classes of social climate determinants: physical features, organizational structure and policies, and the aggregate characteristics of the residents and staff. Specific strategies for improvement within each of these domains may arise from a variety of sources, such as ideas provided by clients and staff and the content of the items on a social climate scale. Ideas for program reorientation can also be pinpointed by information about the association between patients' perceptions of the treatment milieu and their participation in the program. Thus, if patients who participate in more group therapy sessions see the social milieu more positively, we might develop strategies for increasing patients' involvement in group treatment.

Reassessment

After innovations have been implemented, we reassess the social climate to measure the impact of change efforts. This assessment typically takes place after changes have been in operation for a reasonable period of time, such as 6 weeks. When the setting is reevaluated just after innovations have been implemented, we sometimes have identified a temporary decline in clarity or rise in staff control. By scheduling a series of assessments following program change, participants may be able to "fine tune" the innovative program elements; longer-term assessments make it possible to distinguish between stable environmental impact and transient reactions to the change process.

Promoting Change in Treatment Programs

This four-step procedure has been used to improve the social environments of psychiatric as well as alcoholism treatment programs. In one of of our own studies, the WAS showed a lack of clarity and involvement among patients in a psychiatric program located in a small private hospital. Feedback of these findings led to staff discussions and specific modifications. More relevant activities were initiated. Treatment teams took responsibility for handling discipline and explaining their decisions to patients. To ensure clear expectations among patients and consistent staff behavior, program rules and policies were discussed in community meetings. Patients and staff later reported increased support and orientation toward learning new skills and self-understanding; they also saw the milieu as clearer and less rigidly structured (Moos, 1988c).

Milne (1986) conducted a similar study in a psychiatric day hospital. Two baseline assessments showed that patients and staff held similarly unfavorable views of the program; they perceived low levels of involvement, support, spontaneity, and clarity. These findings and subsequent staff discussions led to several changes, including new training programs for staff in anxiety management and behavior therapy and a division of patients into acute and chronic groups who were treated on different days. Following these changes, patients and staff reported significant overall improvements in the treatment environment. The findings were stronger for acute than for chronic patients. These case demonstrations show that formative evaluation and feedback can promote program improvement.

When a treatment setting ceases to function effectively, information about the social climate can identify policies that need to be modified to restore the program to its original therapeutic characteristics. Verinis (1983) studied an alcohol rehabilitation unit that had a high patient retention rate but suddenly experienced an increase in irregular discharges. The WAS showed a concurrent decline in support, spontaneity, and clarity; prior studies have shown that lack of emphasis in these areas is associated with high dropout rates. After staff became aware of the decay in the program environment, they established a more therapeutic atmosphere with significant increases in independence, organization, and clarity. The proportion of irregular discharges declined to its prior level.

Several other studies have focused on alcoholism programs. Eriksen (1987) restructured a short-term alcoholism unit into patient and staff teams and developed a new program based on behavioral and social learning principles. Some of these changes also were implemented in a halfway house. Patients and staff reported increased involvement, autonomy, practical orientation, organization, and clarity; changes in the inpatient program were larger than in the halfway house. In general, new programs based on social learning or behavior modification principles seem to enhance involvement, autonomy, and practical orientation, although sometimes program clarity decreases temporarily (see also Lacoursiere & Bradshaw, 1983).

The data-based feedback process we have described is the essence of formative program evaluation. The social climate measures are easy to administer, and the process does not require technically trained evaluators. The procedure is especially effective in small, stable settings in which participants interact frequently and can exert control over at least some aspects of the intervention program. Participants can focus program change on a few commonly defined areas. This lessens the chance of conflicting goals and makes effective change more likely. After firsthand experience with formative evaluation, clients and program personnel may be more receptive to subsequent research, including an assessment of the program's impact on clients' treatment outcome (Finney & Moos, 1984).

ENRICHING WORK ENVIRONMENTS OF HEALTH CARE STAFF

An intervention program is not only a treatment setting for patients; it is also a work environment for health care staff. To develop an effective treatment setting, the work climate should satisfy staff. Responses from more than 1,600 health care employees to the WES show the special problems in health care facilities. Compared to employees in other work settings, health care staff report less job involvement and less support from co-workers and supervisors. Moreover, health care settings are lacking in autonomy and clarity, are less comfortable physically, and have more work demands and supervisor control. These conditions probably reflect the stressful and emotionally difficult nature of health care and problems associated with large, highly structured organizations (Moos, 1988c).

Variations in work climate affect the morale and performance of health care employees. Staff who see their work as independent and challenging and as characterized by clear and consistent policies and good personal relationships tend to be more satisfied and to perform better. In contrast, staff morale is lower in highly demanding work settings that lack cohesion and autonomy (Moos & Schaefer, 1987). Moreover, work support is associated with changes in student nurses' symptoms as they rotate from one ward to another (Parkes, 1982). A move to a unit that was seen more favorably was associated with a reduction in affective symptoms and an increase in work satisfaction and performance. Comparable connections have been identified between characteristics of work settings and employee morale and performance in other types of work settings (Chapter 6).

Monitoring Changes in Work Environments

Program directors and clinicians can use information about work climate to plan improvements and to monitor the process of organizational change. Wilderman and Mezzelo (1984) examined the effects on work climate of changing a community mental health center from a consultation model to a direct-service model, in which staff spent more time with clients and less with their colleagues. As regularity and structure increased, job clarity and supervisor control increased as well. However, staff cohesion declined, probably because staff members spent much less time with each other.

Quality assurance (QA) programs are being widely instituted in health care settings, but little is known about how they affect staff morale. To examine this issue, Sinclair and Frankel (1982) compared two outpatient mental health programs. They selected one unit of each program to participate in QA activities; they designated the other unit as a control. Contrary to their concern that QA activities might lower morale, there were no negative changes in staff perceptions of the work milieu. In fact, staff in the QA group reported an increase in supervisor support and a decrease in control. Moreover, staff members who provided higher-quality services saw the work climate as more cohesive and independent and less pressured. A well-managed QA program can improve a health care work environment.

Modifying Stressful Work Settings

The assessment and feedback process can provide supervisors and staff with information about the work climate and increase communication among them. It can be used to diagnose problems in a work group, appraise and enhance leadership, identify work groups at risk for organizational dysfunction, facilitate team building, and promote and evaluate a change program (Moos & Billings, in press). We found that this process helped to identify and reduce work stressors among staff in an intensive care unit. Staff were dissatisfied and were showing dysfunctional reactions, such as mild depression and withdrawal from patients. To help understand these problems and identify areas that needed to be changed, a liaison psychiatrist used the real form of the WES to describe the current work climate and the ideal form to describe the staff's preferred work setting.

The WES showed that staff perceived a lack of clarity and organization in the work milieu and relatively low co-worker cohesion and supervisor support as compared to normative data and their own preferences. Group discussion of these findings helped to identify problem areas and guide the staff in developing solutions, which included clarifying specific areas of individual responsibility and establishing regular meetings between nurses and physicians. Staff subsequently felt that the work climate improved, as shown by increases in job involvement and co-worker cohesion, more staff autonomy and clarity, and more emphasis on innovation. Staff morale and the quality of patient care also improved (Koran et al., 1983).

Organizational development theorists believe that employee participation in decision making will reduce role conflict and ambiguity and promote job satisfaction and well-being. Jackson (1983) randomly assigned nursing and clerical employees in a hospital outpatient unit to work situations in which they enjoyed increased participation and control. Employees in the enhanced participation condition reported more autonomy at work and more job satisfaction as well as less role conflict and ambiguity. Employee involvement in decision making may lessen role strains and enhance valued outcomes for both the individual and the organization.

ENRICHING FAMILY ENVIRONMENTS

The assessment and feedback approach can be applied to families as well as to treatment and work settings. As noted earlier, FES may be used to describe families, compare family members' perceptions with each other, and contrast actual and preferred family climates (Moos & Moos, 1986). By conducting a case-by-case analysis of individual FES profiles and of the congruence of perceptions among family members, we showed how an understanding of family functioning can be helpful in treating alcohol problems (Chapter 6). We provide a case example here to show how the FES can depict the social milieu of a family in treatment and how such information can facilitate the therapeutic process and evaluate progress in therapy (Fuhr, Moos, & Dishotsky, 1981).

Changing the Family Environment of the Cartwright Family

Roger and Jody Cartwright were in their late twenties and had been married for 2 years. Mrs. Cartwright had a 9-year-old daughter, Shirley, from a brief prior marriage. Mrs. Cartwright was in close contact with her three older brothers, who were frequent guests living in the Cartwrights' home for several weeks at a time. Mrs. Cartwright sought individual therapy during the breakup of her first marriage a few years earlier. At that time, she reported excessive drinking under stress, problems in relating to men, difficulty in expressing her feelings, and lack of self-confidence.

Subsequently, Mr. and Mrs. Cartwright entered therapy to discuss her drinking problem and explore a lack of warmth in their relationship. Mrs. Cartwright's drinking was triggered by her brothers' demeaning and antagonistic behavior. Rather than venting her anger, she suppressed her feelings and drank heavily until she blew up in a violent rage. Managing their daughter Shirley's behavior also was problematic, because neither parent was effective in setting limits for her. According to the therapist, Mrs. Cartwright undercut her husband's attempts to discipline Shirley, thereby weakening his authority. The couple described a chaotic family life in which Mrs. Cartwright unsuccessfully tried to combine employment and housework, while Mr. Cartwright refused to help with meal preparation or child care.

The Initial FES Profiles

After several counseling sessions, the therapist asked Mr. and Mrs. Cartwright to complete the FES in three ways. Using Form R, they each gave their impressions of the current family environment. Because Mrs. Cartwright's brothers had a significant impact on the family, the Cartwrights also used a separate Form R to describe what the family was like with her brothers present. They then used Form I to indicate how they saw an ideal family milieu.

The picture of the nuclear family provided by the FES (Figure 11.3)

IMPROVING TREATMENT, WORK, AND FAMILY SETTINGS

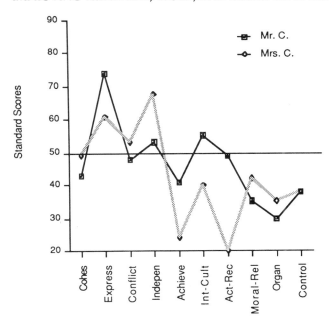

Figure 11.3 Pretherapy family environment for the Cartwright family.

was quite similar to the therapist's impressions. The combination of moderate to high expressiveness and independence and lack of organization and control define a family with little commitment or sense of togetherness. Mr. and Mrs. Cartwright agreed that family activities were poorly planned and disorganized and that family rules and duties were not defined clearly. Mrs. Cartwright reported a lack of family participation in social activities, but Mr. Cartwright disagreed.

The adverse influence of Mrs. Cartwright's brothers was shown clearly by the Cartwrights' description of the family when the brothers were present. Both agreed that cohesion and expressiveness were much lower and that conflict was much higher. The brothers were not on sufficiently good terms with Mr. Cartwright to permit the maintenance of usual family interaction patterns. They were seen as intruders who disrupted the family. The FES Form I showed that the Cartwrights agreed on the change they needed to make in most areas.

Feedback and Planning Change

The therapist's first step in giving feedback to the couple was to point out that they both wanted more cohesion, less conflict, and more cultural and recreational activities. The couple considered several dimensions in tandem in planning changes. In reviewing the items on the FES conflict and organization subscales, Mr. Cartwright recognized that family tension was increased by his lack of help in housework and by the family's scheduling problems and poor planning. This problem was alleviated by a decision to obtain part-time household help. Similarly, the couple knew that their communication was seriously eroded by their difficulty in setting limits for Shirley, as reflected on the FES control subscale. This issue prompted intensive discussion of how Mrs. Cartwright undercut her husband's authority and ventilation of his anger about it.

Feedback of the FES scores with and without Mrs. Cartwright's brothers at home dramatically highlighted their dangerous influence on the couple's relationship. Coincidentally, the Cartwrights moved to a new home at this time. The move helped them to change the way they interacted with Mrs. Cartwright's brothers and to develop more control over Shirley's friends.

The Outcome of Treatment

Three months later, Mr. and Mrs. Cartwright completed the FES Form R for both the nuclear family and extended family, including her brothers. Improvements were substantial, as was expected from the relatively high initial agreement on goals. The Cartwrights described their relationship much more favorably; cohesion and organization were higher and conflict was somewhat lower (Figure 11.4). Moreover, their cultural and family social activities increased, although the couple wanted more change in this area. The system of family control did not change substantially; Mr. and Mrs. Cartwright maintained flexible rules and democratic decision making. Because Mrs. Cartwright's brothers visited less frequently, their disruptive influence became clearer, and she was able to deal with them more assertively.

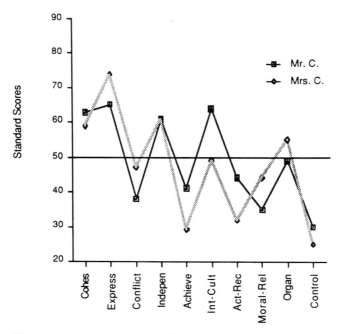

Figure 11.4 Posttherapy family environment for the Cartwright family.

Clinical Applications of Family Evaluations

Such family assessments can help to monitor the progress and outcome of therapy. In this respect, several investigators have found the FES to be a sensitive measure of change during family-oriented crisis intervention and treatment. Bader (1982) studied a group of families before, immediately after, and 2 months after an intensive 1-week residential multiple-family workshop. These families increased significantly in cohesion, expressiveness, and independence immediately after the workshop; they showed additional increases in these three areas at the 2-month follow-up. A matched untreated control group did not change over time. Schreibman and her colleagues (1984) found that a skills training program helped parents manage their child's discipline problems and promoted improvement in family functioning. Trained parents reported increases in family expressiveness and intellectual and social pursuits, along with a decline in target children's problem behaviors. Similarly, Egan (1983) noted that stress management training can help abusive parents to lessen family conflict.

Szapocznik and his co-workers (1983) compared the relative effectiveness of conjoint family therapy, with the entire family present for most sessions, and one-person family therapy, with only one family member present for most sessions. Both conditions were effective in increasing expressiveness and moral-religious emphasis. However, patients in the one-person condition experienced an increase in family cohesion, whereas patients in the conjoint condition reported a decline. According to Szapocznik and his colleagues (1983), the effectiveness of one-person treatment may flow from its positive impact on the patient's internalized view of family cohesion.

Family evaluations can be useful in understanding a clinical problem and providing diagnostic feedback to family members. The FES encourages a clear, practical focus on the client's present family climate. It provides a conceptual framework that can help to train family counselors and to clarify some of the salient aspects of family interaction. In parent training and systems-oriented counseling programs, the FES can be used to identify family strengths and problems. Such information can help clinicians tailor interventions to individual families and evaluate their effects (Brady & Ambler, 1982; Ford, Bashford, & De Witt, 1984).

The FES also can help in matching families with interventions. Pino (1984) identified connections between specific aspects of family climate and different approaches to family therapy. The affective/interpersonal therapies are conceptually connected to the three relationship dimensions, suggesting that intimacy training, self-disclosure, and conflict management training may be most effective in promoting relationship qualities in a family. Methods such as assertiveness and need achievement training, self-esteem training, and family discussions about preferred activities should promote changes in family independence, achievement, and intellectual orientation. Organization and control are conceptually related to behavioral and cognitive modalities and perhaps may be altered most easily by methods such as behavior management and family contracts. More generally, the conceptual congruence between these family climate domains and the domains tapped by our other measures makes it possible to obtain an integrated perspective on a person's overall social context. Such a perspective can promote a better understanding of the links between the family and other important settings in clients' lives.

GENERAL PERSPECTIVES ON IMPROVING SOCIAL SETTINGS

We have described some ways in which treatment, work, and family settings can be monitored and changed. Although our emphasis has been on social climate, we recognize that other domains of environmental factors are important both in their own right and as determinants of social climate. In this regard, we see the environment as a dynamic system composed of four domains: physical and architectural features, policy and program factors, suprapersonal characteristics (aggregate personal characteristics of individuals in a setting), and social climate. By considering these four domains, we can enrich our ideas about social settings and how to alter them.

The Treatment Program as a Dynamic System

We have developed the Multiphasic Environmental Assessment Procedure (MEAP) to assess geriatric and psychiatric treatment programs in terms of these four domains (Moos & Lemke, 1984). The MEAP consists of four main instruments, the content of which reflects the four domains. The Physical and Architectural Features (PAF) checklist taps dimensions such as physical amenities, safety features, and space availability. The Policy and Program Information Form (POLIF) measures dimensions such as policy clarity, resident choice and control, and provisions for privacy. The Resident and Staff Information Form (RESIF) assesses the suprapersonal environment by obtaining information on residents' social backgrounds, degree of diversity, and functional abilities and on staff characteristics. The Sheltered Care Environment Scale (SCES) assesses residents' and staff members' perceptions of the facility social environment.

The MEAP enables evaluation researchers to examine a treatment program as a dynamic system. An overall assessment can alert evaluators that a program fails to accomplish desired objectives, as when clients report that they cannot influence policies even though the facility has several resident committees, a residents' council, and apparent resident participation in decision making. In an organizational development program, Wells and her colleagues (1986) used information from different parts of the MEAP to plan interventions and improve residential facilities for older persons.

Multiphasic procedures also help identify how the four environmental domains influence each other. With the MEAP, we found that residents established more rapport when they were in settings with more physical amenities, better social-recreational aids, and more personal space. These settings also had more socially competent residents and policies that provided more personal choice and control. Residents felt more independent when they were in facilities that provided them with a richer array of social activities and allowed them wider choice in organizing their daily lives and more control over certain aspects of facility policies. Appropriate physical features and program policies can promote more supportive, independence-oriented social climates (Moos & Igra, 1980).

Information about the determinants of social climate can point to specific changes that may produce desired shifts in a treatment program. Vaglum, Friis, and Karterud (1985) noted that larger size, poor staffing, compulsory group treatment activities, and a confrontational staff orientation tended to produce an unsupportive and poorly organized treatment milieu. When structure and policy factors were changed in one program by decreasing its size, reducing the time devoted to compulsory group activities, and changing from a confrontational to a task orientation, the treatment environment showed the expected improvement. Joint changes in physical features and policies can reinforce each other. Thus, cohesion was increased in one of our alcoholism treatment programs by removing television sets from individual rooms and setting up a common viewing area (a physical design innovation) and instituting family-style meals (a policy change).

Important benefits can be derived from the assessment and feedback process. The process exposes staff to new ways of thinking about their program and its policies. Irrespective of the specific changes that may ensue, staff acquire a broader framework for describing their setting. Instead of describing the program in terms of high versus low quality, staff think about it in terms of several dimensions. This cognitive shift facilitates program innovation by providing alternate ways to plan change. Moreover, information obtained from environmental assessment procedures can be used to design new programs as well as to modify and improve existing ones (Moos, Lemke, & David, 1987).

Resistance to Change and Other Problems

The procedures we have described can arouse anger and resistance. One problem is that individuals have different preferences and may disagree about how settings should be altered. Some clients and staff believe that a program should be well organized, whereas others are convinced that too much structure squelches independence and self-reliance. In addition, some patients espouse apparently contradictory preferences, such as drug abusers who prefer a treatment climate oriented toward both spontaneity and staff control. In fact, staff often face the dilemma of trying to create a milieu that fosters self-understanding while simultaneously controlling alcohol and drug use and coping with patients' impulsivity and aggression (Penk & Robinowitz, 1978).

Program modifications that are not shaped to meet patient or staff needs are unlikely to achieve the desired effect. For example, specific but delimited policy changes such as allowing nurses to wear street clothes instead of uniforms, adding part-time clerks to a ward, granting patients the right of access to their hospital record, or using cigarettes as incentives to try to increase constructive activity typically fail to produce major changes in a treatment milieu. More innovative and comprehensive changes are needed to have a substantial impact (Moos, 1988a, 1988c).

A quite different issue is the emergence of unintended consequences. Sometimes temporary problems arise after policies are changed. Patients in two of our studies reported a temporary decline in program clarity after policy shifts were made. The decline pointed to the need for better communication. In addition, the initial changes in our halfway house program led to more structure and an erosion of the quality and spontaneity of personal relationships. The continuing maturation eventually achieved the desired outcome, but a decline in rapport and openness can occur as new policies lead to temporary increases in program structure.

A related problem arises when changes exceed the original goals. Although well-planned changes can be compatible with program goals, the process of change can be hard to control once it is initiated. Policy shifts may elicit changes in staff preferences that create a desire for further program development. Assessment and feedback initiate a dynamic, ongoing process that may alter participants' preferences as well as their views of the current environment.

Another point is that pressures emanating from the broader hospital or social context may make it hard to develop or maintain an innovation. Friis (1981) conducted a 6-year longitudinal study using a Norwegian version of the WAS to monitor a psychiatric program and facilitate its development as a therapeutic community. After some improvements were made, administrative problems in the hospital forced the program to become a closed unit primarily for acute psychotic patients. Subsequently, the treatment environment returned to roughly what it had been before the intervention. Although feedback about the social environment can promote changes, the resulting improvement may not survive structural changes in the larger facility. These problems can be managed, but they highlight the need to understand how to develop successful innovations and find ways to maintain them.

Determinants of Successful Innovations

At least three sets of factors are involved in successful innovations. The first set comprises aspects of the innovation itself, such as the explicitness of the plans and the ease of implementing them. The second set is the methods used to introduce and implement the innovation. Feedback mechanisms that stimulate interaction, problem identification, and participation in decision making are helpful. Ongoing interaction between staff and consultants is better than single workshops or in-service training. Consultants must give people enough time to understand the process of change and to identify and resolve implementation problems.

The third set encompasses the characteristics of the adopting unit, such as an alcoholism treatment program or an adolescent residential center. The organizational climate and level of administrative support are especially salient factors. High staff morale and active backing by managers heighten the chance of success. In this respect, an initial program assessment may help to increase rapport and foster a more comprehensive innovation.

Lacoursiere and Bradshaw (1983) found that active support from hospital administrators was essential in reorganizing a substance abuse program. A host of problems arose from low staff morale, conflicts within the nursing staff, lack of communication among staff members, inadequate assessment of patients, inability to provide effective rehabilitation, and so on. After securing help from the hospital administration and conducting an initial assessment, the investigators developed new staff assessment teams, held weekly meetings of a reorganization planning committee, and implemented several new treatment procedures. Staff members were apprehensive at first, but the continued effort eventually succeeded. After 9 months, staff attitudes had improved, and the new treatment program was judged to be much better than the old one.

Improving social settings is a complex process. Successful innovations often undergo gradual but continual modification during the implementation phase, reflecting a process of mutual adaptation between the advocate of change and the setting in which changes are being made.

12
Implications for Treatment and Program Evaluation

In this chapter, we first review the findings of our research program and discuss their implications for the diagnosis and treatment of alcoholism. We then focus on the integration of theory and evaluation research and consider the different types of theories that may guide an evaluation. Next, we consider aspects of the methodology of evaluation research, including research design, outcome assessment, and cost analyses. We then discuss how the expanded paradigm can help to examine attempts to match patients with appropriate treatments.

Following that, we return to a major theme in Chapter 1: how the expanded paradigm increases the utility of evaluation research findings, especially for shaping the nature of alcoholism treatment. We also consider how the paradigm enhances the role of evaluation researchers. We conclude by noting that more broadly focused evaluations may help to resolve the current crisis in alcoholism treatment.

THE MAJOR FINDINGS

Here we highlight the major findings of our research and evaluate how well we have achieved our aims. In Chapter 1, we outlined two broad objectives. The first was to examine the implementation, process, and outcome of residential treatment for alcoholism; the second was to learn more about the nature and course of treated alcoholism and the factors influencing treatment outcome.

Treatment Implementation, Processes, and Short-Term Outcome

To assess the adequacy of treatment implementation, we measured patients' length of stay and exposure to various treatment components, as well as the quality of the treatment environment (Chapter 2). The latter

IMPLICATIONS FOR TREATMENT AND PROGRAM EVALUATION 221

approach taps the social climate of treatment settings on 10 dimensions that provide a systematic framework for understanding the context of a program. Moreover, this approach assesses treatment both as provided by the program and as received by patients.

When we evaluated the adequacy of treatment implementation against standards developed by Sechrest and his colleagues (1979), we concluded that the five programs varied in important ways and were viable treatment approaches. Patients participated in a variety of treatment components and generally had positive perceptions of their programs. Overall, the programs compared favorably with normative conditions in alcoholism and psychiatric programs.

With considerable effort, we achieved an 87% 6-month follow-up rate and found that treated alcohol abusers who were more difficult to follow had worse treatment outcome (Chapter 3). Our findings underscore the importance of obtaining high follow-up rates in order to portray accurately the extent of patient improvement after alcoholism treatment.

The Impact of Treatment

As is the case in most treatment outcome studies, the patients we studied improved substantially in their drinking behavior and other areas of functioning at the 6-month follow-up as compared to their functioning at intake (Chapter 3). Some targeting of program effects was suggested by the improvement in occupational functioning exhibited by the Salvation Army participants, the enhanced social functioning shown by the halfway house residents, and the substantial increase in abstinence found among the aversion conditioning program clients.

To examine which aspects of treatment programs might be responsible for this improvement, we linked length of stay and several treatment components to treatment outcome (Chapter 4). Three treatment components—therapy sessions, films and lectures on alcoholism, and on-site AA meetings—were associated with positive outcomes in several of the programs, although the strength of these relationships varied. Antabuse was also related to better treatment outcome in the two programs in which it was used, as were worship services and part-time jobs in the Salvation Army program. By concentrating their resources on more effective treatment components, administrators can "fine-tune" programs. More ambitiously, clinicians can develop new programs composed of treatment components that are more strongly linked to positive outcomes for their patient population.

Although many alcoholism program evaluations have found very weak or no treatment effects once patient intake characteristics are controlled, our analyses show that such findings are unduly pessimistic (Chapter 4). We examined treatment in a more differentiated way by analyzing specific treatment elements and aspects of the treatment milieu. These within-program treatment components and perceptions of the treatment environment mediated most of the effects of the treatment programs; in addition, they were significantly related to outcome after the effects of the programs were taken into account.

We also used an analytic technique that did not assign the outcome variance that was jointly explained by patient and treatment variables just to patient variables. This procedure enabled us to identify somewhat stronger effects of treatment (see Figure 4.4). Patient demographic and intake functioning characteristics independently accounted for an average of 7% of the variance in the four main 6-month outcome indices (alcohol consumption, abstinence, physical symptoms, and depression), whereas treatment (program, treatment experiences, and treatment environment) independently explained an average of over 6% in these four indices. Patient intake characteristics and treatment jointly accounted for another 7%. Overall, we were able to explain 12% to 29% of the variance in these four indices of treatment outcome (mean = 21%) by patient and treatment variables combined. These proportions of variance explained by treatment are larger than those accounted for in most evaluations of alcoholism programs and point to a more substantial impact of treatment on outcome, at least over the subsequent 6 months.

Sex and Marital Status

We focused on the role of two important patient characteristics: sex and marital status (Chapter 5). Women and men obtained similar treatment and showed comparable treatment outcome, but they responded differently to specific treatment components. Participation in male-dominated therapy groups was related to better outcome for men as compared to women; in contrast, exposure to films and lectures on alcoholism, a more individually oriented treatment component, was linked to better outcome among women relative to men. For men patients, being married was associated with better outcome, but this was not as true for women, perhaps because their husbands were more likely to be heavy drinkers than were the wives of male patients.

After leaving treatment, married men were more likely to participate in outpatient aftercare, which was related to positive outcome for them. Overall, married men do better after treatment than married or unmarried women do. These findings highlight the need for more research to examine the effects of individually oriented treatment options, special groups for women, or women group therapists in programs with mainly men patients.

The Nature and Course of Treated Alcohol Abuse

Our second broad goal was to learn more about the nature and course of treated alcohol abuse and the factors that influence functioning after treatment. Our findings about the longer-term course of treated alcohol abuse among married patients are relatively optimistic. They highlight the sub-

IMPLICATIONS FOR TREATMENT AND PROGRAM EVALUATION 223

stantial benefits that can flow from successful treatment and natural recovery as well as the significant personal and social costs of continued alcohol abuse.

Remitted and Relapsed Patients

At the 2-year follow-up, about half of the patients were in remission and doing about as well in most areas as demographically matched nonproblem drinking adults (Chapter 8). Of those patients in remission at the 2-year follow-up, 77% of those followed were still in remission 8 years later (another eight had died). Even among those who relapsed in the first 2 years after treatment, 33% who were reassessed were in remission at the 10-year follow-up. In part, these outcomes reflect our focus on patients who returned to families following treatment and who generally had some social and occupational resources on which to base their recovery. In any case, our findings show that many married alcohol abusers can achieve essentially normal lives following treatment.

At the 2-year follow-up, there were only a few differences between the remitted patients and the community controls residing in the same census tracts. Remitted patients were less likely to consume alcohol but were more anxious, used more medications, made more frequent visits to physicians, were more likely to smoke and to have smoking-related symptoms, and were less active socially. Beyond these mainly health-related differences, however, no others emerged in a number of personal and environmental domains. At the 10-year follow-up, most of these differences were no longer apparent; in fact, patients who were remitted at the 10-year follow-up were functioning better than patients who were remitted at the 2-year follow-up.

Other researchers have also reported a positive long-term course for some treated alcoholics. For example, Nordstrom and Berglund (1987) identified 55 men with good social adjustment an average of 21 years after their first hospitalization for alcoholism. The authors speculated that physiological processes associated with aging, including changing reactions to alcohol, may have been important factors in remission. Their findings show that some middle-aged and older alcoholics have the ability to maintain adequate social adjustment.

On the other hand, many of the patients we followed over the 10-year period experienced continuing alcohol problems. During this time, 19 persons died and more than 25% of the surviving patients were divorced. The information we obtained from death certificates and from family members indicated that most of the patients who died were drinking heavily prior to the illness or injury that ended their lives. Moreover, personal and social costs of continued alcohol abuse were evident among the 36 survivors, who were classified as relapsers at the 10-year follow-up. These findings underscore the significant cost of continued alcohol abuse for patients and their families. We believe that the relapsed patients could have improved to the level of functioning shown by the remitted patients; accordingly, the gap between these two groups reflects the potential influence of treatment and natural recovery processes.

The Impact of Life Context Factors

Even though we examined treatment more thoroughly than is done in many evaluations, our analyses of the family sample data showed that treatment variables and patient intake characteristics combined explained an average of only 21% and 17% of the variance in the four main outcome criteria at the 6-month and 2-year follow-ups. Accordingly, we examined the influence of life context factors and coping responses on treatment outcome (Chapter 7). In general, both 2-year and 10-year outcomes were better for those patients whose spouses were functioning better; who returned to families that were more cohesive, expressive, and well organized; and who relied less heavily on avoidance coping strategies. Patients who were in more involving and cohesive work settings tended to show better treatment outcome; however, this finding occurred only among patients not living with their families. Many of these concurrent relationships held in predictive analyses in which 6-month and 2-year predictors were linked to 2-year and 10-year functioning, respectively.

On average, patients' demographic and intake functioning characteristics accounted for 11% of the 2-year and 12% of the 10-year variance in the four main outcome criteria. Concurrent life context factors accounted for average increments of 20% and 17% in the variance of the four criteria at the 2-year and 10-year follow-ups, respectively. Overall, we were able to explain 16% to 53% of the 2-year outcome variance (mean = 31%) and 16% to 49% of the 10-year outcome variance (mean = 29%) in these four indices. When treatment factors were included in the analyses of our overall model, life stressors and family resources accounted for an average increment of 6% of the variance in the four main 6-month outcome criteria. These life context factors, combined with coping responses, explained an additional average of 23% of the variance in these four criteria at the 2-year follow-up. These are important increments over the proportions explained by a model that does not include life context and coping factors.

We were not surprised to find concurrent relationships between life context and coping factors and individual functioning. However, we also found such relationships over time. Life context factors at 6 months predicted an average increment of 10% of the variance in alcohol consumption, physical symptoms, and depression at 2 years, compared to an average of 14% predicted by patient characteristics at intake. Finally, aspects of patients' life contexts at 2 years predicted an average increment of 17% of the variance in 10-year alcohol consumption, physical symptoms, and depression compared to an average of 14% accounted for by patients' intake characteristics. Thus, prior life context factors are as predictive of treatment outcome as are patients' initial sociodemographic characteristics and level of functioning.

These findings point to the need for a fundamental shift in thinking about alcoholism as well as alcoholism treatment programs and their effects. A treatment program is only one of many factors that influence alcohol consumption and related aspects of health and well-being. Current life context factors also shape alcohol abuse and individual mood and behavior. Thus, many of the hard-won gains of treatment programs fade away over time. This is precisely what we should expect on the basis of our knowledge about environmental impact and the diversity of influences to which patients are exposed. Inherent in the belief that a treatment program can promote change is the assumption that other more recent environmental factors can modify such change. Conversely, if life context factors can alter people, so can treatment and aftercare programs.

Spouses and Children

A comprehensive account of the course of alcohol abuse should consider its impact on the family of the alcohol abuser. Accordingly, we focused on the spouses and children of patients who returned to family settings following treatment. At the 2-year and 10-year follow-ups, spouses of remitted patients generally were comparable to spouses of normal-drinking community controls in their functioning and life contexts (Chapter 9). In contrast, spouses living with actively alcoholic partners at the 2-year follow-up were functioning less well and were in more stressful family environments than spouses of remitted patients or spouses of community controls. There was a 39% divorce rate among spouses of relapsed patients in the ensuing 8 years. At the 10-year follow-up, the remaining spouses of relapsed patients also were doing somewhat less well than the other two groups of spouses.

When we examined the determinants of spouse adaptation, we found that the alcoholic partner's overall functioning (not just drinking behavior) had an important influence on the spouse; spouses whose partners were more impaired showed more impairment themselves. In addition, poorer initial spouse functioning, more stressful life events, less family cohesion and expressiveness and more family conflict, and reliance on avoidance coping all contributed to poorer spouse adaptation. To understand spouse functioning more fully, researchers need to look beyond the alcoholic partner's functioning and examine other life stressors and coping resources that affect the spouse. Overall, a stress and coping perspective can be applied to spouses as well as to their patient-partners.

Consistent with the results for spouses, we found that children of patients in remission functioned as well as children in control families; children of relapsed patients showed more emotional and health problems (Chapter 10). In addition, the emotional status of children was related to the physical and social functioning of both their alcoholic and nonalcoholic parents. These findings indicate that alcohol abuse has pervasive effects on spouses and children but that these effects diminish or even disappear entirely when the alcoholic family member is recovering.

In summary, alcohol abuse can follow widely different paths after treatment. Treatment has some positive influence on short-term outcome, but both short-term and long-term outcomes are much more strongly determined by the patient's personal and environmental resources. How well a patient's spouse and children adapt is tied, at least in part, to how well the patient is functioning.

IMPLICATIONS FOR DIAGNOSIS AND TREATMENT

Alcoholism treatment programs are quite successful in achieving cessation or reduction in drinking behavior and improvement in other areas of functioning over the short run, but they often do not maintain these positive changes over time (Maisto & Carey, 1987; Nathan & Skinstad, 1987; Saxe et al., 1983). Patients' life contexts and coping skills play an ongoing role in the posttreatment course of alcohol abuse. These factors typically explain as much or more of the variance in treatment outcome as do an individual's demographic characteristics and initial levels of functioning. Thus, clinicians tend not to focus on the factors that most strongly influence the process of recovery among substance abusers. These factors are thought to be extraneous to treatment, but they continue long after treatment, are more pervasive and intense, and have a stronger impact on outcome (Orford, 1985).

These facts point to a reason for the typical decay of treatment benefits over time. Treatment does not substantially influence the life context and coping factors that are closely linked to the process of remission and relapse (Chapter 7). Thus, our findings show that treatment should be oriented toward strengthening natural recovery processes and improving the life contexts of patients and their ability to manage these contexts (see also Edwards, 1984; Mulford, 1984; Vaillant et al., 1983). In this respect, Miller and Hester (1986) have suggested restructuring treatment to minimize hospitalization and residential care and to focus primarily on intensive outpatient treatment oriented toward the prevention of relapse. Similarly, we believe that residential programs for alcohol abuse can provide a temporary respite that enables patients to recover from the immediate physical and psychological consequences of excessive drinking; however, a more active long-term phase of treatment must follow the patient's return to the community.

The idea of shaping formal interventions to enhance the natural recovery process is supported by research on other substance abuse disorders as well as by studies of the psychosocial outcomes of a diversity of psychiatric and medical conditions (Moos, 1985a; Moos, in press). For example, after studying factors related to abstinence from heroin, Wille

(1983) concluded that treatment for drug dependence must complement natural recovery processes (see also Biernacki, 1986). Orford (1985) came to similar conclusions about the treatment of drug abuse and obesity. Here, we note the implications of these ideas for comprehensive assessment and diagnosis and then briefly describe three treatment approaches that focus on relevant life context and coping factors: family-oriented treatment, coping skills training, and community reinforcement programs.

Comprehensive Assessment and Diagnosis

A biopsychosocial approach to treating alcohol disorders demands the application of biological, psychological, and environmental assessment procedures (Leigh & Reiser, 1985). However, many clinicians focus primarily on demographic factors and the history of alcohol-related symptoms and behavior. They tend to obtain detailed information on patient characteristics that are difficult or impossible to change. In contrast, we recommend more emphasis on identifying potentially alterable characteristics of patients and their environments and on using this information in the treatment process to promote better outcome. In addition, because patients and their spouses and children influence each other, it is important to evaluate the status and functioning of the alcoholic's family and social system.

Clinicians who seek to apply a biopsychosocial perspective need systematic methods of assessing life context and coping factors (for examples, see Billings & Moos, 1983b; Marlatt & Gordon, 1985; Moos & Billings, 1982b; Wanberg & Horn, 1983). Information about current and expected stressors can identify situations that may increase the risk of relapse; information about patients' preferred coping patterns may help clinicians teach patients how to reduce stressors more effectively and maximize the adaptive aspects of a particular coping strategy. Routine evaluations of patients' life contexts, especially their family and work settings, can monitor the outcome of patients' efforts to change their everyday environments.

More comprehensive and conceptually focused measures of life stressors, social resources, and coping responses will enhance the prediction of treatment outcome and facilitate more effective clinical interventions. Accordingly, we are developing a Life Stressors and Social Resources Inventory, which taps ongoing life circumstances and new life events in eight important domains such as physical health, financial, work, spouse/partner, children, and extended family. We are also constructing a Coping Responses Inventory that taps appraisal-focused, problem-focused, and emotion-focused coping responses. These inventories can be used to develop profiles that depict patients' life contexts and coping preferences; they may also have some value in planning and evaluating alcoholism treatment (Moos, 1988).

As Drake and Wallach (1988) note, clinicians who understand hospital and community settings from the patient's perspective are better able to facilitate planning for discharge and aftercare. A patient with a positive family, peer group, or work situation is likely to collaborate in treatment aimed toward discharge and relapse prevention. However, patients without such social resources may subvert discharge planning and aftercare unless the clinician tries to deal with the problematic community living situation. The mutual planning process may also promote a more empathic clinician-patient relationship and reduce the risk that the patient will try to manipulate the alcoholism treatment system.

Most traditional assessment procedures focus on obtaining an accurate diagnosis. In contrast, Hayes, Nelson, and Jarrett (1987) emphasize the "treatment utility of assessment," that is, the extent to which assessment contributes to better treatment outcome, most often by enhancing treatment planning. As an example, an assessment of patients' perceptions of the treatment environment can help to identify patients who see a program in an idiosyncratic way and who might profit from a special peer support group to help integrate them into treatment. An assessment of the family environment can help a family therapist decide whether to focus on communication skills training (if there is low cohesion and expressiveness) or clarification of family rules and structure (if there is low organization and control).

In this respect, program evaluators have placed too much emphasis on the identification of prognostic demographic and intake functioning characteristics. Conceptual and clinical advances await an understanding of the dynamic factors that underlie the connections between pretreatment indices and treatment outcome. Thus, marital and occupational satisfaction are likely to be more relevant than marital and occupational status. More important, personal characteristics, such as a patient's sense of self-efficacy, may predict outcome because they reflect the social contexts in which relapse is likely to occur (Tucker et al., 1985). A high sense of self-efficacy may imply a constellation of life situations that has little "press" toward relapse. More generally, we suspect that personal and demographic resources at treatment intake foreshadow good treatment outcome, primarily because they indicate the presence of stable life context factors that promote recovery.

Family-Oriented Treatment

Our findings point to the pivotal influence of family functioning on treatment outcome. We found that family cohesion, expressiveness, and organization predicted better long-term outcome. However, the five programs we studied had almost no emphasis on family treatment; this was even true for the milieu-oriented and aversion conditioning programs in which many of the patients were married and living with their families. We believe that family-oriented therapy should be considered as a component in the treatment of almost all alcoholic patients who are living with their families; we think it is clinically appropriate for a large proportion of such patients.

Clinicians are developing effective interpersonal or systems approaches and behavioral approaches to family treatment (Hazelrigg, Cooper, & Borduin, 1987); some of these procedures are being used with alcoholic patients. For example, O'Farrell, Cutter, and Floyd (1985) formulated a behavioral marital therapy program to help alcoholic patients and their partners initiate daily caring behaviors, develop communication skills, plan shared recreational activities, and establish structured interactions and written contracts to decrease drinking and alcohol-related interactions. When this program was added to regular outpatient alcoholism treatment, it produced clinically significant improvement in alcoholics' marital relationships, especially among couples who reported moderate levels of positive communication at the outset.

In structuring the initial stages of family treatment, clinicians will need to consider the preexisting quality of family relationships. For example, Ford, Bashford, and De Witt (1984) found that a minimal intervention was sufficient to improve communication skills among moderately cohesive couples, but that a more intensive intervention was needed for couples who initially reported low levels of cohesion. In a treatment program that was specifically directed toward improving the clarity of communication, however, the initial severity of communication problems predicted better outcome (Vannicelli, Gingerich, & Ryback, 1983).

As the specific aspects of family functioning associated with relapse are identified, clinicians can develop targeted treatment programs to change them. This process has proven fruitful in the development of family treatment for schizophrenia and depression. A series of studies found that expressed emotion, involving critical comments by relatives, hostility, and overinvolvement, was a risk factor for relapse. These findings led to the development of educational and counseling programs designed to reduce relatives' criticism and hostility; some of these programs resulted in a sharp decline of relapse rates (Goldstein, Hand, & Hahlweg, 1986).

Coping Skills Training

When stressful life circumstances arise, patients who lack adequate coping skills are vulnerable to resuming alcohol abuse. Thus, we found that patients who relied less on active-cognitive and more on avoidance coping responses experienced poorer short- and long-term treatment outcome. In addition, avoidance coping was associated with more family conflict and less family cohesion, which also predicted poorer outcome. Clinicians and researchers have begun to recognize the central role of inadequate coping skills in alcohol abuse and to develop cognitive and behavioral skills training programs that are showing positive short-term results (Marlatt & Gordon, 1985).

Most coping skills programs emphasize behavioral strategies, but our findings show that cognitive strategies are at least as effective in preventing relapse. In fact, cognitive coping can be used in all kinds of circumstances, including those in which behavioral options are unavailable. It can also serve to facilitate behavioral coping. Oei and Jackson (1982) found that cognitive restructuring was more effective than behavioral social skills training in producing and maintaining social skills and in reducing alcohol consumption; both approaches were more effective than traditional supportive therapy. The authors speculated that maladaptive cognitions prevented patients from using the behavioral responses they had learned in the skills training program.

Shiffman (1985) found that behavioral coping was more responsive to contextual factors such as alcohol consumption, which diminished its use, and depression, which lessened its effectiveness. Cognitive coping strategies can be applied flexibly in many circumstances; they are less under situational control and thus not as likely to be disrupted by increased life stressors or reduced social support as are behavioral responses.

These ideas are consistent with the secondary prevention program formulated by Sanchez-Craig and her colleagues (1987), who noted that problem drinkers who were attempting not to relapse relied on cognitive coping at least as much as on behavioral coping. In fact, cognitive strategies, such as self-reinforcement and reappraisal, were used in close to 90% of the situations in which clients tried to cope with strong urges to drink. Accordingly, Sanchez-Craig and her co-workers (1987) developed an outpatient skills training program for early-stage problem drinkers; they have also applied the program to other client populations, such as drug abusers.

Community-Oriented Treatment Programs

Several researchers have found that integrated treatments that focus on improving alcoholic patients' life contexts and coping skills are especially effective (e.g., Mallams et al., 1982; Page & Badgett, 1984). For example, Fagan and Mauss (1986) designed a rehabilitation program for skid-row alcoholics that focuses primarily on the community reentry and adaptation process. On the whole, clients showed relatively good outcome at follow-up. According to Fagan and Mauss (1986), program success was due mainly to channeling of clients into new friendships, AA, renewed family connections, and employment opportunities.

Azrin and his colleagues have conducted the most extensive research program of this type. Initially, these researchers found that inpatient reinforcement programs were more effective than standard hospital treatment (Azrin, 1976; Hunt & Azrin, 1973). As a next step, Azrin and his colleagues (1982) evaluated an outpatient version of the community reinforcement approach. Patients were randomly assigned to a traditional therapy group; an Antabuse program involving a significant other; or a combined behavior therapy and Antabuse program in which clients were taught drink refusal skills, muscle relaxation, and how to cope with potential relapse-inducing social situations. They were also provided with advice about social and recreational activities and, if needed, marital counseling and help in finding a job.

At a 6-month follow-up, the behavior therapy group was drinking less than either of the other two groups. Single patients responded better to the behavior therapy condition, whereas married patients achieved similar benefits from either Antabuse or behavior therapy. Apparently, the married patients already had some of the resources that the behavior therapy condition was trying to foster. By combining Antabuse with the community reinforcement approach, Azrin and his colleagues developed a comprehensive intervention that addresses each of the three primary facets of the biopsychosocial disorder of alcohol abuse.

Financing Alcoholism Services

Our findings also have policy implications for financing alcoholism and mental health services. Cahalan (1987) has noted that the prospective payment principles embodied in the diagnosis-related group (DRG) approach are problematic for alcoholism, especially when DRG payments are based on an overall average length of stay for alcoholic patients. Application of a DRG for alcohol dependence with a mean length of inpatient stay of 8 days, such as initially proposed by the Health Care Financing Administration, might limit treatment to detoxification services and lead to inadequate treatment for those alcohol abusers who need residential treatment. More important, reimbursement policies need to emphasize outpatient care and to take into account patients' personal and social resources, especially the characteristics of the family and residential settings that influence required treatment intensity and duration.

Some efforts are being made to establish realistic standards and reimbursement policies for substance abuse and mental health services. One approach is to identify different populations of service users and to develop insurance criteria for each group. As we would expect, psychiatric diagnosis is a relatively poor indicator of patients' service needs; patients' personal and social resources should be taken into account to predict treatment needs better (Taube et al., 1984). Comprehensive diagnostic assessment, combined with a focused program of case management, might ensure both availability of needed services and efficient cost control (Goldman & Taube, 1988).

IMPLICATIONS FOR THEORIES TO GUIDE TREATMENT EVALUATIONS

Our study was able to address a number of important issues and to generate implications for alcoholism treatment because it was guided by theory. In fact, there is a growing consensus that program evaluations are more useful when embedded in a theoretical context—when an evaluation tries to explain or generate additional knowledge about some process or phenomenon.

Most theory-driven evaluations are guided by a theory of the treatment process (Bickman, 1986; Chen & Rossi, 1983; Lipsey et al., 1985). However, the expanded paradigm (Figure 1.2) suggests that a theory guiding a treatment evaluation can focus on one or more of at least three broad types of phenomena or processes: the treatment selection process, the treatment process, and the process underlying the disorder being treated. Moreover, the paradigm reflects broad classes of variables that can be considered in examining each process. First, the type and amount of treatment patients obtain is viewed as a function of their demographic characteristics, functioning, and life contexts at intake, as well as factors in the treatment setting. Second, treatment processes are seen as affecting outcome directly as well as indirectly through their influence on life context and coping factors, which may be viewed as instrumental outcomes that are related to the ultimate outcome. Finally, the onset and course of the disorder are viewed as determined by patient characteristics and life context factors, which may influence the course of the disorder even when they are not affected by an intervention.

Program evaluations that focus on one or more of these three processes can be guided by a biopsychosocial model and by any of a number of more specific theories; for example, theories of alcoholism include learning theories, psychodynamic approaches, a theory of self-regulation, and stress and coping theory. We used a stress and coping perspective and information about patients' life contexts to try to explain the treatment process and the subsequent course of alcoholism. Stress and coping theory can also be applied to explain the process of entering treatment, with treatment entry viewed as the outcome of information and help seeking when personal and social resources have been expended. Overall, use of an expanded approach to treatment evaluation may facilitate theory development or help to identify especially promising theoretical approaches. In the following sections, we discuss some theoretical perspectives that can help evaluators focus on treatment selection, treatment processes, and the nature of alcohol abuse.

Theories of Treatment Selection

Theories of alcoholism treatment selection can be divided into three subclasses: theories of treatment entry, theories of program selection and allocation, and theories of within-program treatment selection and allocation. Formal theories in these areas are virtually nonexistent, but some initial conceptual and empirical work has taken place.

Treatment Entry

Drawing on established models of health care utilization, Beckman and Kocel (1982) have begun to develop a model of alcoholism treatment entry that includes patient and life context variables. Their model encompasses

IMPLICATIONS FOR TREATMENT AND PROGRAM EVALUATION

(1) individual predisposing factors such as age, gender, and socioeconomic status; (2) perceptions and beliefs about drinking behavior, alcoholism treatment, and health; (3) personal enabling factors such as alienation and feelings of mastery, as well as the history of drinking behavior and treatment; and (4) social enabling factors such as insurance coverage, proximity to treatment facilities, and support networks. In addition to suggesting foci for future studies, such models may impose some order on the scattered findings generated thus far.

The process of entering treatment can be studied in large-scale general population surveys by comparing problem drinkers who have and have not sought treatment (e.g., Hingson et al., 1982). In addition, smaller-scale studies can help clarify the treatment entry process by tracking individuals who contact referral points in the alcoholism intervention system (such as information and referral centers) and comparing those who do and do not become involved in treatment. We are currently conducting a study of this type. Finally, evaluations of alcoholism treatment can provide new information on the determinants of treatment entry by going beyond asking patients about sources of referral and inquiring about factors such as stressful life situations that precipitated their seeking treatment (Weisner, 1986).

Program Selection and Allocation

In the real world, patients do not select and are not assigned to alcoholism treatment programs at random. Instead, personal and social factors combine to determine program selection and admission. These selection processes produce systematic relationships between patient characteristics and program type. As noted in Chapter 2, patients in the two private programs we studied had more social resources and were functioning better at intake than those in the three public programs.

Program selection processes are most difficult to study at the "between-program" level, given that most treatment evaluations focus either on one program or on two or more treatment conditions to which patients have been randomly assigned. Advances in our understanding of between-program selection and allocation processes are more likely to come from policy-oriented researchers with access to information from multiprogram data bases. Unfortunately, models derived from such data bases are likely to emphasize economic determinants and to gloss over the social and psychological factors that also play a role in determining the program in which a patient is treated.

Within-Program Treatment Selection

Once in a program, different types of patients may receive differential treatment and aftercare. Some patients may find particular treatment components appealing and opt to include them in their treatment regimens. Clinicians may try to individualize treatment to address each patient's specific configuration of problems. These processes can produce systematic relationships between patients' characteristics and the treatment they receive. Such selection and assignment processes can be studied with an expanded paradigm in which both the quantity and quality of treatment are assessed.

To apply a comprehensive model of within-program selection processes, it is also important to assess life context factors prior to treatment. In a study of treatment for depression, we found that depressed patients who experienced more life stressors prior to intake were treated less intensively and were less likely to receive psychoactive medication. We speculated that treatment providers made situational attributions about the cause of depression among patients who report stressful environments and dispositional attributions about the cause of depression among patients in seemingly more benign circumstances. These attributions may lead clinicians to provide brief treatment for patients judged to have reactive depression and longer treatment for patients thought to have dispositional depression (Billings & Moos, 1984b).

Dropout from Treatment. Patient attrition is the most widely studied form of within-program treatment selection in the alcoholism field. Although the expanded paradigm suggests that patient, treatment, and life context factors can be related to dropout, most studies of patient attrition have focused on patients' personal characteristics. It is important to broaden the explanatory network in attrition studies to encompass treatment variables because they may be changed more readily than patient attributes. In this respect, Smart and Gray (1978) found that treatment variables were better predictors of dropout than were patient characteristics. Patients who were more likely to remain in treatment were those who had a medical assessment, had one type of therapy as opposed to a mixture, received medication, and had either a physician or nurse as their primary therapist (see also Fink et al., 1985).

Before terminating treatment prematurely, patients probably weigh the costs and benefits of dropping out versus remaining in treatment. Patients in residential treatment may consider the quality of the family and work settings to which they will return. If these settings are more attractive than treatment, patients may be more likely to terminate treatment. Consistent with this idea, Reynolds and his colleagues (1982) reported that patients who did not complete a treatment regimen saw their families as more cohesive and organized and more concerned with recreational activities and moral-religious issues than did completers. Knowledge of patients' life contexts may help program evaluators to model and predict patients' decisions about leaving or staying in treatment better. It may also help to identify patients for whom early treatment termination may not signal a poor prognosis.

With respect to theoretical content, we need to consider how patient, treatment, and life context factors promote or inhibit patients' *treatment* integration and *social* integration within a program. Most studies of patient attrition focus on variables that hinder treatment integration, such

IMPLICATIONS FOR TREATMENT AND PROGRAM EVALUATION

as a cognitive orientation that slows down learning during treatment, or barriers to quick treatment entry, such as a waiting period.

Treatment integration also can be estimated by identifying the type of treatment milieu a client expects at intake. If a client's expectations are discrepant from the actual program, an orientation before entry could correct them. Similarly, a client could be asked about the treatment he or she expects and appropriate information could be given to counter discrepant expectations. In this regard, Velleman (1984) found that expectations were matched less well for dropouts than for patients who remained in treatment. Similarly, Rees (1985) reported that longer-term patients were more satisfied than dropouts with what a psychiatrist had told them about their problem, its cause, the planned treatment, and the likely outcome.

Velleman's (1984) study also highlights the importance of social integration. Residents of a halfway house who left the program prematurely were more dissatisfied with the level of privacy, felt that opportunities outside the program were better than those in treatment, and rated staff less positively. Staff rated treatment dropouts less positively, liked them less, and spent less time with them. Similarly, we found that men who dropped out of the Salvation Army program saw the treatment milieu as less involving, supportive, clear, and well organized than did those who remained (Chapter 4). With early identification of patients who feel socially remote, treatment staff could take steps to facilitate their integration and thereby reduce attrition.

Participation in Aftercare. We have emphasized the importance of aftercare as an integral part of effective alcoholism treatment (see also Ahles et al., 1983; Ito & Donovan, 1986; Walker et al., 1983), but we know very little about the determinants of participation in aftercare. As in studies of dropout, researchers have focused primarily on patient personal characteristics as predictors; research on aftercare should also consider treatment and life context factors.

We know of only one study relating treatment characteristics and participation in aftercare. Pratt and his colleagues (1977) studied an aftercare reentry group for alcoholic patients. Patients who participated in the group had reported more independence in the social climate of the inpatient program in which they were treated. Attenders also experienced somewhat more emphasis on self-understanding and the expression of anger. Alcoholic patients who see a treatment program as encouraging independence, self-exploration, and the open expression of personal feelings may be more likely to participate in aftercare services offered by that program.

A great deal remains to be learned about why problem drinkers enter treatment and about the factors that determine the programs they select and the treatment they obtain. Naturalistic studies can clarify this issue by examining the relationship of patients' personal and life context characteristics to treatment selection and assignment. Learning more about treatment selection is important in its own right; in addition, more knowledge about these processes may enable us to estimate better between- and within-program treatment effects in naturalistic studies, as described later in this chapter.

Theories of Treatment Processes

A theory of treatment specifies the techniques or procedures to be applied to bring about desired outcomes. In some cases, the theory may indicate the processes or mechanisms through which change can be effected. Treatment theories identify the program components to be examined in an analysis of treatment implementation and treatment processes.

Some treatment theories specify relevant intervening variables or processes that mediate treatment effects. For example, the treatment theory espoused by AA focuses on bringing the client to accept an "alcoholic" identity and to acknowledge loss of control over drinking behavior. Evaluations of programs guided by AA principles could be strengthened by measuring these intervening variables. A process analysis could indicate if outcome is better for clients who see themselves as "alcoholics" who have lost control over drinking. By examining the influence of AA on intervening factors and the ultimate outcome of abstinence, the evaluation could probe both the program's effects and its underlying theory. If the ultimate outcome is not being achieved, the evaluator can try to isolate whether this is due to a failure of treatment to affect relevant intervening variables or a failure of theory, that is, a positive outcome is not achieved even though relevant intervening variables are affected.

Another pattern the evaluator might uncover is that the ultimate outcome is achieved even though the presumed relevant intervening variables are not affected in the manner expected. Such findings point to the need to modify the theory. For example, Beck and his colleagues (1979) developed a cognitive theory of depression: people who attribute the causes of stressful life circumstances to internal, stable, and global factors are more likely to become depressed. They also developed a cognitive theory of treatment, which posits that changes in these "depressogenic" attributions will help to alleviate depression. Subsequently, several controlled evaluations showed that cognitive treatment led to significant improvement in depression. When evaluation researchers measured the presumed mediators of improvement, however, they found that patients treated with noncognitive approaches (such as behavioral skills training or antidepressant medication) showed as much change in cognitive attributions as did patients in cognitive treatment. These process-oriented studies are leading to new causal mediational models of the role of cognition in the etiology and course of depression (Hollon et al., 1987).

If the treatment theory is not well articulated, the evaluator can help treatment providers specify the process of treatment by using a "cause map" (Lipsey & Pollard, 1989; Weick & Bougon, 1986). A cause map graphically depicts treatment providers' beliefs about cause-effect relationships in their program. Providers describe their beliefs about important program features, aspects of patients, aspects of treatment providers and their activities, and theories of how positive outcomes are achieved. When a consensus regarding key program features is reached, providers are asked to specify pairs or small sets of program variables that influence each other. From these causal attributions, an evaluator pieces together the overall causal network, encompassing the program's operations and effects. This approach also reveals the extent of agreement among treatment providers about the nature of the treatment model.

Theories of the Nature and Course of the Disorder

Theories of alcohol abuse fall into at least two classes: etiologic theories and relapse theories. Etiologic theories specify the factors responsible for the onset and persistence of a disorder, whereas relapse theories point to factors responsible for the resumption of the disorder after remission. Both classes of theories focus on factors that may cause maladaptive states and the conditions that alter individual vulnerability to such causal agents.

Some etiologic theories may be extended to explain relapses. For example, stress and coping theory may help to explain the process of remission and relapse after treatment as well as the development of alcohol abuse. Other aspects of relapse theories may stand somewhat apart from etiological considerations. Thus, Marlatt and Gordon (1985) focus on cognitive and behavioral reactions to "slips" or failures to maintain control over drinking behavior once control has been achieved. Either type of theory can guide the identification of patient and life context factors that may influence outcome.

In contrast to the paucity of theories of treatment selection, many theories of alcohol abuse are available to guide alcoholism treatment evaluations. These theories cut across a number of disciplines and include genetic and physiological theories (e.g., Tarter et al., 1985) and sociocultural theories (Jessor et al., 1968; Seeman & Anderson, 1983). In fact, Blane and Leonard (1987) have compiled a volume devoted only to various psychological theories of alcohol abuse. Whenever an evaluation focuses on multiple treatment programs with divergent treatment philosophies, a theory of the disorder provides a way to guide the multisite research within a single theoretical perspective—something not possible if the different treatment processes were modeled.

Our evaluation of five divergent residential treatment programs was guided by a stress and coping theory of alcoholism. Our findings imply that life stressors are a significant component of one or more of the combinations of factors that may produce alcohol abuse or precipitate relapse. However, stressors alone are neither necessary nor sufficient to lead to either alcohol abuse or relapse. Personal and social resources must also be considered. This complex, interactive situation implies that the influence of any one set of factors, such as stressors, is likely to be modest.

Given the multivariate nature of alcohol abuse and the heterogeneity of alcohol abusers, one theory of this disorder may never provide a full explanatory account. Instead, we may need several theories to account for the range and intensity of symptoms found in the entire population of alcohol-abusing and alcohol-dependent persons. These theories would specify different combinations of factors that could lead to or perpetuate alcohol abuse.

THE METHODOLOGY OF EVALUATION RESEARCH

Having considered some implications of the expanded paradigm for theories to guide the selection of variables in evaluation research, we turn to the methodological implications of the paradigm. We focus on implications for research design, outcome assessment, and cost analyses.

Research Design

A basic methodological question that evaluators face is whether to use an experimental or a naturalistic research design. For many, the answer is obvious—choose a true experiment with random assignment of patients to treatment or control conditions.

Experimental Designs

Random assignment to experimental conditions provides estimates of treatment effects that have high internal validity, that is, one can be reasonably confident that an observed treatment effect is a causal one. For this reason, experiments have been described as the "Cadillacs" of research designs for program evaluations (Hatry, Winnie, & Fisk, 1973). Like Cadillacs, experiments are expensive and best suited to travel on straight "superhighways" that are "paved" with strong logistical support. They typically focus on a single research question: How effective is the treatment package, on average?

It is possible to extend this analogy further. An additional feature of Cadillacs is that they are equipped with a "cruise control" that allows the driver to sit back and let the car drive itself. The driver is not required to use this feature, but it is very seductive. Because experiments, whether or not they are grounded in a theory, generate estimates of treatment effects that have high internal validity, many evaluators are content to sit back and let the research design rather than theoretical propositions drive their studies (Chen & Rossi, 1983). The "pride of ownership" derived from employing the Cadillac of research designs may reinforce this tendency.

It is possible for experimental evaluations to examine a theory of treatment or of the focal problem or disorder. However, evaluators using ex-

IMPLICATIONS FOR TREATMENT AND PROGRAM EVALUATION 239

perimental designs often must devote the bulk of their finite resources to fulfilling the logistical demands of implementing and monitoring a true experiment in a field setting. Consequently, fewer resources are available to develop a theoretical framework, construct or select measures to tap relevant variables, obtain data on more representative samples, and conduct multivariate analyses to probe theoretical implications. In short, a Cadillac can be fitted with special equipment for "off the road" excursions, but this equipment adds additional costs to an already expensive vehicle.

When theoretical propositions (or the effects of within-group treatment differences such as length of stay) are examined within the context of an experiment, *non*experimental (correlational) methods typically are employed. For example, Rossi and his coworkers (1980) used an experimental design to determine that a program providing monetary aid to newly released prisoners had no significant impact on recidivism. Using correlational causal modeling techniques, they found that the monetary aid had a direct "effect" of reducing property crime but an indirect effect of increasing property crime by decreasing the incentive to obtain employment. These two counteracting forces resulted in no significant overall impact for the program. On the basis of these correlational findings, Rossi and his colleagues suggested changes in the program to reduce the employment disincentive.

Some evaluators may feel distressed at the prospect of coupling an experiment with exploratory approaches to data analysis. They can take comfort from the way in which the father of experimental methods, R.A. Fisher, sought to explain wheat yield in terms of bushels per acre.

> He found that after he controlled variety, and fertilizer, there was considerable variation from year to year. . . . Now Fisher set himself on the trail of the residual variation. . . . [H]e started reading the records of the plots and found weeds a possible factor. He considered the nature of each species of weed and found that the response of specific weed varieties to rainfall and cultivation accounted for much of the cycle. But the large trends were not explained until he showed that the upsurge of weeds after 1875 coincided with a school-attendance act which removed cheap labor from the fields, and another cycle that coincided with the retirement of a superintendent who made weed removal his personal concern.(Edwards & Cronbach, 1952, p. 58)

Fisher's actions are consistent with our approach of analyzing the influence of life context on treatment outcome. As we noted earlier (Moos, Finney, & Cronkite, 1980), "farmers do not apply fertilizer to their crops and then retire from the field to await the harvest without thought to cultivation, irrigation, insect management, and weed control," and "astute agricultural researchers, like Fisher, would not attempt to evaluate the impact of fertilizer without taking into account . . . subsequent environmental events" (p. 350). Farmers and Fisher provide good role models for alcoholism treatment providers and evaluators.

Another benefit of embedding an experimental evaluation in a theoretical framework relates to the original purpose of using an experimental design. Random assignment probabilistically equates experimental groups on preexisting characteristics, but it does not remove the within-group relationships of patient characteristics, life context factors, or treatment variations to outcome. By controlling for variables that are related to outcome within treatment groups (such as in an analysis of covariance), the evaluator can generate more powerful estimates of between-group treatment effects (Boruch & Gomez, 1979; Chen & Rossi, 1983).

Naturalistic Designs

But what of the evaluator who decides to use a naturalistic design in order to study other important processes or issues in addition to treatment effects, or to enhance external validity? How is he or she to estimate the effects of treatment in the absence of random assignment of patients to experimental groups? In this situation, theory is crucial (Cordray, 1986).

In principle, either of two approaches can be used to achieve unbiased estimates of treatment effects in naturalistic studies (Cronbach, 1982): apply a valid theory of treatment selection or a theory of the disorder. When the variables that determine either treatment selection or posttreatment functioning are controlled, the effects of treatment can be gauged without bias. It is not sufficient to match persons on or statistically adjust for a few demographic or pretreatment functioning variables. Instead, a valid theory of either treatment selection or the course of the disorder is required to identify the relevant variables to be assessed and controlled. By estimating treatment effects from both treatment selection and posttreatment functioning models, an evaluator can determine the consistency of the treatment effect estimates that are generated. If the findings are similar, the evaluator can be more confident of having accurately estimated the treatment effect.

Given the current level of knowledge about the determinants of treatment selection and of posttreatment functioning in the substance abuse and mental health fields, no model of either process is likely to produce unbiased estimates of treatment effects. In most situations, the more pragmatic approach is to use theory to guide nonexperimental analyses whose findings may buttress a logical argument regarding the effect of the intervention. At its best, such an approach would proceed in two stages. First, treatment implementation analyses guided by program theory (and/or normative or ideal standards—see Sechrest et al., 1979) would be applied to establish that a viable, reasonably strong intervention had been offered. This stage of the analysis "rules in" the intervention as a plausible explanation of postintervention "effects" (Cordray, 1986).

In the second stage, the three-step analysis outlined by Baron and Kenny (1986) could be used to examine a treatment process theory in more detail. The linkages between treatment received and presumed mediating variables would be analyzed first to see if the intervention produced the intermediate changes thought to be necessary to achieve the

IMPLICATIONS FOR TREATMENT AND PROGRAM EVALUATION

ultimate outcomes. Then, the linkages between mediators and the ultimate outcomes would be examined. Finally, one would determine if the initial treatment effect was reduced or eliminated when the mediating variables specified by the treatment process theory were controlled. To the extent that the analyses support the causal chain specified by the theory, one has more confidence that the treatment is exerting an impact.

Assessing Treatment Outcome

Our findings and the expanded paradigm have a number of implications for the measurement of outcome criteria. The multidimensionality of alcohol abuse necessitates broad-spectrum diagnoses and intervention programs; outcome indices should encompass the major aspects of patients' alcohol-related, physical, psychological, and social functioning. In addition, the full influence of treatment can be gauged more accurately when outcome indices also focus on patients' family members and social contexts. We want to underscore two additional issues here: the timing of outcome assessment and the congruence between outcome indices and treatment emphases.

In the traditional paradigm, outcomes are often measured long after participation in the intervention because the evaluation is geared toward finding out whether the program succeeded in some ultimate sense. Given a focus on intervening life context factors, however, it is apparent that to test "the effect of a program on a distant variable that is subject to dozens of other influences invites a negative report" (Cronbach, 1982, p. 223).

In contrast, assessing treatment outcome at program termination and at two or more follow-ups should identify both immediate treatment effects and the extent to which they are altered by patients' posttreatment experiences. A treatment component might improve psychological functioning within the protective confines of a residential program but not prepare patients to cope with the stressors of daily life. Similarly, a multipoint assessment of outcome enables an evaluator to identify lagged or "sleeper" effects. Training in role skills may lead to long-term improvement even though it has little immediate benefit. Assessments at the end of treatment help evaluators identify changes that occurred during treatment; later follow-ups help estimate the maintenance and generalization of such changes.

A related issue is the importance of matching outcome indicators to treatment components. For example, the effectiveness of family and group therapy might be evaluated on indicators of family and interpersonal functioning, whereas the efficacy of aversion conditioning might be tested by the ability to maintain abstinence or nonproblem drinking. We noted earlier that clients treated in the halfway house program, which emphasized individual and group counseling, did better than expected in social functioning but showed just average improvement in drinking-related outcome (Chapter 4). By conceptualizing a program as a group of treatment components linked to different outcome indicators, evaluators may be able to estimate treatment effects more precisely.

Cost Analyses

The demand for accountability in health care delivery has increased the use of cost analyses in program evaluations. Cost analyses fall into three major categories. Cost-effectiveness analysis compares the costs in different programs of achieving the same outcome—for example, one person who is abstinent for 12 months. Cost-benefit analysis tries to place a monetary value both on the resources expended or foregone to have a patient participate in a treatment program and on the benefits of treatment. Finally, cost-utility analysis recognizes that programs have multiple effects; different stakeholders (such as treatment providers, patients, patients' relatives) weight specific outcome dimensions, which are then combined to yield a global index (Levin, 1987).

Cost analyses are an important new aspect of the expanding paradigm of evaluation research. Like other aspects of the paradigm, they can enhance the utility of evaluation findings (Levin, 1987; McCrady et al., 1986). By focusing not only on the effects of program alternatives but also on the cost of resources needed to achieve them, such analyses provide decision makers with important information. Cost analyses can also point to positive but modest program effects that represent large benefits relative to costs. For example, low-cost outpatient alcoholism treatment may produce only a small proportion of remissions over a 6-month interval; nevertheless, it may prove cost effective when its full benefits, such as increased time at work, greater productivity, and reduced marital violence, are taken into account.

The press for cost analyses should increase the extent to which some of the other aspects of the expanded paradigm are included in program evaluations. The effort to identify the cost of units of service should increase the data available on patient participation in specific treatment components, which will facilitate treatment implementation and treatment process analyses. On the benefits side, efforts to identify the broader benefits of treatment may enhance the likelihood of an analysis of the impact of alcoholism treatment on a diverse array of outcome criteria and on patients' families.

THE EXPANDED PARADIGM AND RESEARCH ON PATIENT-TREATMENT MATCHING

In evaluations of alcoholism treatment programs, much of the variance in outcome measures typically remains unexplained after the "main effects" of patient, treatment, and even life context factors have been examined. Consequently, many reports of such evaluations end with a call for re-

IMPLICATIONS FOR TREATMENT AND PROGRAM EVALUATION

search on matching patients and treatments. At best, any single treatment approach, like any specific etiological factor, is only one component of a combination of factors that may produce remission. Other combinations of factors, some without any treatment element, also may produce remission. A particular treatment approach is likely to be effective only in combination with specific personal and environmental characteristics of patients. As such, its main or linear effects are likely to be modest.

Theory and Patient-Treatment Matching

Only a few studies in the alcoholism field have identified significant patient-treatment interaction effects, perhaps because most of the other research has lacked guidance from appropriate theory. McLachlan (1974) used conceptual systems theory to identify alcoholic patients' cognitive abilities and styles and to characterize different degrees of "structure" in inpatient treatment and aftercare. Although no main effects were found for patient conceptual level or treatment structure, there was an important interaction effect. Of patients matched with both inpatient and aftercare services (i.e., low conceptual level patients with structured treatments; high conceptual level patients with less structured treatments), 77% were rated as recovered at a 12- to 16-month follow-up. For mismatched patients, however, only 38% were in the recovered category.

Studies of patient-treatment matching, like treatment evaluations in general, tend to be more useful when embedded in a theoretical framework (Finney & Moos, 1986). Like the etiologic theories for many health disorders, etiologic theories of alcohol abuse have progressed from "formistic" (either-or) and "mechanistic" (single cause) stages to more complex "contextual" (context-dependent) and "organistic" (interactive) stages (Schwartz, 1982). The trend in alcoholism etiologic theories to develop more complex, interactive perspectives bodes well for studies of patient-treatment matching. Mechanistic or single-cause theories tend to produce prescriptions for a single treatment approach. The movement toward more organistic theories may make it easier to formulate theoretical implications for differential treatment. Instead of piecing together differential treatment prescriptions from two or more etiologic theories, researchers and practitioners may be able to develop more systematic and powerful prescriptive treatments from a single, integrated theoretical system.

As an example, stress and coping theory suggests one approach to matching patients with treatments. Alcohol abusers can be assessed to determine how much of their distress is a result of internally or externally imposed demands. If a patient is distressed because of self-imposed performance standards, he or she can be taught self-reinforcement and relaxation skills. If the patient's distress is due to pressures in the environment, he or she can be taught assertive coping responses to try to alleviate those pressures (Abrams, 1983).

When well-developed theories are not readily available, exploratory analyses can play an important role in the search for effective prescriptive treatment approaches. Such analyses can trigger fruitful theoretical insights and yield findings that can be examined more rigorously in a later study. The work of McLellan and his colleagues (McLellan, Luborsky, et al., 1983; McLellan, Woody, et al., 1983) illustrates the productive application of this process.

In the first stage of their research, they tried unsuccessfully to identify patient-treatment interactions among drug- and alcohol-abusing patients assigned to one of six inpatient or outpatient treatment programs. However, the severity of patients' psychiatric disorders predicted poorer outcome across programs. This finding led the researchers to explore patient-treatment interactions at different levels of psychiatric impairment. Patients with less severe psychiatric problems did well in each program, whereas patients with more severe psychiatric problems consistently did poorly. However, patients who had psychiatric problems of intermediate severity (60% of the sample) seemed to respond differentially to different types of treatment.

McLellan, Woody, and their co-workers (1983) used these results to design and prospectively evaluate a patient-treatment matching system. For example, they assigned patients with psychiatric and employment problems of intermediate severity to one of several inpatient programs, but not to an outpatient program. They tried to assign every new patient to an appropriate treatment condition; only 53% of the patients (62% of the alcohol-dependent patients) could be matched, however. The major reason for mismatched patients was lack of an available slot in the appropriate program (27% of mismatches). Only 13% of the patients refused or were unable to accept the assigned treatment program.

Compared to the mismatched alcohol-dependent patients, the matched patients had better 6-month outcomes in multiple areas: family relations, employment, medical condition, legal status, and drug abuse. These results illustrate the promise of patient-treatment matching. They also suggest that patient-treatment matching may be a complex process involving higher-order interactions among multiple variables, such as psychiatric severity, stressors and resources in different life areas, and treatment modality.

Treatment, Life Context Factors, and Patient-Treatment Matching

The expanded evaluation paradigm has other implications for matching efforts and for evaluating the effectiveness of differential treatment. With respect to treatment implementation, the paradigm points to the need to determine how well distinctive differential treatments are actually realized at the aggregate or program level (Skinner, 1981b). At the individual patient level, the strength of each treatment should be ensured so that an appropriate test of the matching hypothesis can be conducted. For ex-

IMPLICATIONS FOR TREATMENT AND PROGRAM EVALUATION

ample, if learning new skills (such as coping with relapse-inducing situations) or concepts (such as an "alcoholic" self-identity) is part of the treatment, the evaluator should establish that individual patients acquire them. The evaluator will probably need to consider differences in patients' information-processing abilities and coping styles. In short, some *within*-treatment matching of patient characteristics with therapeutic and treatment delivery efforts may be necessary to ensure adequate aggregate treatment implementation, a precondition for a powerful test of differential effectiveness *between* treatments for different patient types.

Finally, information on life context factors may enhance attempts to match patients and treatments. For example, among young adults who are not physically dependent on alcohol, the outcome of programs oriented toward abstinence versus moderate drinking might vary with the extent of social pressure to drink encountered by the patients (Polich et al., 1981). Moreover, the impact of matching patients' cognitive levels and treatment structure might be strengthened by changing the structure of patients' life contexts. Procedures such as those employed by Azrin and his associates (1982) in their community reinforcement program could increase the organization of the life contexts of low conceptual level clients. In addition, data on life context factors can be incorporated in process analyses, so that researchers can begin to understand *why* (through what causal mechanisms) patient-treatment interactions occur.

THE UTILITY OF TREATMENT EVALUATIONS

As we have shown, one important benefit from applying the expanded paradigm is the enhanced usefulness of findings from evaluation research. The findings can be used "instrumentally" to develop and improve intervention programs as well as "conceptually" to change how people think about programs and their impacts and/or the disorder the programs are intended to remedy (Weiss, 1978).

Developing and Improving Programs

An implementation assessment may reveal that all the components of an apparently strong treatment program have not been delivered, that treatment activity is not of high quality, or that clients do not attend to or comprehend all treatment components. Efforts can then be made to remedy the situation. In Chapter 11, we described some data-based feedback procedures to accomplish such program changes. Similarly, if process analyses identify especially effective treatment components, more resources can be concentrated on them and less effective components can be deemphasized.

In addition, evaluations that consider life context and coping factors may yield information that can help to identify high-risk patients and develop new intervention strategies. As we noted earlier, intervention programs can focus on promoting social support in family and other community settings, enhancing personal resources such as self-reliance and resourcefulness, and teaching cognitive and behavioral coping skills to help clients deal with stressful situations more effectively.

Determining the Generalizability of Findings

Much of the literature on evaluation research design has emphasized internal validity, or the confidence with which we can infer a causal relationship between treatment and outcome (Cook & Campbell, 1979). However, Cronbach and his colleagues (1980) have argued that external validity—"the validity of inferences that go beyond the data—is the crux in social action" (p. 231). Decision makers need to know to what extent the results of an evaluation can be expected to generalize to new situations in which the program may be implemented.

Traditionally, discussions of how to estimate the generalizability of evaluation findings have reflected a "similarity" approach. In other words, to decide whether reported findings might generalize to a new situation, program managers compare the patients, treatment context, and treatment providers in the reported research and the projected site. However, the ability to make such comparisons is constrained by the sparse information on these topics usually provided in research reports. In addition, one often has no way of knowing if the patient variables on which data are reported (such as demographic characteristics) actually influence the outcome of a given treatment approach.

Knowledge of the causal mechanisms through which the treatment exerts its effects provides a much sounder basis from which to draw inferences of generalizability. By knowing the causal process involved, a treatment provider can gauge if that process (1) can be replicated in a particular setting with a particular staff and (2) addresses specific deficits or draws on specific resources possessed by the patients in the new program. If both conditions are met, the provider has more confidence that the reported effects will generalize to the proposed site. Regarding this approach to generalizability evaluation, Weiss (1972) concluded that "it is in probing the theoretical premises of the program that evaluation can ultimately become most practical"(p. 84).

Changing Concepts about the Program or the Disorder Being Treated

Information obtained from program evaluations may help to expand and refine how treatment providers and program administrators conceive of the intervention or the disorder to which it is directed. With respect to thinking about interventions, two characteristics are apparent in the expanded paradigm shown in Figure 1.2. First, treatment is the central focus, as is appropriate for an evaluation. Second, treatment is in the context of multiple prior and subsequent patient and life context factors. "It is the individual's day-to-day world and the decisions he or she makes to accommodate to it or to change it that are primary, and it is within that framework that expert treatment plays its modest role" (Orford, 1985, p. 269).

By putting treatment in proper perspective, the expanded paradigm provides program administrators and clinicians more realistic expectations about the impact they may have on their clients. If communicated effectively to funding sources, such expectations should provide a more rational baseline for judging program effectiveness. In addition, realistic expectations about therapeutic impact should give treatment providers more satisfaction from patients' modest and time-constrained improvements.

Another important conceptual use of evaluation findings (Weiss, 1978) is to shape or reorient how policymakers and program developers think about the problem or behavior that required the intervention in the first place. For a long time, alcohol abuse was thought to be a chronic condition with "internal" determinants. However, the Rand Corporation's evaluation of alcoholism treatment (Polich et al., 1981) provided new descriptive information on the natural course of treated alcoholism. Consistent with earlier findings on generally untreated problem drinkers, the Rand researchers discovered that the drinking behavior of many severely symptomatic alcoholics fluctuated widely over time. Such findings suggest that individual alcoholics may be responding to environmental factors such as social pressure to drink, social controls over drinking, and life stressors and social resources. As we noted earlier, such findings provide some basis for optimism that treatment programs can have at least short-term impacts.

Enhancing the Role of Evaluation Researchers

It is traditional to view the utility of research findings or of an evaluation model from the perspective of the consumer of the research. However, the expanded paradigm also has utility for evaluation researchers themselves. In the summative paradigm, evaluators perform an ill-fated role as judge, attempting to monitor how well a program meets externally determined performance standards. The psychological bankruptcy of this isolated judgmental role led Patton (1978, p. 49) to comment that "to evaluate is to do unto others as you would *not* have them do unto you." In contrast, the expanded paradigm allows evaluators to play more fulfilling "instrumental" and "conceptual" roles. We have indicated how the expanded paradigm affords evaluators the opportunity to act as change agents by generating findings that can be used to reformulate programs. The conceptual utility of findings that can be generated within the expanded framework also allows evaluators to help educate administrators and staff (Cronbach et al., 1980).

Evaluators stand at the interface between a treatment program and the external administrative and societal context. Their role is distinct from that of clinicians who provide direct treatment services and from administrators who manage programs. By shaping evaluation foci and using their expertise about treatment program and conceptual and theoretical issues, evaluators can foster communication between clinicians and administrators and help both to fulfill their functions better. These active roles give evaluators more stable short-term rewards, enhance the intellectual challenge of their work, and enable them to contribute to the development of effective treatment programs as well as to the advancement of basic knowledge in the behavioral and social sciences (Moos & Finney, 1985b).

CONCLUSION

After surveying the state of alcoholism treatment, Edwards (1980) argued that "the potential and meaning of what is in many ways a crisis, should not be lost." He noted that "the whole alcoholism treatment field now has about it a great sense of potential for change and movement" (p. 319). Adherence to an oversimplified biomedical model of alcoholism and an atheoretical paradigm of evaluation research has contributed to this crisis; a broader biopsychosocial orientation and reliance on an expanded paradigm of evaluation research can help to resolve it.

The expanded paradigm reflects an increased emphasis on the implementation and process of treatment. In addition, it considers life context factors by embedding an evaluation in a theory of the treatment process or of the disorder. As such, it can help to isolate sources of program failure and of decay in treatment gains and to formulate ways to improve treatment. This evaluation paradigm affords the opportunity for greater insight into the mechanisms through which treatment exerts its effects, better understanding of other factors that contribute to recovery and relapse, and an enriched data base with which to develop more effective treatment programs oriented toward clients' normal life situations. Movement in these directions should benefit both individual patients and society in the effort to reduce alcohol abuse and its harmful effects.

References

Abrams, D. B. (1983). Psycho-social assessment of alcohol and stress interactions: Bridging the gap between laboratory and treatment outcome research. In L. A. Pohrecky & J. Brick (Eds.), *Stress and alcohol use* (pp. 61–86). New York: Elsevier.

Adler, R., & Raphael, B. (1983). Children of alcoholics. *Australian and New Zealand Journal of Psychiatry, 17,* 3–8.

Ahles, T. A., Schlundt, D. G., Prue, D. M., & Rychtarik, R. G. (1983). Impact of aftercare arrangements on the maintenance of treatment success in abusive drinkers. *Addictive Behaviors, 8,* 53–58.

Albrecht, O. L., & Higgins, P. C. (1977). Rehabilitation success: The interrelationships of multiple criteria. *Journal of Health and Social Behavior, 18,* 36–45.

American Psychiatric Association (1987). *Diagnostic and statistical manual of mental disorders* (3rd ed., rev.). Washington, DC: American Psychiatric Association.

Aneshensel, C. S., Frerichs, R. R., & Clark, V. A. (1981). Family roles and sex differences in depression. *Journal of Health and Social Behavior, 22,* 379–393.

Annis, H. M. (1980). Treatment of alcoholic women. In G. Edwards & M. Grant (Eds.), *Alcoholism treatment in transition* (pp. 128–139). Baltimore: University Park Press.

Annis, H. M., & Liban, C. B. (1980). Alcoholism in women: Treatment modalities and outcomes. In O. Kalant (Ed.), *Research advances in alcohol and drug problems* (Vol. 5, pp. 385–422). New York: Plenum.

Armor, D., Polich, J., & Stambul, H. (1978). *Alcoholism and treatment.* New York: Wiley.

Azrin, N. H. (1976). Improvements in the community-reinforcement approach to alcoholism. *Behavior Research and Therapy, 14,* 339–348.

Azrin, N. H., Sisson, R. W., Meyers, R., & Godley, M. (1982). Alcoholism treatment by disulfiram and community reinforcement therapy. *Journal of Behavioral Therapy and Experimental Psychiatry, 13,* 105–112.

Babor, T. F., Dolinsky, Z., Rounsaville, B., & Jaffe, J. (1988). Unitary versus multidimensional models of alcoholism treatment outcome: An empirical study. *Journal of Studies on Alcohol, 49,* 167–177.

Babor, T., Mendelson, J., Uhly, B., & Souza, E. (1980). Drinking patterns in experimental and barroom settings. *Journal of Studies on Alcohol, 41,* 635–651.

Babor, T. F., Stephens, R. S., & Marlatt, G. A. (1987). Verbal report methods in clinical research on alcoholism: Response bias and its minimization. *Journal of Studies on Alcohol, 48,* 410–424.

Bader, E. (1982). Redecisions in family therapy: A study of change in an intensive family therapy workshop. *Transactional Analysis Journal, 12,* 27–38.

Baer, P. E., Garmezy, L. B., McLaughlin, R. J., Pokorny, A. D., & Wernick, M. J. (1987). Stress, coping, family conflict, and adolescent alcohol use. *Journal of Behavioral Medicine, 10,* 449–466.

Baron, R. M., & Kenny, D. A. (1986). The moderator-mediator variable distinction in social psychological research: Conceptual, strategic, and statistical considerations. *Journal of Personality and Social Psychology, 51,* 1173–1182.

Barr, H. L., Antes, D., Ottenberg, D. J., & Rosen, A. (1984). Mortality of treated alcoholics and drug addicts: The benefits of abstinence. *Journal of Studies on Alcohol, 45,* 440–452.

Beardslee, W. R., Bemporad, J., Keller, M. B., & Klerman, G. L. (1983). Children of parents with major affective disorder: A review. *American Journal of Psychiatry, 140,* 825–832.

Beck, A. T., Rush, A. J., Shaw, B. F., & Emery, G. (1979). *Cognitive therapy of depression: A treatment manual.* New York: Guilford Press.

Beckman, L. J. (1975). Women alcoholics: A review of social and psychological studies. *Journal of Studies on Alcohol, 36,* 797–824.

Beckman, L. J., & Amaro, H. (1984). Patterns of women's use of alcohol treatment agencies. In S. C. Wilsnack & L. J. Beckman (Eds.), *Alcohol problems in women* (pp. 319–348). New York: Guilford Press.

Beckman, L. J., & Amaro, H. (1986). Personal and social difficulties faced by women and men entering alcoholism treatment. *Journal of Studies on Alcohol, 47,* 135–145.

Beckman, L. J., & Kocel, K. M. (1982). The treatment-delivery system and alcohol abuse in women: Social policy implications. *Journal of Social Issues, 38,* 139–151.

Bell, M. (1983). The perceived social environment of a therapeutic community for drug abusers. *International Journal of Therapeutic Communities, 4,* 262–270.

Bell, M. (1985). Three therapeutic communities for drug abusers: Differences in treatment environments. *Journal of the Addictions, 20,* 1523–1531.

Bell, M., & Ryan, E. (1985). Where can therapeutic community ideals be realized? An examination of three treatment environments. *Hospital and Community Psychiatry, 36,* 1286–1291.

Benson, C. S., & Heller, K. (1987). Factors in the current adjustment of young, adult daughters of alcoholic and problem-drinking fathers. *Journal of Abnormal Psychology, 96,* 305–312.

REFERENCES

Berglund, M., & Tunving, K. (1985). Assaultive alcoholics 20 years later. *Acta Psychiatrica Scandinavica, 71,* 141–147.

Bergstrom, B., Ohlin, H., Lindblom, P. E., & Wadstein, J. (1982). Is disulfiram implantation effective? *Lancet, 1,* 49–50.

Bickman, L. (1986). The functions of program theory. In L. Bickman (Ed.), *Using program theory in evaluation: New directions for program evaluation* (Vol. 33, pp. 5–18). San Francisco: Jossey-Bass.

Biernacki, P. (1986). *Pathways from heroin addiction: Recovery without treatment.* Philadelphia: Temple University Press.

Billings, A., Cronkite, R., & Moos, R. (1983). Social environmental factors in unipolar depression: Comparisons of depressed patients and nondepressed controls. *Journal of Abnormal Psychology, 92,* 119–133.

Billings, A., Cronkite, R., & Moos, R. (1985). Difficulty of follow-up and post-treatment functioning among depressed patients. *Journal of Affective Disorders, 8,* 9–16.

Billings, A., & Moos, R. (1982a). Family environments and adaptation: A clinically applicable typology. *American Journal of Family Therapy, 10,* 26–38.

Billings, A., & Moos, R. (1982b). Social support and functioning among community and clinical groups: A panel model. *Journal of Behavioral Medicine, 5,* 295–311.

Billings, A., & Moos, R. (1982c). Work stress and the stress-buffering roles of work and family resources. *Journal of Occupational Behavior, 3,* 215–232.

Billings, A., & Moos, R. (1983a). Comparisons of children of depressed and non-depressed parents: A social-environmental perspective. *Journal of Abnormal Child Psychology, 11,* 463–485.

Billings, A., & Moos, R. (1983b). Psychosocial processes of recovery among alcoholics and their families: Implications for clinicians and program evaluators. *Addictive Behaviors, 8,* 205–218.

Billings, A., & Moos, R. (1984a). Chronic and nonchronic unipolar depression: The differential role of environmental stressors and resources. *Journal of Nervous and Mental Disease, 172,* 65–75.

Billings, A., & Moos, R. (1984b). Treatment experiences of adults with unipolar depression: The influence of patient and life context factors. *Journal of Consulting and Clinical Psychology, 52,* 119–131.

Billings, A., & Moos, R. (1985a). Life stressors and social resources affect post-treatment outcomes among depressed patients. *Journal of Abnormal Psychology, 94,* 140–153.

Billings, A., & Moos, R. (1985b). Psychosocial processes of remission in unipolar depression: Comparing depressed patients with matched community controls. *Journal of Consulting and Clinical Psychology, 53,* 314–325.

Billings, A., & Moos, R. (1986). Children of parents with unipolar depression: A controlled 1-year follow-up. *Journal of Abnormal Child Psychology, 14,* 149–166.

Blane, H. T., & Leonard, K. E. (Eds.) (1987). *Psychological theories of drinking and alcoholism.* New York: Guilford Press.

Blumberg, L., Shipley T. E., Jr., & Shandler, I. W. (1973). *Skid row and its alternatives: Research and recommendations from Philadelphia.* Philadelphia: Temple University Press.

Blume, S. B. (1980). Researchers on women and alcohol. In *Alcoholism and alcohol abuse among women: Research issues* (NIAAA Research Monograph No. 1, U.S. Department of Health, Education, and Public Welfare Publication No. ADM-80-835). Washington, DC: U.S. Government Printing Office.

Boruch, R. F., & Gomez, H. (1979). Measuring impact: Power theory in social program evaluation. In L. Datta & R. Perloff (Eds.), *Improving evaluations* (pp. 139–170). Beverly Hills, CA: Sage.

Bourne, P. G., & Light, E. (1979). Alcohol problems in blacks and women. In J. H. Mendelson & N. K. Mello (Eds.), *The diagnosis and treatment of alcoholism* (pp. 83–123). New York: McGraw-Hill.

Brady, C. A., & Ambler, J. (1982). Use of group educational techniques with remarried couples. In J. Hansen & L. Messinger (Eds.), *Therapy with remarriage families* (pp. 145–157). Rockville, MD: Aspen Publications.

Braiker, H. B. (1982). The diagnosis and treatment of alcoholism in women. In *Special population issues* (NIAAA Alcohol and Health Monograph No. 14, U.S. Department of Health and Human Services Publication No. ADM-82-1193). Washington, DC: U.S. Government Printing Office.

Brissett, D., Laundergan, J. C., & Kammeier, M. L. (1981). Reflections on the treatment process by nonabstinent alcoholics. *International Journal of the Addictions, 16*, 407–413.

Bromet, E. J., Ed, V., & May, S. (1984). Family environments of depressed outpatients. *Acta Psychiatrica Scandinavica, 69*, 197–200.

Brown, S. (1985). Reinforcement expectancies and alcoholism treatment outcome after a one-year follow-up. *Journal of Studies of Alcohol, 46*, 304–308.

Brownell, K. D. (1984). Behavioral, psychological, and environmental predictors of obesity and success at weight reduction. *International Journal of Obesity, 8*, 543–550.

Brownell, K. D., Marlatt, G. A., Lichtenstein, E., & Wilson, G. T. (1986). Understanding and preventing relapse. *American Psychologist, 41*, 765–782.

Burling, T. A., & Ziff, D. C. (1988). Tobacco smoking: A comparison between alcohol and drug abuse inpatients. *Addictive Behaviors, 13*, 185–190.

Caddy, G. R., & Block, T. (1985). Individual differences in response to treatment. In M. Galizio & S. A. Maisto (Eds.), *Determinants of substance abuse: Biological, psychological, and environmental factors* (pp. 317–362). New York: Plenum.

Cahalan, D. (1987). *Understanding America's drinking problem: How to combat the hazards of alcohol.* San Francisco: Jossey-Bass.

Callan, V. J., & Jackson, D. (1986). Children of alcoholic fathers and recovered alcoholic fathers: Personal and family functioning. *Journal of Studies on Alcohol, 47*, 180–182.

Carpenter, P. (1984). The use of intergenerational family ratings: Methodological and interpretive considerations. *Journal of Clinical Psychology, 40*, 505–512.

Cartwright, A. (1985). Is treatment an effective way of helping clients resolve difficulties associated with alcohol? In N. Heather, I. Robertson, & P. Davies (Eds.), *The misuse of alcohol: Crucial issues in dependence treatment and prevention* (pp. 117–134). New York: New York University Press.

Chaney, E. F., & Roszell, D. K. (1985). Coping in opiate addicts maintained on methadone. In S. Shiffman & T. A. Wills (Eds.), *Coping and substance use* (pp. 267–293). New York: Academic Press.

REFERENCES

Chen, H., & Rossi, P. H. (1983). Evaluating with sense: The theory-driven approach. *Evaluation Review, 7,* 283–302.
Choquette, K. A., Hesselbrock, M. N., & Babor, T. F. (1985). Discriminative control of alcoholics' drinking by the drinking situation. *Journal of Studies on Alcohol, 46,* 412–417.
Clair, D., & Genest, M. (1987). Variables associated with the adjustment of offspring of alcoholic fathers. *Journal of Studies on Alcohol, 48,* 345–355.
Clausen, J. A. (1983). Sex roles, marital roles and response to mental disorder. In J. Greenley (Ed.), *Research in community and mental health* (Vol. 3, pp. 165–208). Greenwich, CT: JAI Press.
Clausen, J. A. (1986). A 15- to 20-year follow-up of married adult psychiatric patients. In L. Erlenmeyer-Kimling & N. E. Miller (Eds.), *Life-span research on the prediction of psychopathology* (pp. 175–194). Hillsdale, NJ: Erlbaum.
Clausen, J. A., Pfeffer, N. G., & Huffine, C. L. (1982). Help-seeking in severe mental illness. In D. Mechanic (Ed.), *Psychosocial epidemiology: Symptoms, illness behavior, and help seeking* (pp. 135–155). New York: Neale Watson.
Cloninger, C. R., Bohman, M., & Sigvardsson, S. (1981). Inheritance of alcohol abuse. *Archives of General Psychiatry, 38,* 861–868.
Cohler, B., Gallant, D., Grunebaum, H., & Kaufman, C. (1983). Social adjustment among schizophrenic, depressed and well mothers and their school-aged children. In H. Morrison (Ed.), *Children of depressed parents: Risk, identification, and intervention* (pp. 65–97). New York: Grune & Stratton.
Condiotti, M. M., & Lichtenstein, E. (1981). Self-efficacy and relapse in smoking cessation programs. *Journal of Consulting and Clinical Psychology, 49,* 648–658.
Cook, T. D., & Campbell, D. T. (1979). *Quasi-experimentation: Design and analysis issues for field settings.* Chicago: Rand-McNally.
Cooke, R., & Rousseau, D. (1984). Stress and strain from family roles and work role expectations. *Journal of Applied Psychology, 69,* 252–260.
Cooper, A. M., Sobell, M. B., Maisto, S. A., & Sobell, L. C. (1980). Criterion intervals for pretreatment drinking measures in treatment evaluation. *Journal of Studies on Alcohol, 41,* 1186–1195.
Cooper, M. L., Russell, M., & George, W. H. (1988). Coping expectancies and alcohol abuse: A test of social learning formulations. *Journal of Abnormal Psychology, 97,* 218–230.
Coppotelli, H. C., & Orleans, C. T. (1985). Partner support and other determinants of smoking cessation maintenance among women. *Journal of Consulting and Clinical Psychology, 53,* 455–460.
Cordray, D. S. (1986). Quasi-experimental analysis: A mixture of methods and judgment. In W. K. Trochim (Ed.), *Advances in quasi-experimental design and analysis: New directions for program evaluation* (No. 31, pp. 9–27). San Francisco: Jossey-Bass.
Cosper, R. (1979). Drinking as conformity: A critique of sociological literature on occupational differences in drinking. *Journal of Studies on Alcohol, 40,* 868–891.
Costello, R. M. (1975a). Alcoholism treatment and evaluation: In search of methods. *International Journal of the Addictions, 10,* 251–275.

Costello, R. M. (1975b). Alcoholism treatment and evaluation: In search of methods. II. Collation of two-year follow-up studies. *International Journal of the Addictions, 10,* 857–867.

Costello, R. M. (1980). Alcoholism treatment effectiveness: Slicing the outcome variance pie. In G. Edwards & M. Grant (Eds.), *Alcoholism treatment in transition* (pp. 113–127). Baltimore: University Park Press.

Costello, R. M., Baillargeon, J. G., & Tiller, D. (1979). Formative program evaluation and milieu therapy with alcohol abusers. *Journal of Clinical Psychology, 35,* 449–453.

Cox, W. M. (1987). Personality theory and research. In H. Blane & K. Leonard (Eds.), *Psychological theories of drinking and alcoholism* (pp. 55–89). New York: Guilford Press.

Coyne, J. C., Kessler, R. C., Tal, M., Turnbull, J., & Wortman, C. B. (1987). Living with a depressed person. *Journal of Consulting and Clinical Psychology, 55,* 347–352.

Cronbach, L. J. (1982). *Designing evaluations of educational and social programs.* San Francisco: Jossey-Bass.

Cronbach, L. J., Ambron, S. R., Dornbusch, S. M., Hess, R. D., Hornik, R. C., Phillips, D. C., Walker, D. F., & Weiner, S. S. (1980). *Toward reform of program evaluation.* San Francisco: Jossey-Bass.

Cronkite, R. C., & Moos, R. H. (1980). The determinants of posttreatment functioning of alcoholic patients: A conceptual framework. *Journal of Consulting and Clinical Psychology, 48,* 305–316.

Cronkite, R., & Moos, R. (1984). The role of predisposing and moderating factors in the stress-illness relationship. *Journal of Health and Social Behavior, 25,* 372–393.

Dahlgren, L. (1979). Female alcoholics: IV. Marital situation and husbands. *Acta Psychiatrica Scandinavica, 59,* 59–69.

Daniels, D., Moos, R. H., Billings, A. G., & Miller, J. J. III (1987). Psychosocial risk and resistance factors among children with chronic illness, healthy siblings, and healthy controls. *Journal of Abnormal Child Psychology, 15,* 295–308.

deBlois, C. S., & Stewart, M. A. (1983). Marital histories of women whose first husbands were alcoholic or antisocial. *British Journal of Addiction, 78,* 205–213.

De Soto, C. B., O'Donnell, W. E., Allred, L. J., & Lopes, C. E. (1985). Symptomatology in alcoholics in various stages of abstinence. *Alcoholism: Clinical and Experimental Research, 9,* 505–512.

Deutsch, C. (1982). *Broken bottles, broken dreams: Understanding and helping the children of alcoholics.* New York: Columbia University Press.

Doherty, E. G. (1978). Are differential discharge criteria used for men and women psychiatric inpatients? *Journal of Health and Social Behavior, 9,* 107–116.

Dohrenwend, B. S., & Martin, J. L. (1979). Personal versus situational determination of anticipation and control of the occurrence of stressful life events. *American Journal of Community Psychology, 7,* 453–468.

Douglas, J. J., & Nutter, C. P. (1986). Treatment-related change in sex roles of addicted men and women. *Journal of Studies on Alcohol, 47,* 201–206.

Drake, R. E., & Vaillant, G. E. (1988). Predicting alcoholism and personality disorder in a 33-year longitudinal study of children of alcoholics. *British Journal of Addiction, 83,* 799–807.

Drake, R. E., & Wallach, M. A. (1988). Mental patients' attitudes toward hospitalization: A neglected aspect of hospital tenure. *American Journal of Psychiatry, 145,* 29–34.
Drew, L. R. (1968). Alcoholism as a self-limiting disease. *Quarterly Journal of Studies on Alcohol, 29,* 957–967.
Duckitt, A., Brown, D., Edwards, G., Oppenheimer, E., Sheehan, M., & Taylor, C. (1985). Alcoholism and the nature of outcome. *British Journal of Addiction, 80,* 153–162.
Dunn, N. J., Jacob, T., Hummon, N., & Seilhamer, R. A. (1987). Marital stability in alcoholic-spouse relationships as a function of drinking pattern and location. *Journal of Abnormal Psychology, 96,* 99–107.
Dwoskin, J., Gordis, E., & Dorph, D. (1979). Life-table analysis of treatment outcome following 185 consecutive alcoholism halfway house discharges. *Alcoholism: Clinical and Experimental Research, 3,* 334–340.
Edwards, A. L., & Cronbach, L. J. (1952). Experimental design for research in psychotherapy. *Journal of Clinical Psychology, 8,* 51–59.
Edwards, D., Yarvis, R., Swaback, D., Mueller, D., & Wagman, W. (1979). Developing comparison groups for community mental health: The utility of community surveys. *American Journal of Community Psychology, 7,* 123–127.
Edwards, G. (1980). Alcoholism treatment: Between guesswork and uncertainty. In G. Edwards & M. Grant (Eds.), *Alcoholism treatment in transition* (pp. 307–320). Baltimore: University Park Press.
Edwards, G. (1984). Drinking in longitudinal perspective: Career and natural history. *British Journal of Addiction, 79,* 175–183.
Edwards, G., Kyle, E., Nicholls, P., & Taylor, C. (1978). Alcoholism and correlates of mortality: Implications for epidemiology. *Journal of Studies on Alcohol, 39,* 1607–1617.
Edwards, G., Oppenheimer, E., Duckitt, A., Sheehan, M., & Taylor, C. (1983). What happens to alcoholics? *Lancet, 2* 269–271.
Egan, K. J. (1983). Stress management and child management with abusive parents. *Journal of Clinical Child Psychology, 12,* 292–299.
Einhorn, H. J., & Hogarth, R. M. (1986). Judging probable cause. *Psychological Bulletin, 99,* 3–19.
El-Guebaly, N., Offord, D. R., Sullivan, K. T., & Lynch, G. W. (1978). Psychosocial adjustment of the offspring of psychiatric inpatients: The effect of alcoholic, depressive, and schizophrenic parentage. *Canadian Psychiatric Association Journal, 23,* 281–290.
Elkins, R. L. (1980). Covert sensitization treatment of alcoholism: Contributions of successful conditioning to subsequent abstinence. *Addictive Behaviors, 5,* 67–89.
Ellis, A. S., & Krupinski, J. (1964). The evaluation of a treatment programme for alcoholics: A follow-up study. *Medical Journal of Australia, 1,* 8–13.
Ellsworth, R. B. (1979). Does follow-up loss reflect poor outcome? *Evaluation and the Health Professions, 2,* 419–437.
Emery, R. E., Weintraub, S., & Neale, J. M. (1982). Effects of marital discord on the school behavior of children of schizophrenic, affectively disordered, and normal parents. *Journal of Abnormal Child Psychology, 10,* 215–228.
Emrick, C. D. (1974). A review of psychologically oriented treatment of alcoholism. I. The use and interrelationships of outcome criteria and drinking be-

havior following treatment. *Quarterly Journal of Studies on Alcohol, 35,* 523–549.

Emrick, C. (1975). A review of psychologically oriented treatment of alcoholism: II. The relative effectiveness of different treatment approaches and the effectiveness of treatment versus no treatment. *Journal of Studies on Alcohol, 36,* 88–108.

Enos, D. M., & Handal, P. J. (1986). The relation of parental marital status and perceived family conflict to adjustment in white adolescents. *Journal of Consulting and Clinical Psychology, 54,* 820–824.

Eriksen, L. (1987). Ward atmosphere changes during restructuring of an alcoholism treatment center: A quasi-experimental study. *Addictive Behaviors, 12,* 33–42.

Etringer, B. D., Gregory, V. R., & Lando, H. A. (1984). Influence of group cohesion on the behavioral treatment of smoking. *Journal of Consulting and Clinical Psychology, 52,* 1080–1086.

Fagan, R. W., & Mauss, A. L. (1986). Social margin and social reentry: An evaluation of a rehabilitation program for skid-row alcoholics. *Journal of Studies on Alcohol, 47,* 413–425.

Fairchild, H., & Wright, C. (1984). A social-ecological assessment and feedback intervention of an adolescent treatment agency. *Adolescence, 19,* 263–275.

Feuerstein, M., Sult, S., & Houle, M. (1985). Environmental stressors and chronic low back pain: Life events, family and work environment. *Pain, 22,* 295–307.

Fink, E., Longabaugh, R., McCrady, B., Stout, R., Beattie, M., Ruggieri-Authelet, A., & McNeill, D. (1985). Effectiveness of alcoholism treatment in partial vs. inpatient settings: Twenty-four month outcomes. *Addictive Behaviors, 10,* 235–248.

Finney, J., & Moos, R. (1984). Environmental assessment and evaluation research: Examples from mental health and substance abuse programs. *Evaluation and Program Planning, 7,* 151–167.

Finney, J. W., & Moos, R. H. (1986). Matching patients with treatments: Conceptual and methodological issues. *Journal of Studies on Alcohol, 47,* 122–134.

Finney, J., & Moos, R. (1989). Theory and method in program evaluation. *Evaluation and Program Planning, 12,* 307–316.

Finney, J., Moos, R., & Chan, D. (1981). Length of stay and program component effects in the treatment for alcoholism: A comparison of two techniques for process analysis. *Journal of Consulting and Clinical Psychology, 49,* 120–131.

Finney, J., Moos, R., Cronkite, R., & Gamble, W. (1983). A conceptual model of the functioning of married persons with impaired partners: Spouses of alcoholic patients. *Journal of Marriage and the Family, 45,* 23–34.

Finney, J., Moos, R., & Mewborn, R. (1980). Posttreatment experiences and treatment outcome of alcoholic patients six months and two years after hospitalization. *Journal of Consulting and Clinical Psychology, 48,* 17–29.

Fitzgerald, J. L., & Mulford, H. A. (1981). Social attributes, problem drinking and alcoholism treatment contacts: Labeling versus social etiology. *Journal of Studies on Alcohol, 42,* 403–413.

Fitzgerald, J. L., & Mulford, H. A. (1985). An experimental test of telephone

aftercare contacts with alcoholics. *Journal of Studies on Alcohol, 46,* 418–424.
Folkman, S., & Lazarus, R. S. (1980). An analysis of coping in a middle-aged community sample. *Journal of Health and Social Behavior, 21,* 219–239.
Folkman, S., & Lazarus, R. S. (1986). Stress processes and depressive symptomatology. *Journal of Abnormal Psychology, 95,* 107–113.
Fondacaro, M. R., & Moos, R. H. (1987). Social support and coping: A longitudinal analysis. *American Journal of Community Psychology, 15,* 653–673.
Ford, J. D., Bashford, M. B., & DeWitt, K. N. (1984). Three approaches to marital enrichment: Toward optimal matching of participants and interventions. *Journal of Sex and Marital Therapy, 10,* 41–48.
Friedman, S., Jeger, A., & Slotnick, R. (1982). Social ecological assessment of mental health treatment environments: Towards self-evaluation. *Psychological Reports, 50,* 631–638.
Friis, S. (1981). From enthusiasm to resignation in a therapeutic community: A process evaluation of a mental hospital ward with the Ward Atmosphere Scale (WAS). *Journal of the Oslo City Hospitals, 31,* 51–54.
Fuhr, R., Moos, R., & Dishotsky, N. (1981). The use of family assessment and feedback in ongoing family therapy. *American Journal of Family Therapy, 9,* 24–36.
Gabrielli, W. F., & Plomin, R. (1985). Drinking behavior in the Colorado adoptee and twin sample. *Journal of Studies on Alcohol, 46,* 24–31.
Geisbrecht, N. (1983). Stakes in conformity and the "normalization" of deviants: Accounts by former and current skid row inebriates. *Journal of Drug Issues, 13,* 299–322.
Gentry, W. D. (1984). *Handbook of behavioral medicine.* New York: Guilford Press.
Gilbert, F. S. (1988). The effect of type of aftercare follow-up on treatment outcome among alcoholics. *Journal of Studies on Alcohol, 49,* 149–159.
Goldman, H. H., & Taube, C. A. (1988). High users of outpatient mental health services: II. Implications for practice and policy. *American Journal of Psychiatry, 145,* 24–28.
Goldstein, M. J., Hand, I., & Hahlweg, K. (1986). *Treatment of schizophrenia: Family assessment and intervention.* Berlin: Springer-Verlag.
Gomberg, E. S., & Lisansky, J. M. (1984). Antecedents of alcohol problems in women. In S. C. Wilsnack & L. J. Beckman (Eds.), *Alcohol problems in women* (pp. 233–259). New York: Guilford Press.
Gorman, J., & Rooney, J. (1979). The influence of Al-Anon on the coping behavior of wives of alcoholics. *Journal of Studies on Alcohol, 40,* 1030–1038.
Halikas, J. A., Lyttle, M. O., & Morse, C. L. (1984). Skid row alcoholism: An objective definition for use in detoxification and treatment planning. *Journal of Clinical Psychiatry, 45,* 214–216.
Hall, R. L., Hesselbrock, V. M., & Stabenau, J. R. (1983). Familial distribution of alcohol use: II. Assortative mating of alcoholic probands. *Behavior Genetics, 13,* 373–382.
Hanna, E. (1978). Attitudes toward problem drinkers. *Journal of Studies on Alcohol, 39,* 98–109.
Harburg, E., Davis, D., Cummings, K. M., & Gunn, R. (1981). Negative affect, alcohol consumption and hangover symptoms among normal drinkers in a small community. *Journal of Studies on Alcohol, 42,* 998–1012.

Harford, T. C. (1978). Contextual drinking patterns among men and women. In F. Seixas (Ed.), *Currents in alcoholism* (Vol. 4, pp. 287–296). New York: Grune & Stratton.

Harford, T. C. (1984). Situational factors in drinking: A developmental perspective on drinking contexts. In P. M. Miller & T. D. Nirenberg (Eds.), *Prevention of alcohol abuse* (pp. 119–156). New York: Plenum.

Hatry, H. P., Winnie, R. E., & Fisk, D. M. (1973). *Practical program evaluation for state and local government officials*. Washington, DC: Urban Institute.

Hattie, J. A., Sharpley, C. F., & Rogers, H. J. (1984). Comparative effectiveness of paraprofessional and professional helpers. *Psychological Bulletin, 95*, 534–541.

Hayes, S. C., Nelson, R. O., & Jarrett, R. B. (1987). The treatment utility of assessment: A functional approach to evaluating assessment quality. *American Psychologist, 42*, 963–974.

Hazelrigg, M. D., Cooper, H. M., & Borduin, C. M. (1987). Evaluating the effectiveness of family therapies: An integrative review and analysis. *Psychological Bulletin, 101*, 428–442.

Hesselbrock, M. N., Meyer, R. E., & Keener, J. J. (1985). Psychopathology in hospitalized alcoholics. *Archives of General Psychiatry, 42*, 1050–1055.

Hill, M. J., & Blane, H. T. (1967). Evaluation of psychotherapy with alcoholics: A critical review. *Quarterly Journal of Studies on Alcohol, 28*, 76–104.

Hingson, R., Mangione, T., Meyers, A., & Scotch, N. (1982). Seeking help for drinking problems: A study in the Boston Metropolitan Area. *Journal of Studies on Alcohol, 43*, 273–288.

Hirsch, B., Moos, R., & Reischl, T. (1985). Psychosocial adjustment of adolescent children of a depressed, arthritic, or normal parent. *Journal of Abnormal Psychology, 94*, 154–164.

Hirsch, B., & Reischl, T. (1985). Social networks and developmental psychopathology: A comparison of adolescent children of a depressed, arthritic, or normal parent. *Journal of Abnormal Psychology, 94*, 272–281.

Holahan, C. J., & Moos, R. (1981). Social support and psychological distress: A longitudinal analysis. *Journal of Abnormal Psychology, 90*, 365–370.

Holahan, C. J., & Moos, R. (1987a). The personal and contextual determinants of coping strategies. *Journal of Personality and Social Psychology, 52*, 946–955.

Holahan, C. J., & Moos, R. (1987b). Risk, resistance, and psychological distress: A longitudinal analysis with adults and children. *Journal of Abnormal Psychology, 96*, 3–13.

Hollon, S. D., DeRubeis, R. J., & Evans, M. D. (1987). Causal mediation of change in treatment for depression: Discriminating between nonspecificity and noncausality. *Psychological Bulletin, 102*, 139–149.

Hull, J. G. (1981). A self-awareness model of the causes and effects of alcohol consumption. *Journal of Abnormal Psychology, 90*, 586–600.

Hull, J. G., Young, R. D., & Jouriles, E. (1986). Applications of the self-awareness model of alcohol consumption: Predicting patterns of use and abuse. *Journal of Personality and Social Psychology, 51*, 790–796.

Hunt, G., & Azrin, N. H. (1973). A community-reinforcement approach to alcoholism. *Behavior Research and Therapy, 11*, 91–104.

Istavan, J., & Matarazzo, J. D. (1984). Tobacco, alcohol, and caffeine use: A review of their interrelationships. *Psychological Bulletin, 95*, 301–326.

Ito, J. R., & Donovan, D. M. (1986). Aftercare in alcoholism treatment: A review. In W. R. Miller & N. Heather (Eds.), *Treating addictive behaviors: Processes of change* (pp. 435–452). New York: Plenum.

Jackson, J. (1954). The adjustment of the family, the crisis of alcoholism. *Quarterly Journal of Studies on Alcohol, 15,* 562–586.

Jackson, S. (1983). Participation in decision making as a strategy for reducing job-related strain. *Journal of Applied Psychology, 68,* 3–19.

Jacob, T. (1986). Alcoholism: A family interaction perspective. In C. Rivers (Ed.), *Nebraska Symposium on Motivation, 34.* Lincoln: University of Nebraska Press.

Jacob, T., Dunn, N. J., & Leonard, K. (1983). Patterns of alcohol abuse and family stability. *Alcoholism: Clinical and Experimental Research, 7,* 382–385.

Jacob, T., & Leonard, K. (1986). Psychosocial functioning in children of alcoholic fathers, depressed fathers, and control fathers. *Journal of Studies on Alcohol, 47,* 373–380.

Jacob, T., & Seilhamer, R. A. (1987). Alcoholism and family interaction. In T. Jacob (Ed.), *Family interaction and psychopathology: Theories, methods and findings* (pp. 535–580). New York: Plenum.

Jacobson, G. R. (1982). The role of shelter facilities in the treatment of alcoholics. In E. M. Pattison & E. Kaufman (Eds.), *Encyclopedic handbook of alcoholism* (pp. 894–906). New York: Gardner Press.

Jacobson, N. S., Follette, W. C., & Revenstorf, D. (1984). Psychotherapy outcome research: Methods for reporting variability and evaluating clinical significance. *Behavior Therapy, 15,* 336–352.

Janis, I. L. (1983). The role of social support in adherence to stressful decisions. *American Psychologist, 38,* 143–160.

Jessor, R., Graves, T. D., Hanson, R. C., & Jessor, S. L. (1968). *Society, personality, and deviant behavior: A study of a tri-ethnic community.* New York: Holt, Rinehart and Winston.

Jessor, R., & Jessor, S. L. (1977). *Problem behavior and psychosocial development: A longitudinal study of youth.* New York: Academic Press.

Johnson, S., & Garzon, S. R. (1978). Alcoholism and women. *American Journal of Drug and Alcohol Abuse, 5,* 107–122.

Jones, S., & Lanyon, R. (1981). Relationship between adaptive skills and outcome of alcoholism treatment. *Journal of Studies on Alcohol, 42,* 521–525.

Judge, J. J. (1971). Alcoholism treatment at the Salvation Army: A new Men's Social Service Center program. *Quarterly Journal of Studies on Alcohol, 32,* 462–467.

Kammeier, M. L., & Conley, J. J. (1979). Toward a system for prediction of posttreatment abstinence and adaptation. In M. Galanter (Ed.), *Currents in alcoholism* (Vol. 6, pp. 111–119). New York: Grune & Stratton.

Kanter, R. M. (1977). Some effects of proportions on group life: Skewed sex ratios and responses to token women. *American Journal of Sociology, 82,* 965–990.

Katz, L. (1964). The Salvation Army Men's Social Service Center. I. Program. *Quarterly Journal of Studies on Alcohol, 25,* 324–332.

Katz, L. (1966). The Salvation Army Men's Social Service Center. II. Results. *Quarterly Journal of Studies on Alcohol, 27,* 636–647.

Kauffman, C., Grunebaum, H., Cohler, B., & Gamer, E. (1979). Superkids: Competent children of psychotic mothers. *American Journal of Psychiatry, 136,* 1398–1402.

Kaufman, E., & Pattison, E. M. (1982). The family and alcoholism. In E. M. Pattison & E. Kaufman (Eds.), *Encyclopedic handbook of alcoholism* (pp. 663–672). New York: Gardner Press.

Kazdin, A. E., & Wilson, G. T. (1978). Criteria for evaluating psychotherapy. *Archives of General Psychiatry, 35,* 407–416.

Killen, J. D., Maccoby, N., & Taylor, C. B. (1984). Nicotine gum and self-regulation training in smoking relapse prevention. *Behavior Therapy, 15,* 234–248.

Kirk, S., & Masi, J. (1978). Aftercare for alcoholics: Services of community mental health centers. *Journal of Studies on Alcohol, 39,* 545–547.

Kissin, B., & Hanson, M. (1982). The bio-psycho-social perspective in alcoholism. In J. Solomon (Ed.), *Alcoholism and clinical psychiatry* (pp. 1–19). New York: Plenum.

Klein, D. N., Clark, D. C., Dansky, L., & Margolis, E. T. (1988). Dysthymia in the offspring of parents with primary unipolar affective disorder. *Journal of Abnormal Psychology, 97,* 265–274.

Knop, J., Teasdale, T. W., Schulsinger, F., & Goodwin, D. W. (1985). A prospective study of young men at high risk for alcoholism: School behavior and achievement. *Journal of Studies on Alcohol, 46,* 273–278.

Kobasa, S., & Puccetti, M. (1983). Personality and social resources in stress resistance. *Journal of Personality and Social Psychology, 45,* 839–850.

Kohn, M., & Schooler, C. (1983). *Work and personality: An inquiry into the impact of social stratification.* Norwood, NJ: Ablex.

Koran, L., Moos, R., Moos, B., & Zasslow, M. (1983). Changing hospital work environments: An example of a burn unit. *General Hospital Psychiatry, 5,* 7–13.

Kotler, P., & Wingard, D. L. (1989). The effect of occupational, marital and parental roles on mortality. The Alameda County Study. *American Journal of Public Health, 79,* 607–612.

Krantz, S., & Moos, R. (1987). Functioning and life context among spouses of remitted and nonremitted depressed patients. *Journal of Consulting and Clinical Psychology, 55,* 353–360.

Krueger, D. W. (1981). Stressful life events and the return to heroin use. *Journal of Human Stress, 7,* 3–8.

Kurtines, W., Ball, L., & Wood, G. (1978). Personality characteristics of longterm recovered alcoholics: A comparative analysis. *Journal of Consulting and Clinical Psychology, 46,* 971–977.

Lacoursiere, R., & Bradshaw, S. (1983). Problems in a treatment program for substance misuse: The process of reorganizing into assessment teams and modules. *Journal of Studies on Alcohol, 44,* 647–664.

La Porte, D. J., McLellan, A. T., Erdlen, F. R., & Parente, R. J. (1981). Treatment outcome as a function of follow-up difficulty in substance abusers. *Journal of Consulting and Clinical Psychology, 49,* 112–119.

Lazarus, R., & Folkman, S. (1984). *Stress, appraisal, and coping.* New York: Springer-Verlag.

Leaf, P., & Bruce, M. (1987). Gender differences in the use of mental health-

REFERENCES

related services: A re-examination. *Journal of Health and Social Behavior, 28,* 171–183.

Leff, J., & Vaughn, C. (1985). *Expressed emotion in families: Its significance for mental illness.* New York: Guilford.

Leigh, H., & Reiser, M. F. (1985). *The patient: Biological, psychological, and social dimensions of medical practice* (2nd ed.). New York: Plenum.

Levin, H. M. (1987). *Cost-effectiveness: A primer.* Beverly Hills, CA: Sage.

Lichtenstein, E. (1982). The smoking problem: A behavioral perspective. *Journal of Consulting and Clinical Psychology, 50,* 804–819.

Lindbeck, V. (1975). *The woman alcoholic* (Public Affairs Pamphlet No. 529). New York: Public Affairs Committee.

Lindsay, J. S. B. (1986). The general hospital and the therapeutic community in North Queensland. *International Journal of Therapeutic Communities, 7,* 129–138.

Link, B. G., Dohrenwend, B. P., & Skodol, A. E. (1986). Socio-economic status and schizophrenia: Noisome occupational characteristics as a risk factor. *American Sociology Review, 51,* 242–258.

Linsky, A. S., Straus, M. A., & Colby, J. P. (1985). Stressful events, stressful conditions and alcohol problems in the United States: A partial test of Bales's theory. *Journal of Studies on Alcohol, 46,* 72–80.

Lipsey, M. W., Crosse, S., Dunkle, J., Pollard, J., & Stobart, G. (1985). Evaluation: The state of the art and the sorry state of the science. In D. S. Cordray (Ed.), *Utilizing prior research in evaluation planning: New directions for program evaluation* (Vol. 27, pp. 7–28). San Francisco, CA: Jossey-Bass.

Lipsey, M. W., & Pollard, J. A. (1989). Driving toward theory in program evaluation: More models to choose from. *Evaluation and Program Planning, 12,* 317–328.

Litman, G. K. (1986). Women and alcohol problems. *British Journal of Addiction, 81,* 601–603.

Litman, G. K., Eiser, J., Rawson, N., & Oppenheim, A. (1979). Towards a typology of relapse: Differences in relapse precipitants and coping behaviours between alcoholic relapsers and survivors. *Behaviour, Research and Therapy, 17,* 89–94.

Lowenstein, A. (1984). Coping with stress: The case of prisoners' wives. *Journal of Marriage and the Family, 46,* 699–708.

Ludwig, A. M. (1985). Cognitive processes associated with "spontaneous" recovery from alcoholism. *Journal of Studies on Alcohol, 46,* 53–58.

Lutz, M., Appelt, H., & Cohen, R. (1980). Belastungsfaktoren in den familien alkoholkranker und depressiver frauen aus der sicht der ehemanner. *Social Psychiatry, 15,* 137–144.

MacDonald, j. G. (1987). Predictors of treatment outcome for alcoholic women. *International Journal of the Addictions, 22,* 235–248.

Mackenzie, A., Allen, R. P., & Funderburk, F. R. (1986). Mortality and illness in male alcoholics: An 8-year follow-up. *International Journal of the Addictions, 21,* 865–882.

Mackenzie, A., Funderburk, F. R., Allen, R. P., & Stefan, R. L. (1987). The characteristics of alcoholics frequently lost to follow-up. *Journal of Studies on Alcohol, 48,* 119–123.

Maisto, S. A., & Carey, K. B. (1987). Treatment of alcohol abuse. In T. D. Nirenberg & S. A. Maisto (Eds.), *Developments in the assessment and treatment of addictive behaviors* (pp. 173–211). Norwood, NJ: Ablex.

Maisto, S. A., Sobell, L. C., Sobell, M. B., & Sanders, B. (1985). Effects of outpatient treatment for problem drinkers. *American Journal of Drug and Alcohol Abuse, 11*, 131–149.

Malcolm, M. T., Madden, J. S., & Williams, A. E. (1974). Disulfiram implantation critically evaluated. *British Journal of Psychiatry, 125*, 485–489.

Mallams, J. H., Godley, M. D., Hall, G. M., & Meyers, R. J. (1982). A social-systems approach to resocializing alcoholics in the community. *Journal of Studies on Alcohol, 43*, 1115–1123.

Mandell, W. (1979). A critical overview of evaluations of alcoholism treatment. *Alcoholism: Clinical and Experimental Research, 3*, 315–323.

Markowitz, M. (1984). Alcohol misuse as a response to perceived powerlessness in the organization. *Journal of Studies on Alcohol, 45*, 225–227.

Marlatt, G. A., & Gordon, J. R. (Eds.) (1985). *Relapse prevention: Maintenance strategies in addictive behavior change.* New York: Guilford Press.

May, S. J., & Kuller, L. H. (1975). Methodological approaches in the evaluation of alcoholism treatment: A critical review. *Preventive Medicine, 4*, 464–481.

Mayer, J., & Meyerson, D. (1970). Characteristics of outpatient alcoholics in relation to change in drinking, work, and marital status during treatment. *Quarterly Journal of Studies on Alcohol, 31*, 889–897.

McCabe, R. J. R. (1986). Alcohol-dependent individuals sixteen years on. *Alcohol and Alcoholism, 21*, 85–91.

McCrady, B. S., Longabaugh, R., Fink, E., Stout, R., Beattie, M., & Ruggieri-Authelet, A. (1986). Cost-effectiveness of alcoholism treatment in partial hospital versus inpatient settings after brief inpatient treatment: Twelve month outcomes. *Journal of Consulting and Clinical Psychology, 54*, 708–713.

McLachlan, J. (1974). Therapy strategies, personality orientation, and recovery from alcoholism. *Canadian Psychiatric Association Journal, 19*, 25–30.

McLellan, A. T., Luborsky, L., Woody, G. E., O'Brien, C. P., & Kron, R. (1981). Are the "addiction-related" problems of substance abusers really related? *Journal of Nervous and Mental Disease, 169*, 232–239.

McLellan, A. T., Luborsky, L., Woody, G. E., O'Brien, C. P., & Druley, K. A. (1983). Predicting response to alcohol and drug abuse treatments: Role of psychiatric severity. *Archives of General Psychiatry, 40*, 620–625.

McLellan, A. T., Woody, G. E., Luborsky, L., O'Brien, C. P., & Druley, K. A. (1983). Increased effectiveness of substance abuse treatment: A prospective study of patient-treatment "matching." *Journal of Nervous and Mental Disease, 171*, 597–605.

Menaghen, E., & Mervis, E. (1984). Coping with occupational problems: The limits of individual efforts. *Journal of Health and Social Behavior, 25*, 406–423.

Mendelson, J. H., Miller, K. D., Mello, N. K., Pratt, H., & Schmitz, R. (1982). Hospital treatment for alcoholism: A profile of middle income Americans. *Alcoholism: Clinical and Experimental Research, 6*, 377–383.

Merikangas, K. R. (1982). Assortative mating for psychiatric disorders and psychological traits. *Archives of General Psychiatry, 39*, 1173–1180.

Merikangas, K. R., Bromet, E. J., & Spiker, D. G. (1983). Assortative mating,

REFERENCES

social adjustment, and course of illness in primary affective disorder. *Archives of General Psychiatry, 40*, 795–800.

Merikangas, K. R., Weissman, M. M., Prusoff, B. A., Pauls, D. L., & Leckman, J. F. (1985). Depressives with secondary alcoholism: Psychiatric disorders in offspring. *Journal of Studies on Alcohol, 46*, 199–204.

Mermelstein, R., Cohen, S., Lichtenstein, E., Baer, J. S., & Kamarck, T. (1986). Social support and smoking cessation and maintenance. *Journal of Consulting and Clinical Psychology, 54*, 447–453.

Miller, W. R. (1983). Controlled drinking: A history and a critical review. *Journal of Studies on Alcohol, 44*, 68–83.

Miller, W. R., & Hester, R. K. (1980). Treating the problem drinker. In W. R. Miller (Ed.), *The addictive behaviors: Treatment of alcoholism, drug abuse, smoking, and obesity* (pp. 11–141). New York: Pergamon Press.

Miller, W. R., & Hester, R. K. (1986). Inpatient alcoholism treatment: Who benefits? *American Psychologist, 41*, 794–805.

Miller, W. R., Taylor, C. A., & West, J. C. (1980). Focused versus broad-spectrum behavior therapy for problem drinkers. *Journal of Consulting and Clinical Psychology, 48*, 590–601.

Milne, D. (1986). Planning and evaluating innovations in nursing practice by measuring the ward atmosphere. *Journal of Advanced Nursing, 11*, 203–210.

Mink, I. T., & Nihira, K. (1986). Family lifestyles and child behaviors: A study of direction of effects. *Developmental Psychology, 22*, 610–616.

Mitchell, R., Cronkite, R., & Moos, R. (1983). Stress, coping and depression among married couples. *Journal of Abnormal Psychology, 92*, 433–448.

Mitchell, R. E., & Hodson, C. A. (1983). Coping with domestic violence: Social support and psychological health among battered women. *American Journal of Community Psychology, 11*, 629–654.

Mitchell, R. E., & Hodson, C. A. (1986). Coping and social support among battered women: An ecological perspective. In S. Hobfoll (Ed.), *Stress, social support, and women* (pp. 153–169). New York: Hemisphere.

Moos, R. H. (1974). *Evaluating treatment environments*. New York: Wiley.

Moos, R. H. (Ed.) (1984). *Coping with physical illness: New directions*. New York: Plenum.

Moos, R. (1985a). Evaluating social resources in community and health care contexts. In P. Karoly (Ed.), *Measurement strategies in health psychology* (pp. 433–459). New York: Wiley.

Moos, R. (1985b). The Background and Follow-up Information Forms. In D. J. Lettieri, J. E. Nelson, & M. A. Sayers (Eds.), *NIAAA treatment handbook series: Vol. II. Alcoholism treatment assessment research instruments* (pp. 261–274) (DHHS Publication No. ADM 85-1380). Washington, DC: U.S. Government Printing Office.

Moos, R. H. (1986a). *Coping with life crises: An integrated approach*. New York: Plenum.

Moos, R. H. (1986b). Work as a human context. In M. S. Pallak & R. O. Perloff (Eds.), *Psychology and work: Productivity, change, and employment* (pp. 13–19). Washington, DC: American Psychological Association.

Moos, R. H. (1986c). *Work Environment Scale manual: Second edition*. Palo Alto, CA: Consulting Psychologists Press.

Moos, R. H. (1987a). Growth-promoting aspects and interconnections of school, work, and family settings. *Psychological Assessment, 3*, 3–26.

Moos, R. H. (1987b). *The Social Climate Scales: A user's guide*. Palo Alto, CA: Consulting Psychologists Press.

Moos, R. H. (1988a). *Community-Oriented Programs Environment Scale manual: Second edition*. Palo Alto, CA: Consulting Psychologists Press.

Moos, R. (1988b). Life stressors and coping resources influence health and well-being. *Psychological Assessment, 4,* 133–158.

Moos, R. H. (1988c). *Ward Atmosphere Scale manual: Second edition*. Palo Alto, CA: Consulting Psychologists Press.

Moos, R. (in press). Life stressors, social resources, and the treatment of depression. In J. Becker & A. Kleinman (Eds.), *Advances in mood disorders: Vol. I. Psychological aspects*. New York: Erlbaum.

Moos, R., & Billings, A. (1982a). Children of alcoholics during the recovery process: Alcoholic and matched control families. *Addictive Behaviors, 7,* 155–163.

Moos, R., & Billings, A. (1982b). Conceptualizing and measuring coping resources and processes. In L. Goldberger & S. Breznitz (Eds.), *Handbook of stress: Theoretical and clinical aspects* (pp. 212–230). New York: Macmillan.

Moos, R., & Billings, A. (in press). Understanding and improving work climates. In J. W. Jones, B. D. Steffy, & D. W. Bray (Eds.), *Applying psychology in business: The manager's handbook*. Lexington, MA: Lexington Books.

Moos, R., Cronkite, R., Billings, A., & Finney, J. (1984). *Health and Daily Living Form manual*. Palo Alto, CA: Social Ecology Laboratory, Stanford University and Veterans Administration Medical Center.

Moos, R., & Finney, J. (1985b). New directions in program evaluation: Implications for expanding the role of alcoholism researchers. In B. McCrady, N. Noel, & T. Nirenberg (Eds.), *Future directions in alcohol abuse treatment research* (Research Monograph No. 15, pp. 173–203). Washington, DC: National Institute on Alcohol Abuse and Alcoholism.

Moos, R., Finney, J., & Chan, D. (1981). The process of recovery from alcoholism: I. Comparing alcoholic patients and matched community controls. *Journal of Studies on Alcohol, 42,* 383–402.

Moos, R. H., Finney, J. W., & Cronkite, R. C. (1980). The need for a paradigm shift in evaluations of treatment outcome: Extrapolations from the Rand research. *British Journal of Addiction, 75,* 347–350.

Moos, R., Finney, J., & Gamble, W. (1982). The process of recovery from alcoholism: II. Comparing spouses of alcoholic patients and spouses of matched community controls. *Journal of Studies on Alcohol, 43,* 888–909.

Moos, R., & Fuhr, R. (1982). The clinical use of social-ecological concepts: The case of an adolescent girl. *American Journal of Orthopsychiatry, 52,* 111–122.

Moos, R., & Igra, A. (1980). Determinants of the social environment of sheltered care settings. *Journal of Health and Social Behavior, 21,* 88–98.

Moos, R., & Lemke, S. (1984). Supportive residential settings for older people. In I. Altman, M. P. Lawton, & J. Wohlwill (Eds.), *Elderly people and the environment* (pp. 159–190). New York: Plenum.

Moos, R., Lemke, S., & David, T. (1987). Priorities for design and management in residential settings for the elderly. In V. Regnier & J. Pynoos (Eds.), *Housing the aged: Design directives and policy considerations* (pp. 179–205). New York: Elsevier.

REFERENCES

Moos, R., & Moos, B. (1984). The process of recovery from alcoholism: III. Comparing family functioning in alcoholic and matched control families. *Journal of Studies on Alcohol, 45,* 111–118.

Moos, R., & Moos, B. (1986). *Family Environment Scale manual: Second edition.* Palo Alto, CA: Consulting Psychologists Press.

Moos, R., & Schaefer, J. (1986). Life transitions and crises: A conceptual overview. In R. Moos (Ed.), *Coping with life crises: An integrated approach* (pp. 3–28). New York: Plenum.

Moos, R., & Schaefer, J. (1987). Evaluating health care work settings: A holistic conceptual framework. *Psychology and Health, 1,* 97–122.

Mosher, L., & Menn, A. (1978). Lower barriers in the community: The Soteria model. In L. I. Stein & M. A. Test (Eds.), *Alternatives to mental hospital treatment* (pp. 75–113). New York: Plenum.

Mulford, H. A. (1977). Stages in the alcoholic process: Toward a cumulative nonsequential index. *Journal of Studies on Alcohol, 38,* 563–583.

Mulford, H. A. (1984). Rethinking the alcohol problem: A natural processes model. *Journal of Drug Issues, 14,* 31–43.

Nace, E. P. (1982). Therapeutic approaches to the alcoholic marriage. *Psychiatric Clinics of North America, 5,* 543–564.

Nathan, P. E. (1986). Outcomes of treatment for alcoholism: Current data. *Annals of Behavioral Medicine, 8,* 40–46.

Nathan, P. E., & Skinstad, A.-H. (1987). Outcomes of treatment for alcohol problems: Current methods, problems, and results. *Journal of Consulting and Clinical Psychology, 55,* 332–340.

National Institute on Alcohol Abuse and Alcoholism (1987). *Sixth special report to the U.S. Congress on alcohol and health.* Washington, DC: U.S. Department of Health and Human Services.

Neuberger, O. W., Hasha, N., Matarazzo, J. D., Schmitz, R. E., & Pratt, H. H. (1981). Behavioral-chemical treatment of alcoholism: An outcome replication. *Journal of Studies on Alcohol, 42,* 806–810.

Ng, M. L., Tam, Y. K., & Luk, S. L. (1982). Evaluation of different forms of community meeting in a psychiatric unit in Hong Kong. *British Journal of Psychiatry, 140,* 491–497.

Nihira, K., Mink, I. T., & Meyers, C. E. (1985). Home environment and development of slow learning adolescents: Reciprocal relations. *Developmental Psychology, 21,* 784–794.

Noel, N. E., McCrady, B. S., Stout, R. L., & Fisher-Nelson, H. (1987). Predictors of attrition from an outpatient alcoholism treatment program for couples. *Journal of Studies on Alcohol, 48,* 229–235.

Nordstrom, G., & Berglund, M. (1986). Successful adjustment in alcoholism: Relationships between causes of improvement, personality, and social factors. *Journal of Nervous and Mental Disease, 174,* 664–668.

Nordstrom, G., & Berglund, M. (1987). Ageing and recovery from alcoholism. *British Journal of Psychiatry, 151,* 382–388.

Nylander, I., & Rydelius, P. A. (1982). A comparison between children of alcoholic fathers from excellent versus poor social conditions. *Acta Paediatrica Scandinavica, 71,* 809–813.

O'Connor, A., & Daly, J. (1985). Alcoholics: A twenty year follow-up study. *British Journal of Psychiatry, 146,* 645–647.

Oei, T. P. S., & Jackson, P. (1982). Social skills and cognitive behavioral approaches to the treatment of problem drinking. *Journal of Studies on Alcohol, 43,* 532–547.

O'Farrell, T. J., Cutter, H. S. G., & Floyd, F. J. (1985). Evaluating behavioral marital therapy for male alcoholics: Effects on marital adjustment and communication from before to after treatment. *Behavior Therapy, 16,* 147–167.

O'Farrell, T. J., Harrison, R. H., & Cutter, H. S. G. (1981). Marital stability among wives of alcoholics: An evaluation of three explanations. *British Journal of Addiction, 76,* 175–189.

Ogborne, A. C. (1988). Bridging the gap between the two cultures of alcoholism research and treatment. *British Journal of Addiction, 83,* 729–733.

Ogborne, A. C., Sobell, M. B., & Sobell, L. C. (1985). The significance of environmental factors for the design and the evaluation of alcohol treatment programs. In M. Galizio & S. A. Maisto (Eds.), *Determinants of substance abuse: Biological, psychological, and environmental factors* (pp. 363–382). New York: Plenum.

Ojehagen, A., Skjaerris, A., & Berglund, M. (1988). Prediction of posttreatment drinking outcome in a 2-year out-patient alcoholic treatment program: A follow-up study. *Alcoholism: Clinical and Experimental Research, 12,* 46–51.

Orford, J. (1985). *Excessive appetites: A psychological view of addictions.* New York: Wiley.

Orford, J., Guthrie, S., Nicholls, P., Oppenheimer, E., Egert, S., & Hensman, C. (1975). Self-reported coping behavior of wives of alcoholics and its association with drinking outcome. *Journal of Studies on Alcohol, 36,* 1255–1267.

Orford, J., & Harwin, J. (Eds.) (1982). *Alcohol and the family.* London: Croom Helm.

Orford, J., Oppenheimer, E., Egert, S., Hensman, C., & Guthrie, S. (1976). The cohesiveness of alcoholism-complicated marriages and its influence on treatment outcome. *British Journal of Psychiatry, 128,* 318–339.

Ornstein, P., & Cherepon, J. A. (1985). Demographic variables as predictors of alcoholism treatment outcome. *Journal of Studies on Alcohol, 46,* 425–432.

Page, R. D., & Badgett, S. (1984). Alcoholism treatment with environmental support contracting. *American Journal of Drug and Alcohol Abuse, 10,* 589–605.

Paolino, T., & McCrady, B. (1977). *The alcoholic marriage: Alternative perspectives.* New York: Grune & Stratton.

Parker, D., & Brody, J. (1982). Risk factors for alcoholism and alcohol problems among employed women and men. In *Occupational alcoholism: A review of research* (NIAAA Research Monograph No. 8; pp. 99–127). Washington, DC: U.S. Government Printing Office.

Parker, D., Parker, E., Wolz, M., & Harford, T. (1980). Sex roles and alcohol consumption: A research note. *Journal of Health and Social Behavior, 21,* 43–48.

Parkes, K. (1982). Occupational stress among student nurses: A natural experiment. *Journal of Applied Psychology, 67,* 784–796.

Parkes, K. (1986). Coping in stressful episodes: The role of individual differences, environmental factors, and situational characteristics. England: University of Oxford. *Journal of Personality and Social Psychology, 51,* 1277–1292.

REFERENCES

Patterson, E., Charles, H., Woodward, W., Roberts, W., & Penk, W. (1981). Differences in measures of personality and family environments among black and white alcoholics. *Journal of Consulting and Clinical Psychology, 49,* 1–9.

Pattison, E. M. (1976). A conceptual approach to alcoholism treatment goals. *Addictive Behaviors, 1,* 177–192.

Patton, M. Q. (1978). *Utilization-focused evaluation.* Beverly Hills, CA: Sage.

Pemberton, D. A. (1967). A comparison of the outcome of treatment in female and male alcoholics. *British Journal of Psychiatry, 113,* 367–373.

Penk, W., & Robinowitz, R. (1978). Drug users' views of psychosocial aspects of their treatment environment. *Drug Forum, 7,* 129–143.

Penk, W., Robinowitz, R., Kidd, R., & Nisle, A. (1979). Perceived family environments among ethnic groups of compulsive heroin users. *Addictive Behavior, 4,* 297–309.

Penk, W. E., Uebersax, J. S., Charles, H. L., & Andrews, R. H. (1981). Psychological aspects of data loss in outcome research. *Evaluation Review, 5,* 392–396.

Perri, M. G. (1985). Self-change strategies for the control of smoking, obesity, and problem drinking. In S. Shiffman & T. A. Wills (Eds.), *Coping and substance use.* New York: Academic Press.

Perri, M. G., McAdoo, W. G., Spevak, P. A., & Newlin, D. B. (1984). Effect of a multicomponent maintenance program on long-term weight loss. *Journal of Consulting and Clinical Psychology, 52,* 480–481.

Peters, L. C., & Esses, L. M. (1985). Family environment as perceived by children with a chronically ill parent. *Journal of Chronic Disease, 38,* 301–308.

Pino, C. J. (1984). Family diagnosis and treatment planning and multi-modal family therapy and personalized family enrichment. *Family Therapy, 11,* 175–183.

Piotrkowski, C. (1979). *Work and the family system: A naturalistic study of working class and lower middle class families.* New York: Free Press.

Piotrkowski, C., & Katz, M. (1982). Indirect socialization of children: The effects of mothers' jobs on academic behaviors. *Child Development, 53,* 1520–1529.

Plomin, R., & DeFries, J. (1985). *Origins of individual differences in infancy: The Colorado Adoption Project.* New York: Academic Press.

Polich, J. M., Armor, D. J., & Braiker, H. B. (1981). *The course of alcoholism: Four years after treatment.* New York: Wiley.

Pratt, R., Linn, M., Carmichael, J., & Webb, N. (1977). The alcoholic's perception of the ward as a predictor of aftercare attendance. *Journal of Clinical Psychology, 33,* 915–918.

Price, R. A., Chen, K., Cavalli-Sforza, L. L., & Feldman, M. W. (1981). Models of spouse influence and their application to smoking behavior. *Social Biology, 28,* 14–29.

Pullen, G. P. (1982). The 17 day community. *International Journal of Therapeutic Communities, 2,* 115–126.

Rees, D. W. (1985). Health beliefs and compliance with alcoholism treatment. *Journal of Studies on Alcohol, 46,* 517–524.

Reich, W., Earls, F., & Powell, J. (1988). A comparison of the home and social environments of children of alcoholic and non-alcoholic parents. *British Journal of Addiction, 83,* 831–839.

Reynolds, F. D., O'Leary, M., & Walker, R. D. (1982). Family environment as a predictor of alcoholism treatment outcome. *International Journal of the Addictions, 17,* 341–354.

Riley, D. M., Sobell, L. C., Leo, G. I., Sobell, M. B., & Klajner, E. (1987). Behavioral treatment of alcohol problems: A review and a comparison of behavioral and non-behavioral studies. In W. M. Cox (Ed.), *Treatment and prevention of alcohol problems: A resource manual* (pp. 73–115). New York: Academic Press.

Rimmer, J. (1982). The children of alcoholics: An exploratory study. *Children and Youth Services Review, 4,* 365–373.

Roberts, K. S., & Brent, E. E. (1982). Physician utilization and illness patterns in families of alcoholics. *Journal of Studies on Alcohol, 43,* 119–128.

Roberts, M., Floyd, F., O'Farrell, T., & Cutter, H. (1985). Marital interactions and the duration of alcoholic husbands' sobriety. *American Journal of Drug and Alcohol Abuse, 11,* 303–313.

Roehl, J. E., & Okun, M. A. (1984). Depression symptoms among women reentering college: The role of negative life events and family social support. *Journal of College Student Personnel, 25,* 251–254.

Roghmann, K., Roberts, J., Smith, T., Wells, S., & Wersinger, R. (1981). Alcoholics' versus nonalcoholics' use of services of a health maintenance organization. *Journal of Studies on Alcohol, 42,* 312–322.

Rollnick, S. (1982). Staff-patient perceptions of the helpfulness of an alcoholism treatment program: An exploratory study of treatment relationships. *International Journal of the Addictions, 17,* 513–521.

Room, R. (1980). Treatment-seeking populations and larger realities. In G. Edwards & M. Grant (Eds.), *Alcoholism treatment in transition* (pp. 205–224). Baltimore: University Park Press.

Roosa, M. W., Sandler, I. N., Gehring, M., Beals, J., & Cappo, L. (1988). The Children of Alcoholics Life-Events Schedule: A stress scale for children of alcohol-abusing parents. *Journal of Studies on Alcohol, 49,* 422–429.

Rosenberg, H. (1983). Relapsed versus non-relapsed alcohol abusers: Coping skills, life events, and social support. *Addictive Behaviors, 8,* 183–186.

Rosenthal, D., Teague, M., Retish, P., West, J., & Vessell, R. (1983). The relationship between work environment attributes and burnout. *Journal of Leisure Research, 15,* 125–135.

Rossi, P. H., Berk, R. A., & Lenihan, K. J. (1980). *Money, work and crime: Some experimental results.* New York: Academic Press.

Russell, M., Henderson, C., & Blume, S. B. (1985). *Children of alcoholics: A review of the literature.* Buffalo: New York State Division of Alcoholism and Alcohol Abuse, Research Institute on Alcoholism.

Ryan, E., & Bell, M. (1983). Follow-up of a psychoanalytically oriented long-term treatment program for schizophrenic inpatients. *American Journal of Orthopsychiatry, 53,* 730–739.

Ryan, E., Bell, M., & Metcalf, J. (1982). The development of a rehabilitation psychology program for schizophrenics: Changes in the treatment environment. *Rehabilitation Psychology, 27,* 67–85.

Rydelius, P. (1981). Children of alcoholic fathers: Their social adjustment and their health status over twenty years. *Acta Paediatrica Scandinavica, 70,* Suppl. 286, 1–89.

Sanchez-Craig, M., & Walker, K. (1982). Teaching coping skills to chronic alcoholics in a coeducational halfway house: I. Assessment of programme effects. *British Journal of Addiction, 77,* 35–50.

REFERENCES

Sanchez-Craig, M., Wilkinson, D. A., & Walker, K. (1987). Theory and methods for secondary prevention of alcohol problems: A cognitively based approach. In W. M. Cox (Ed.), *Treatment and prevention of alcohol problems: A resource manual* (pp. 287-331). New York: Academic Press.

Saxe, L., Dougherty, D., Esty, K., & Fine, M. (1983). *The effectiveness and costs of alcoholism treatment* (Health Technology Case Study 22). Washington, DC: Office of Technology Assessment.

Schneewind, K., Beckman, M., & Engfer, A. (1983). *Eltern und kinder: Umwelteinflusse auf das familiare verhalten*. Stuttgart, West Germany: Kollhammer.

Schreibman, L., Kogel, R., Mills, D., & Burke, J. (1984). Training parent-child interactions. In E. Schopler & G. Mesibov (Eds.), *The effects of autism on the family* (pp. 187-205). New York: Plenum.

Schuckit, M. A., Schwei, M. G., & Gold, E. (1986). Prediction of outcome in inpatient alcoholics. *Journal of Studies on Alcohol, 47*, 151-155.

Schwab-Backman, N., Appelt, H., & Rist, F. (1981). Sex-role identification in women alcoholics and depressives. *Journal of Studies on Alcohol, 42*, 654-660.

Schwartz, G. E. (1982). Testing the biopsychosocial model: The ultimate challenge facing behavioral medicine? *Journal of Consulting and Clinical Psychology, 50*, 1040-1053.

Schwartz, M. A., & Wiggins, O. P. (1986). Systems and the structuring of meaning: Contributions to a biopsychosocial medicine. *American Journal of Psychiatry, 143*, 1213-1221.

Sechrest, L., West, S., Phillips, M., Redner, R., & Yeaton, W. (1979). Some neglected problems in evaluation research: Strength and integrity of treatments. In L. Sechrest, S. West, M. Phillips, R. Redner, & W. Yeaton (Eds.), *Evaluation studies review annual* (Vol. IV, pp. 15-35). Beverly Hills, CA: Sage.

Seeman, M., & Anderson, C. S. (1983). Alienation and alcohol: The role of work, mastery, and community in drinking behavior. *American Sociological Review, 48*, 60-77.

Sheehan, J. J., Wieman, R. J., & Bechtel, J. E. (1981). Follow-up of a twelve-month treatment program for chronic alcoholics. *International Journal of the Addictions, 16*, 233-241.

Shiffman, S. (1984). Coping with temptations to smoke. *Journal of Consulting and Clinical Psychology, 52*, 261-267.

Shiffman, S. (1985). Coping with temptations to smoke. In S. Shiffman & T. A. Wills (Eds.), *Coping and substance use* (pp. 223-242). New York: Academic Press.

Shiffman, S. (1986). A cluster-analytic classification of smoking relapse episodes. *Addictive Behaviors, 11*, 295-307.

Siegel, C., Alexander, M. J., & Lin, S. (1984). Severe alcoholism in the mental health sector: II. Effects of service utilization on readmission. *Journal of Studies on Alcohol, 45*, 510-516.

Sinclair, C., & Frankel, M. (1982). The effect of quality assurance activities on the quality of mental health services. *Quality Review Bulletin, 8*, 7-15.

Sjoberg, L., & Samsonowitz, V. (1985). Coping strategies and relapse in alcohol abuse. *Drug and Alcohol Dependence, 15*, 283-301.

Skinner, H. A. (1981a). Assessment of alcohol problems: Basic principles, critical issues, and future trends. In Y. Israel, F. B. Glaser, H. Kallant, R. E.

Popham, W. Schmidt, & R. G. Smart (Eds.), *Research advances in alcohol and drug problems* (Vol. 6, pp. 319–369). New York: Plenum.

Skinner, H. A. (1981b). Different strokes for different folks. In R. E. Meyer, B. C. Glueck, J. E. O'Brien, T. F. Babor, J. H. Jaffe, & J. R. Stabenau (Eds.), *Evaluation of the alcoholic: Implications for research, theory, and treatment* (pp. 349–367). Rockville, MD: National Institute on Alcohol Abuse and Alcoholism.

Slater, E., & Haber, J. (1984). Adolescent adjustment following divorce as a function of familial conflict. *Journal of Consulting and Clinical Psychology, 52,* 920–921.

Smart, R. G., & Gray, G. (1978). Multiple predictors of dropout from alcoholism treatment. *Archives of General Psychiatry, 35,* 363–367.

Smith, E. M., Cloninger, C. R., & Bradford, B. S. (1983). Predictors of mortality in alcoholic women: A prospective follow-up study. *Alcoholism: Clinical and Experimental Research, 7,* 237–243.

Smolensky, W., Martin, D., Lorimor, R., & Forthofer, R. (1980). Leisure behavior and attitudes toward leisure of alcoholics and non-alcoholics. *Journal of Studies on Alcohol, 41,* 293–299.

Snowden, L. R. (1984). Treatment participation and outcome in a program for problem drinker-drivers. *Evaluation and Program Planning, 7,* 65–71.

Sobell, L. C., Sobell, M. B., & Maisto, S. A. (1984). Follow-up attrition in alcohol treatment studies: Is "no news" bad news, good news or no news? *Drug and Alcohol Dependence, 13,* 1–7.

Sokolow, L., Welte, J., Hynes, G., & Lyons, J. (1980). Treatment-related differences between male and female alcoholics. *Focus on Women, 1,* 42–56.

Spiegel, D., & Wissler, T. (1983). Perceptions of family environment among psychiatric patients and their wives. *Family Process, 22,* 537–547.

Spiegel, D., & Wissler, T. (1986). Family environment as a predictor of psychiatric rehospitalization. *American Journal of Psychiatry, 143,* 56–60.

Steiner, H. (1982). The sociotherapeutic environment of a child psychosomatic ward (or, Is pediatrics bad for your mental health?). *Child Psychiatry and Human Development, 13,* 71–78.

Steiner, H., Haldipur, C., & Stack, L. (1982). The acute admission ward as a therapeutic community. *American Journal of Psychiatry, 139,* 897–901.

Steinglass, P. (1980). A life history model of the alcoholic family. *Family Process, 19,* 211–226.

Steinglass, P. (1981). The alcoholic family at home: Patterns of interaction in dry, wet, and transitional stages of alcoholism. *Archives of General Psychiatry, 38,* 578–584.

Steinglass, P., & Robertson, A. (1983). The alcoholic family. In B. Kissin & H. Begleiter (Eds.), *The pathogenesis of alcoholism: Vol. VI. Psychosocial factors* (pp. 243–307). New York: Plenum.

Stiffman, A. R., Jung, K. G., & Feldman, R. A. (1986). A multivariate risk model for childhood behavior problems. *American Journal of Orthopsychiatry, 56,* 204–211.

Strug, D. L., & Hyman, M. M. (1981). Social networks of alcoholics. *Journal of Studies on Alcohol, 42,* 855–884.

Szapocznick, J., Kurtines, W., Foote, F., Perez-Vidal, A., & Hervis, O. (1983). Conjoint versus one person family therapy: Some evidence for the effectiveness of conducting family therapy through one person. *Journal of Consulting and Clinical Psychology, 51,* 889–899.

REFERENCES

Tarter, R. Alterman, A., & Edwards, K. (1985). Vulnerability to alcoholism in men: A behavior/genetic perspective. *Journal of Studies on Alcohol, 46,* 329–356.

Taube, C. A., Lee, E. S., & Forthofer, R. N. (1984). Diagnosis-related groups for mental disorders, alcoholism, and drug abuse: Evaluation and alternatives. *Hospital and Community Psychiatry, 35,* 452–455.

Terry, K., Sobieski, J., Dunne, K., & Steiner, H. (1984). A comparison of staff and patient perceptions of a child and adolescent psychosomatic unit and a pediatric unit. *Child Psychiatry and Human Development, 14,* 230–248.

Thoits, P. A. (1983). Multiple identities and psychological well-being: A reformulation and test of the social isolation hypothesis. *American Sociological Review, 48,* 174–187.

Thoits, P. A. (1986). Multiple identities: Examining gender and marital status differences in distress. *American Sociological Review, 51,* 259–272.

Thom, B. (1984). A process approach to women's use of alcohol services. *British Journal of Addiction, 79,* 377–382.

Thomson, B., & Vaux, A. (1986). The importation, transmission, and moderation of stress in the family system. *American Journal of Community Psychology, 14,* 39–57.

Timmer, S. G., Veroff, J., & Colten, M. E. (1985). Life stress, helplessness and the use of alcohol and drugs to cope. In S. Shiffman, & T. A. Wills (Eds.), *Coping and substance use.* New York: Academic Press.

Tuchfeld, B. (1981). Spontaneous remission in alcoholics: Empirical observations and theoretical implications. *Journal of Studies on Alcohol, 42,* 626–641.

Tuchfeld, B. S., Lipton, W. L., & Lile, E. A. (1983). Social involvement and the resolution of alcoholism. *Journal of Drug Issues, 13,* 323–332.

Tucker, J. A., Vuchinich, R. E., & Harris, C. V. (1985). Determinants of substance abuse relapse. In M. Galizio & S. A. Maisto (Eds.), *Determinants of substance abuse: Biological, psychological, and environmental factors* (pp. 383–421). New York: Plenum.

Vaglum, P., Friis, S., & Karterud, S. (1985). Why are the results of milieu therapy for schizophrenic patients contradictory? An analysis based on four empirical studies. *The Yale Journal of Biology and Medicine, 58,* 349–361.

Vaillant, G. E. (1983). *The natural history of alcoholism: Causes, patterns, and paths to recovery.* Cambridge, MA: Harvard University Press.

Vaillant, G. E., Clark, W., Cyrus, C., Milofsky, E. S., Kopp, J., Wulsin, V. W., & Mogielnicki, N. P. (1983). Prospective study of alcoholism treatment: Eight-year follow-up. *American Journal of Medicine, 75,* 455–463.

Vaillant, G. E., & Milofsky, E. S. (1982). The etiology of alcoholism: A prospective viewpoint. *American Psychologist, 37,* 494–503.

Van Dijk, W. K., & Van Dijk-Koffeman, A. (1973). A follow-up study of 211 treated male alcohol addicts. *British Journal of Addiction, 68,* 3–24.

Vannicelli, M. (1978). Impact of aftercare in the treatment of alcoholics: A cross-lagged panel analysis. *Journal of Studies on Alcohol, 39,* 1875–1886.

Vannicelli, M. (1984). Treatment outcome of alcoholic women: The state of the art in relation to sex bias and expectancy effects. In S. C. Wilsnack & L. J. Beckman (Eds.), *Alcohol problems in women* (pp. 369–412). New York: Guilford Press.

Vannicelli, M., Gingerich, S., & Ryback, R. (1983). Family problems related to the treatment and outcome of alcoholic patients. *British Journal of Addiction, 78,* 193–204.

Vaughn, C. E., Snyder, K. S., Jones, S., Freeman, W. B., & Falloon, I. R. H. (1984). Family factors in schizophrenic relapse. *Archives of General Psychiatry, 41,* 1169–1177.

Velleman, R. (1984). The engagement of new residents: A missing dimension in the evaluation of halfway houses for problem drinkers. *Journal of Studies on Alcohol, 45,* 251–259.

Verbrugge, L. (1985). Gender and health: An update on hypotheses and evidence. *Journal of Health and Social Behavior, 26,* 156–182.

Verhaest, S. (1983). The assessment of the maturation of a therapeutic community. *International Journal of Therapeutic Communities, 4,* 183–195.

Verinis, J. S. (1983a). Agreement between alcoholics and relatives when reporting follow-up status. *International Journal of the Addictions, 18,* 891–894.

Verinis, J. S. (1983b). Ward atmosphere as a factor in irregular discharge for an alcohol rehabilitation unit. *International Journal of the Addictions, 18,* 895–899.

Vuchinich, R. E., & Tucker, J. A. (1988). Contributions from behavioral theories of choice to an analysis of alcohol abuse. *Journal of Abnormal Psychology, 97,* 181–195.

Walker, R. D., Donovan, D. M., Kivlahan, D. R., & O'Leary, M. R. (1983). Length of stay, neuropsychological performance, and aftercare: Influences on alcohol treatment outcome. *Journal of Consulting and Clinical Psychology, 51,* 900–911.

Wanberg, K. W., & Horn, J. L. (1983). Assessment of alcohol use with multidimensional concepts and measures. *American Psychologist, 38,* 1055–1069.

Ward, D. (1981). The influence of family relationships on social and psychological functioning: A follow-up study. *Journal of Marriage and the Family, 43,* 807–815.

Ward, D. A., Bendel, R. B., & Lange, D. (1982). A reconsideration of environmental resources and the posttreatment functioning of alcoholic patients. *Journal of Health and Social Behavior, 23,* 310–317.

Watson, C. G., & Pucel, J. (1985). Consistency of posttreatment alcoholics' drinking patterns. *Journal of Consulting and Clinical Psychology, 53,* 679–683.

Weick, K. E., & Bougon, M. G. (1986). Organization as cognitive maps. In H. P. Simms, Jr. & D. A. Gioia (Eds.), *The thinking organization* (pp. 102–135). San Francisco: Jossey-Bass.

Weisner, C. (1986). The social ecology of alcohol treatment in the United States. In M. Galanter (Ed.), *Recent developments in alcoholism (Vol. 5, pp. 203–243).* New York: Plenum.

Weiss, C. H. (1972). *Evaluation research: Methods of assessing program effectiveness.* Englewood Cliffs, NJ: Prentice-Hall.

Weiss, C. H. (Ed.) (1978). *Using social research in public policy making.* Lexington, MA: D. C. Heath.

Weissman, M. (1983). The depressed mother and her rebellious adolescent. In H. Morrison (Ed.), *Children of depressed parents: Risk, identification, and intervention* (pp. 99–113). New York: Grune & Stratton.

Wells, L., Singer, C., & Polgar, A. (1986). *To enhance quality of life in institutions: An empowerment model in long-term care: A partnership of residents, staff, and families.* Toronto: University of Toronto Press.

Wells-Parker, E., Miles, S., & Spencer, B. (1983). Stress experiences and drinking histories of elderly drunken-driving offenders. *Journal of Studies on Alcohol, 44*, 429–437.

Wendt, R., Mosher, L., Matthews, S., & Menn, A. (1983). Comparison of two treatment environments for schizophrenia. In J. G. Gunderson, O. A. Will, & L. R. Mosher (Eds.), *Principles and practice of milieu therapy* (pp. 17–33). New York: Aronson.

Werner, E. E. (1986). Resilient offspring of alcoholics: A longitudinal study from birth to age 18. *Journal of Studies on Alcohol, 47*, 34–40.

West, M. O., & Prinz, R. J. (1987). Parental alcoholism and childhood psychopathology. *Psychological Bulletin, 102*, 204–218.

Wetzel, J. (1978). Depression and dependence upon unsustaining environments. *Clinical Social Work Journal, 6*, 75–89.

Whitehead, P. C., & Simpkins, J. (1983). Occupational factors in alcoholism. In B. Kissin & H. Begleiter (Eds.), *The pathogenesis of alcoholism: Vol. 6. Psychosocial factors* (pp. 405–496). New York: Plenum.

Wiens, A. N., & Menustik, C. E. (1983). Treatment outcome and patient characteristics in an aversion therapy program for alcoholism. *American Psychologist, 38*, 1089–1096.

Wilderman, R., & Mezzelo, J. (1984). Paving the road to financial security: The direct service model. *Mental Health Administration, 2*, 184–194.

Wille, R. (1983). Processes of recovery from heroin dependence: Relationship to treatment, social changes and drug use. *Journal of Drug Issues, 13*, 333–342.

Wilsnack, R. W., Wilsnack, S. C., & Klassen, A. D., Jr. (1984). Women's drinking and drinking problems. Patterns from a 1981 national survey. *American Journal of Public Health, 74*, 1231–1238.

Wilsnack, S. C. (1982). Alcohol abuse and alcoholism in women. In E. M. Pattison & E. Kaufman (Eds.), *Encylopedic handbook of alcoholism* (pp. 718–735). New York: Gardner Press.

Wilsnack, S. C., & Beckman, L. J. (1984). *Alcohol problems in women.* New York: Guilford Press.

Wilson, G. T. (1985). Psychological prognostic factors in the treatment of obesity. In J. Hirsch & T. B. Van Itallie (Eds.), *Recent advances in obesity research* (Vol. IV). London: Libbey.

Wiseman, J. P. (1979). *Stations of the lost: The treatment of skid row alcoholics.* Chicago: University of Chicago Press.

Wiseman, J. (1980). The "home treatment": The first steps in trying to cope with an alcoholic husband. *Family Relations, 29*, 541–549.

Wiseman, J. (1980). Sober comportment: Patterns and perspectives on alcohol addiction. *Journal of Studies on Alcohol, 42*, 106–126.

Wiseman, J. P. (1982). Skid row alcoholics: Treatment, survival, and escape. In E. M. Pattison & E. Kaufman (Eds.), *Encyclopedic handbook of alcoholism* (pp. 946–953). New York: Gardner Press.

Wolin, S., Bennett, L., Noonan, D., & Teitelbaum, M. (1980). Disrupted family rituals: A factor in the intergenerational transmission of alcoholism. *Journal of Studies on Alcohol, 41*, 199–214.

Yahr, H. T. (1988). A national comparison of public- and private-sector alcoholism treatment delivery system characteristics. *Journal of Studies on Alcohol, 49*, 233–239.

Yeaton, W. H., & Sechrest, L. (1981). Critical dimensions in the choice and maintenance of successful treatments: Strength, integrity, and effectiveness. *Journal of Consulting and Clinical Psychology, 49,* 156–167.

Zucker, R. A., & Gomberg, E. S. L. (1986). Etiology of alcoholism reconsidered: The case for a biopsychosocial process. *American Psychologist, 41,* 783–793.

Zweben, A. (1986). Problem drinking and marital adjustment. *Journal of Studies on Alcohol, 47,* 167–172.

Author Index

Abrams, D. B., 105, 243, 249
Adler, R., 180, 249
Ahles, T. A., 62, 235, 249
Albrecht, O. L., 42, 249
Alexander, M. J., 269
Allen, R. P., 261
Allred, L. J., 254
Alterman, A., 185, 270, 271
Amaro, H., 74, 83, 84, 85, 250
Ambler, J., 215, 252
Ambron, S. R., 254
American Psychiatric Association, 7, 249
Anderson, C. S., 91, 237, 269
Andrews, R. H., 267
Aneshensel, C. S., 83, 249
Annis, H.M., 74, 75, 249
Antes, D., 250
Appelt, H., 177, 261, 269
Armor, D. J., 8, 44, 50, 89, 114, 249, 267
Azrin, N. H., 230, 231, 249, 258

Babor, T. F., 23, 24, 37, 41, 90, 113, 250, 253
Bader, E., 215, 250
Badgett, S., 230, 266
Baer, J. S., 263
Baer, P. E., 185, 250
Baillargeon, J. G., 28, 254
Ball, L., 135, 260
Baron, R. M., 240, 250
Barr, H. L., 148, 250
Bashford, M. B., 215, 229, 257
Beals, J., 268
Beardslee, W. R., 157, 189, 250
Beattie, M., 256, 262

Bechtel, J. E., 269
Beck, A. T., 236, 250
Beckman, L. J., 73, 74, 83, 84, 85, 232, 250, 273
Beckman, M., 269
Bell, M., 202, 203, 206, 250, 268
Bemporad, J., 250
Bendel, R. B., 116, 272
Bennett, L., 273
Benson, C. S., 188, 250
Berglund, M., 72, 151, 163, 223, 251, 265, 266
Bergstrom, B., 25, 251
Berk, R. A., 268
Bible, 11
Bickman, L., 232, 251
Biernacki, P., 152, 153, 227, 251
Billings, A. G., 51, 96, 98, 103–105, 107, 116, 131, 153, 182, 189, 191, 211, 227, 234, 251, 254, 264
Blane, H. T., 4, 237, 251, 258
Block, T., 43, 252
Blumberg, L., 63, 251
Blume, S. B., 74, 75, 179, 251, 268
Bohman, M., 179, 253
Borduin, C. M., 229, 258
Boruch, R. F., 240, 252
Bougon, M. G., 236, 272
Bourne, P. G., 74, 252
Bradford, B. S., 270
Bradshaw, S., 209, 219, 260
Brady, C. A., 215, 252
Braiker, H. B., 8, 44, 75, 89, 252, 267
Brent, E. E., 159, 268
Brissett, D., 28, 252

275

Brody, J., 90, 122, 266
Bromet, E. J., 98, 176, 252, 262
Brown, D., 255
Brown, S., 130, 252
Brownell, K. D., 130, 153, 252
Bruce, M., 74, 260
Burke, J., 269
Burling, T. A., 141, 252

Caddy, G. R., 43, 252
Cahalan, D., 3, 231, 252
Callan, V. J., 183, 252
Campbell, D. T., 253
Cappo, L., 268
Carey, K. B., 226, 261
Carmichael, J., 267
Carpenter, P., 97, 252
Cartwright, A., 4, 252
Cavalli-Sforza, L. L., 267
Chan, D., 61, 139, 256, 264
Chaney, E. F., 124, 252
Charles, H. L., 267
Chen, H., 9, 232, 238, 240, 253
Chen, K., 267
Cherepon, J. A., 43, 66, 266
Choquette, K. A., 90, 253
Clair, D., 188, 253
Clark, D. C., 260
Clark, V. A., 83, 249
Clark, W., 271
Clausen, J. A., 85, 253
Cloninger, C. R., 179, 253, 270
Cohen, R., 177, 261
Cohen, S., 263
Cohler, B., 189, 253, 260
Colby, J. P., 261
Colten, M. E., 90, 271
Condiotti, M. M., 131, 253
Conley, J. J., 75, 259
Cook, T. D., 253
Cooke, R., 196, 253
Cooper, A. M., 44, 253
Cooper, H. M., 229, 258
Cooper, M. L., 130, 253
Coppotelli, H. C., 130, 253
Cordray, D. S., 240, 253
Cosper, R., 91, 253
Costello, R. M., 27, 28, 43, 62, 66, 72, 253, 254
Cox, W. M., 84, 254
Coyne, J. C., 176, 254
Cronbach, L. J., 9, 18, 24, 239, 240, 241, 254, 255
Cronkite, R. C., 51, 85, 98, 103, 107, 116, 126, 132, 176, 178, 239, 251, 254, 256, 263, 264
Crosse, S., 261
Cummings, K. M., 257
Cutter, H. S. G., 229, 266, 268
Cyrus, C., 271

Dahlgren, L., 76, 82, 254
Daly, J., 147, 265
Daniels, D., 193, 254
Dansky, L., 260
David, T., 217, 264
Davis, D., 257
deBlois, C. S., 175, 254
DeFries, J., 185, 267
DeRubeis, R. J., 258
De Soto, C. B., 135, 254
Deutsch, C., 179, 180, 254
De Witt, K. N., 215, 229, 257
Dishotsky, N., 212, 257
Doherty, E. G., 85, 254
Dohrenwend, B. P., 145, 261
Dohrenwend, B. S., 106, 254
Dolinsky, Z., 37, 250
Donovan, D. M., 235, 259, 272
Dornbusch, S. M., 254
Dorph, D., 255
Dougherty, D., 269
Douglas, J. J., 74, 254
Drake, R. E., 179, 180, 227, 254, 255
Drew, L. R., 150, 255
Druley, K. A., 262
Duckitt, A., 41, 255
Dunkle, J., 261
Dunn, N. J., 142, 176, 255, 259
Dunne, K., 271
Dwoskin, J., 39, 255

Earls, F., 267
Ed, V., 98, 252
Edwards, A. L., 239, 255
Edwards, D., 137, 153, 255
Edwards, G., 146, 147, 226, 248, 255
Edwards, K., 185, 270, 271
Egan, K. J., 215, 255
Egert, S., 266
Einhorn, H. J., 41, 255
Eiser, J., 261
El-Guebaly, N., 191, 255
Elkins, R. L., 25, 255
Ellis, A. S., 62, 255
Ellsworth, R. B., 50, 255
Emery, G., 250
Emery, R. E., 157, 189, 194, 255
Emrick, C. D., 4, 41, 75, 255, 256
Engfer, A., 269
Enos, D. M., 194, 256
Erdlen, F. R., 260
Eriksen, L., 209, 256
Esses, L. M., 188, 267
Esty, K., 269
Etringer, B. D., 34, 256
Evans, M. D., 258

Fagan, R. W., 63, 65, 66, 230, 256
Fairchild, H., 207, 256
Falloon, I. R. H., 272

AUTHOR INDEX

Feldman, M. W., 267
Feldman, R. A., 193, 270
Feuerstein, M., 104, 256
Fine, M., 269
Fink, E., 113, 234, 256, 262
Finney, J. W., 9, 61, 112, 116, 139, 141, 145, 161, 166, 173, 210, 239, 243, 248, 256, 264
Fisher-Nelson, H., 265
Fisk, D. M., 238, 258
Fitzgerald, J. L., 22, 62, 256
Floyd, F. J., 229, 266, 268
Folkman, S., 11, 106, 132, 257, 260
Follette, W. C., 137, 259
Fondacaro, M. R., 107, 108, 257
Foote, F., 270
Ford, J. D., 215, 229, 257
Forthofer, R. N., 270, 271
Frankel, M., 210, 269
Freeman, W. B., 272
Frerichs, R. R., 83, 249
Friedman, S., 207, 257
Friis, S., 217, 218, 257, 271
Fuhr, R., 197, 212, 257, 264
Funderburk, F. R., 261

Gabrielli, W. F., 179, 257
Gallant, D., 253
Gamble, W., 161, 256, 264
Gamer, E., 260
Garmezy, L. B., 250
Garzon, S. R., 85, 259
Gehring, M., 268
Geisbrecht, N., 65, 257
Genest, M., 188, 253
Gentry, W. D., 7, 257
George, W. H., 253
Gilbert, F. S., 62, 257
Gingerich, S., 122, 229, 271
Godley, M. D., 249, 262
Gold, E., 72, 269
Goldman, H. H., 231, 257
Goldstein, M. J., 229, 257
Gomberg, E. S. L., 6, 74, 257, 274
Gomez, H., 240, 252
Goodwin, D. W., 260
Gordis, E., 255
Gordon, J. R., 8, 11, 130, 153, 227, 229, 237, 262
Gorman, J., 160, 169, 257
Graves, T. D., 259
Gray, G., 62, 234, 270
Gregory, V. R., 34, 256
Grunebaum, H., 253, 260
Gunn, R., 257
Guthrie, S., 266

Haber, J., 194, 270
Hahlweg, K., 229, 257
Haldipur, C., 206, 270

Halikas, J. A., 63, 257
Hall, G. M., 262
Hall, R. L., 175, 257
Hand, I., 229, 257
Handal, P. J., 194, 256
Hanna, E., 85, 257
Hanson, M., 6, 10, 260
Hanson, R. C., 259
Harburg, E., 90, 257
Harford, T. C., 83, 90, 258, 266
Harris, C. V., 271
Harrison, R. H., 266
Harwin, J., 157, 158, 266
Hasha, N., 265
Hatry, H. P., 238, 258
Hattie, J. A., 34, 258
Hayes, S. C., 228, 258
Hazelrigg, M. D., 229, 258
Heller, K., 188, 250
Henderson, C., 179, 268
Hensman, C., 266
Hervis, O., 270
Hess, R. D., 254
Hesselbrock, M. N., 42, 90, 253, 258
Hesselbrock, V. M., 175, 257
Hester, R. K., 4, 41, 58, 61, 226, 263
Higgins, P. C., 42, 249
Hill, M. J., 4, 258
Hingson, R., 233, 258
Hirsch, B., 190, 197, 258
Hodson, C. A., 178, 263
Hogarth, R. M., 41, 255
Holahan, C. J., 97, 104, 107, 193, 258
Hollon, S. D., 236, 258
Horn, J. L., 227, 272
Hornick, R. C., 254
Houle, M., 104, 256
Huffine, C. L., 85, 253
Hull, J. G., 11, 136, 151, 258
Hummon, N., 255
Hunt, G., 230, 258
Hyman, M. M., 151, 270
Hynes, G., 270

Igra, A., 217, 264
Istavan, J., 141, 258
Ito, J. R., 235, 259

Jackson, D., 183, 252
Jackson, J., 121, 259
Jackson, P., 230, 265
Jackson, S., 211, 259
Jacob, T., 136, 142, 144, 158, 176, 191, 255, 259
Jacobson, G. R., 63, 64, 259
Jacobson, N. S., 137, 259
Jaffe, J., 37, 250
Janis, I. L., 130, 259
Jarrett, R. B., 228, 258
Jeger, A., 207, 257

AUTHOR INDEX

Jessor, R., 90, 237, 259
Jessor, S. L., 90, 259
Johnson, S., 259
Jones, S., 123, 259, 272
Jouriles, E., 151, 258
Judge, J. J., 63, 259
Jung, K. G., 193, 270

Kamarck, T., 263
Kammeier, M. L., 28, 75, 252, 259
Kanter, R. M., 84, 259
Karterud, S., 217, 271
Katz, L., 63, 65, 259
Katz, M., 197, 267
Kauffman, C., 189, 260
Kaufman, C., 253
Kaufman, E., 158, 260
Kazdin, A. E., 137, 260
Keener, J. J., 258
Keller, M. B., 250
Kenny, D. A., 240, 250
Kessler, R. C., 254
Kidd, R. 267
Killen, J. D., 131, 260
Kirk, S., 62, 260
Kissin, B., 6, 10, 260
Kivlahan, D. R., 272
Klajner, E., 268
Klassen, A. D. Jr., 273
Klein, D. N., 189, 260
Klerman, G. L., 250
Knop, J., 180, 260
Kobasa, S., 104, 260
Kocel, K. M., 232, 250
Kogel, R., 269
Kohn, M., 108, 197, 260
Kopp, J., 271
Koran, L., 211, 260
Kotler, P., 146, 260
Krantz, S., 177, 260
Kron, R., 262
Krueger, D. W., 152, 260
Krupinsky, J., 62, 255
Kuller, L. H., 4, 262
Kurtines, W., 135, 154, 260, 270
Kyle, E., 255

Lacoursiere, R., 209, 219, 260
Lando, H. A., 34, 256
Lange, D., 116, 272
Lanyon, R., 123, 259
La Porte, D. J., 50, 260
Laundergan, J. C., 28, 252
Lazarus, R., 11, 106, 132, 257, 260
Leaf, P., 74, 260
Leckman, J. F., 263
Lee, E. S., 271
Leff, J., 132, 157, 261
Leigh, H., 227, 261
Lemke, S., 216, 217, 264

Lenihan, K. J., 268
Leo, G. I., 268
Leonard, K. E., 142, 176, 191, 237, 251, 259
Levin, H. M., 242, 261
Liban, C. B., 74, 249
Lichtenstein, E., 130, 131, 252, 253, 261, 263
Light, E., 252
Lile, E. A., 142, 271
Lin, S., 269
Lindbeck, V., 75, 83, 261
Lindblom, P. E., 25, 251
Lindsay, J. S. B., 206, 261
Link, B. G., 145, 261
Linn, M., 267
Linsky, A. S., 74, 90, 261
Lipsey, M. W., 232, 236, 261
Lipton, W. L., 142, 271
Lisansky, J. M., 74, 257
Litman, G. K., 84, 123, 261
Longabaugh, R., 256, 262
Lopes, C. E., 254
Lorimor, R., 270
Lowenstein, A., 178, 261
Luborsky, L., 262
Ludwig, A. M., 91, 261
Luk, S. L., 202, 265
Lutz, M., 177, 261
Lynch, G. W., 255
Lyons, J., 270
Lyttle, M. O., 257

Maccoby, N., 260
MacDonald, J. G., 74, 261
Mackenzie, A., 46, 146, 261
Madden, J. S., 25, 262
Maisto, S. A., 44, 46, 226, 253, 261, 262, 270
Malcolm, M. T., 25, 262
Mallams, J. H., 230, 262
Mandell, W., 4, 18, 21, 38, 262
Mangione, T., 258
Margolis, E. T., 260
Markowitz, M., 90, 262
Marlatt, G. A., 8, 11, 130, 153, 227, 229, 237, 250, 252, 262
Martin, D., 270
Martin, J. L., 106, 254
Masi, J., 62, 260
Matarazzo, J. D., 141, 258, 265
Matthews, S., 273
Mauss, A. L., 63, 65, 66, 230, 256
May, S. J., 4, 98, 252, 262
Mayer, J., 116, 262
McAdoo, W. G., 267
McCabe, R. J. R., 147, 163, 262
McCrady, B. S., 50, 158, 159, 242, 256, 262, 265, 266
McLachlan, J., 243, 262

AUTHOR INDEX

McLaughlin, R. J., 250
McLellan, A. T., 37, 41, 42, 260, 262
McNeil, D., 256
Mello, N. K., 262
Menaghen, E., 107, 262
Mendelson, J. H., 22, 250, 262
Menn, A., 202, 265, 273
Menustik, C. E., 40, 76, 273
Merikangas, K. R., 175, 176, 193, 262, 263
Mermelstein, R., 152, 263
Mervis, E., 107, 262
Metcalf, J., 202, 268
Mewborn, R., 112, 256
Meyer, R. E., 258
Meyers, A., 258
Meyers, C. E., 194, 265
Meyers, R. J., 249, 262
Meyerson, D., 116, 262
Mezzelo, J., 210, 273
Miles, S., 90, 272
Miller, J. J., III, 254
Miller, K. D., 262
Miller, W. R., 4, 34, 41, 58, 61, 140, 226, 263
Mills, D., 269
Milne, D., 209, 263
Milofsky, E. S., 135, 271
Mink, I. T., 194, 263, 265
Mitchell, R. E., 98, 107, 176, 178, 263
Mogielnicki, N. P., 271
Moos, B. S., 92, 96, 98, 116, 139, 185, 193, 195, 212, 260, 265
Moos, R. H., 9, 12, 22, 23, 26, 28, 29, 35, 51, 61, 84, 85, 92, 96–98, 100, 103, 104, 105, 106, 107, 108, 112, 116, 126, 131, 132, 139, 141, 145, 153, 161, 168, 176–178, 182, 185, 189, 190, 191, 193–195, 197, 198, 202, 206, 209, 210, 211, 212, 216–218, 226, 227, 234, 239, 243, 248, 251, 254, 256–258, 260, 263, 264
Morse, C. L., 257
Mosher, L., 202, 265, 273
Mueller, D., 255
Mulford, H. A., 11, 22, 62, 85, 134, 226, 256, 265

Nace, E. P., 159, 265
Nathan, P. E., 4, 38, 43, 66, 226, 265
National Institute on Alcohol Abuse and Alcoholism, 3, 41, 265
Neale, J. M., 157, 189, 255
Nelson, R. O., 228, 258
Neuberger, O. W., 39, 43, 265
Newlin, D. B., 267
Ng, M. L., 202, 265
Nicholls, P., 255, 266
Nihira, K., 194, 263, 265
Nisle, A., 267
Noel, N. E., 76, 83, 265

Noonan, D., 273
Nordstrom, G., 151, 223, 265
Nutter, C. P., 74, 254
Nylander, I., 179, 265

O'Brien, C. P., 262
O'Connor, A., 147, 265
O'Donnell, W. E., 254
Oei, T. P. S., 230, 265
O'Farrell, T. J., 175, 229, 266, 268
Offord, D. R., 255
Ogborne, A. C., 4, 151, 266
Ohlin, H., 25, 251
Ojehagen, A., 72, 266
Okun, M. A., 97, 268
O'Leary, M. R., 267, 272
Oppenheim, A., 261
Oppenheimer, E., 255, 266
Orford, J., 8, 12, 122, 157, 158, 160, 169, 226, 227, 266
Orleans, C. T., 130, 253
Ornstein, P., 43, 66, 266
Ottenberg, D. J., 250

Page, R. D., 230, 266
Paolino, T., 158, 159, 266
Parente, R. J., 260
Parker, D., 74, 90, 122, 266
Parker, E., 266
Parkes, K., 108, 266
Patterson, E., 97, 267
Pattison, E. M., 43, 158, 260, 267
Patton, M. Q., 267
Pauls, D. L., 263
Pemberton, D. A., 75, 267
Penk, W. E., 46, 97, 218, 267
Perez-Vidal, A., 270
Perri, M. G., 105, 131, 267
Peters, L. C., 188, 267
Pfeffer, N. G., 85, 253
Phillips, D. C., 254
Phillips, M., 269
Pino, C. J., 215, 267
Piotrkowski, C., 194, 197, 267
Plomin, R., 179, 185, 257, 267
Pokorny, A. D., 250
Polgar, A., 272
Polich, J. M., 8, 26, 27, 44, 46, 62, 89, 114, 249, 267
Pollard, J. A., 236, 261
Powell, J., 267
Pratt, H. H. 262
Pratt, R., 235, 265, 267
Price, R. A., 83, 267
Prinz, R. J., 180, 273
Prue, D. M., 249
Prusoff, B. A., 263
Puccetti, M., 104, 260
Pucel, J., 44, 89, 272
Pullen, G. P., 206, 267

Raphael, B., 180, 249
Rawson, N., 261
Redner, R., 269
Rees, D. W., 235, 267
Reich, W., 180, 267
Reischl, T., 190, 197, 258
Reiser, M. F., 227, 261
Retish, P., 268
Revenstorf, D., 137, 259
Reynolds, F. D., 234, 267
Riley, D. M., 36, 268
Rimmer, J., 192, 268
Rist, F., 269
Roberts, J., 268
Roberts, K. S., 158, 268
Roberts, M., 166, 268
Roberts, W., 267
Robertson, A., 136, 270
Robinowitz, R., 218, 267
Roehl, J. E., 97, 268
Rogers, H. J., 34, 258
Roghmann, K., 140, 268
Rollnick, S., 28, 268
Room, R., 3, 268
Rooney, J., 160, 169, 257
Roosa, M. W., 180, 268
Rosen, A., 250
Rosenberg, H., 151, 268
Rosenthal, D., 103, 268
Rossi, P. H., 9, 238–240, 253, 268
Roszell, D. K., 124, 252
Rounsaville, B., 37, 250
Rousseau, D., 196, 253
Ruggieri-Authelet, A., 256, 262
Rush, A. J., 250
Russell, M., 179, 253, 268
Ryan, E., 202, 203, 206, 250, 268
Ryback, R., 122, 229, 271
Rychtarik, R. G., 249
Rydelius, P. A., 179, 265, 268

Samsonowitz, V., 124, 269
Sanchez-Craig, M., 25, 230, 268, 269
Sanders, B., 262
Sandler, I. N., 268
Saxe, L., 3, 4, 36, 41, 226, 269
Schaefer, J. A., 106, 210, 265
Schlundt, D. G., 249
Schmitz, R. E., 262, 265
Schneewind, K., 197, 269
Schooler, C., 108, 197, 260
Schreibman, L., 215, 269
Schuckit, M. A., 72, 269
Schulsinger, F., 260
Schwab-Bakman, N., 269
Schwartz, G. E., 10, 243, 269
Schwartz, M. A., 7, 269
Schwei, M. G., 72, 269
Scotch, N., 258
Sechrest, L., 25, 26, 221, 240, 269, 273
Seeman, M., 91, 237, 269

Seilhamer, R. A., 136, 144, 255, 259
Shandler, I. W., 251
Sharpley, C. F., 34, 258
Shaw, B. F., 250
Sheehan, J. J., 61, 269
Sheehan, M., 255
Shiffman, S., 130, 131, 230, 269
Shipley, T. E., Jr., 251
Siegel, C., 62, 269
Sigvardsson, S., 179, 253
Simpkins, J., 116, 273
Sinclair, C., 210, 269
Singer, C., 272
Sisson, R. W., 249
Sjoberg, L., 124, 269
Skinner, H. A., 24, 269, 270
Skinstad, A. -H., 4, 226, 265
Skjaerris, A., 72, 266
Skodol, A. E., 145, 261
Slater, E., 194, 270
Slotnick, R., 207, 257
Smart, R. G., 62, 234, 270
Smith, E. M., 148, 270
Smith, T., 268
Smolensky, W., 142, 270
Snowden, L. R., 41, 42, 270
Snyder, K. S., 272
Sobell, L. C., 46, 50, 51, 253, 262, 266, 268, 270
Sobell, M. B., 46, 151, 253, 262, 266, 268, 270
Sobieski, J., 271
Sokolow, L., 74, 75, 83, 84, 85, 270
Souza, E., 250
Spevak, P. A., 267
Spencer, B., 90, 272
Spiegel, D., 98, 132, 153, 270
Spiker, D. G., 176, 262
Stabenow, J. R., 175, 257
Stack, L., 206, 270
Stambul, H., 114, 249
Stefan, R. L., 261
Steiner, H., 206, 270, 271
Steinglass, P., 136, 176, 270
Stephens, R. S., 23, 250
Stewart, M. A., 175, 254
Stiffman, A. R., 193, 197, 270
Stobart, G., 261
Stout, R. L., 256, 262, 265
Straus, M. A., 261
Strug, D. L., 151, 270
Sullivan, K. T., 255
Sult, S., 104, 256
Swaback, D., 255
Szapocznik, J., 215, 270

Tal, M., 254
Tam, Y. K., 202, 265
Tarter, R., 185, 237, 270, 271
Taube, C. A., 231, 257, 271
Taylor, C., 255

AUTHOR INDEX

Taylor, C. A., 34, 263
Taylor, C. B., 260
Teague, M., 268
Teasdale, T. W., 260
Teitelbaum, M., 273
Terry, K., 207, 271
Thoits, P. A., 74, 83, 271
Thom, B., 84, 85, 271
Thomson, B., 98, 271
Tiller, D., 28, 254
Timmer, S. G., 90, 271
Tuchfeld, B. S., 65, 71, 90, 142, 271
Tucker, J. A., 130, 228, 271, 272
Tunving, K., 163, 251
Turnbull, J., 254

Uebersax, J. S., 267
Uhly, B., 250

Vaglum, P., 217, 271
Vaillant, G. E., 71, 134, 135, 146, 152, 154, 179, 180, 226, 254, 271
Van Dijk, W. K., 114, 271
Van Dijk-Koffeman, A., 114, 271
Vannicelli, M., 62, 74, 75, 90, 122, 229, 271
Vaughn, C. E., 132, 157, 261, 272
Vaux, A., 98, 271
Velleman, R., 235, 272
Verbrugge, L., 74, 272
Verhaest, S., 202, 272
Verinis, J. S., 24, 209, 272
Veroff, J., 90, 271
Vessell, R., 268
Vuchinich, R. E., 130, 271, 272

Wadstein, J., 25, 251
Wagman, W., 255
Walker, D. F., 254
Walker, K., 25, 268, 269
Walker, R. D., 235, 267, 272
Wallach, M. A., 227, 255
Wanberg, K. W., 227, 272
Ward, D. A., 116, 129, 272
Watson, C. G., 44, 89, 272
Webb, N., 267
Weick, K. E., 236, 272
Weiner, S. S., 254
Weintraub, S., 157, 255

Weisner, C., 233, 272
Weiss, C. H., 272
Weissman, M. M., 190, 263, 272
Wells, L., 216, 272
Wells, S., 268
Wells-Parker, E., 90, 272
Welte, J., 270
Wendt, R., 202, 273
Werner, E. E., 180, 273
Wernick, M. J., 250
Wersinger, R., 268
West, J. C., 34, 263, 268
West, M. O., 180, 273
West, S., 269
Wetzel, J., 97, 273
Whitehead, P. C., 116, 273
Wieman, R. J., 269
Wiens, A. N., 40, 76, 273
Wiggins, O. P., 7, 269
Wilderman, R., 210, 273
Wilkinson, D. A., 269
Wille, R., 152, 226, 273
Williams, A. E., 25, 262
Wilsnack, R. W., 74, 76, 82, 273
Wilsnack, S. C., 73, 75, 76, 273
Wilson, G. T., 130, 137, 252, 260, 273
Wingard, D. L., 146, 260
Winnie, R. E., 238, 258
Wiseman, J. P., 63, 66, 116, 136, 144, 151, 159, 160, 174, 176, 273
Wissler, T., 98, 132, 153, 270
Wolin, S., 183, 273
Wolz, M., 266
Wood, G., 135, 260
Woodward, W., 267
Woody, G. E., 262
Wortman, C. B., 254
Wright, C., 207, 256
Wulsin, V. W., 271

Yahr, H. T., 18, 21, 273
Yarvis, R., 255
Yeaton, W. H., 25, 269, 273
Young, R. D., 151, 258

Zasslow, M., 260
Ziff, D. C., 141, 252
Zucker, R. A., 6, 274
Zweben, A., 136, 159, 274

Subject Index

Abstinence
  change pretreatment to six-month follow-up, 38
  measurement
    pretreatment, 37, 112
    at six-month follow-up, 37
    one-month rates at the two-year follow-up
  relation to other areas of functioning, 41–43, 112–13
  six-month rates, 39–40, Figure 3.1
Aftercare, 62
  gender differences. See Gender
  intensity, 125
  and outcome, 62–63
  participation in, 235–36
Aims of the research, 5. See also Objectives of the research
Alcohol consumption
  change pretreatment to six-month follow-up, 38, Figure 3.1
  fluctuations in, 89, 116, 144
  measurement of, 37
  pretreatment, 37
  relation to other areas of functioning, 41–43, 51, 112–13
  self-report accuracy, 23–24
  and tension-reduction, 11
Alcoholics Anonymous
  participation and gender, 79–80
  participation and marital status, 79–80
  participation and treatment outcome, 58, 60, 62, 65, Table 4.1
Alcoholism treatment
  compared to no treatment, 40–41
  financing, 231
  diagnosis-related group, 231
  and gender, 74
  and marital status, 74
  as societal response, 3
  two tiers, 38
Antabuse and treatment outcome, 57, 58, 60, Table 4.1
Antianxiety medications and treatment outcome, 60
Anxiety. See Mood and health status
Appraisal. See Coping responses
Attrition. See Dropping out of treatment
Aversion conditioning patients
  characteristics, 21–22
  intake functioning, 38–40
  six-month follow-up functioning, 38–40
Aversion conditioning program
  booster sessions and outcome, 62
  description, 20, 32
    COPES profile, 32, Figure 2.3
  patient characteristics, 21–22
  staff, 20
  outcome, 56–57, Figure 4.3
Aversion conditioning treatment and abstinence rates, 40

Background characteristics. See Social background characteristics; Patient characteristics
Background Information Form (BIF), 22
Biopsychosocial perspective, 6–7, 248
  in diagnosis, 227
  match with expanded evaluation paradigm, 7, 232, 248

SUBJECT INDEX

Black-box approach, 7–9, 36, 71, 88,
    Figure 1.1. *See also* Traditional
    evaluation paradigm
  and questions left unanswered, 9

Children of alcoholics, 179, 225
  comparison with children of controls,
    182–83, Table 10.1
  comparison with children of depressed
    parents, 191–94
  determinants of functioning, 185–88,
    196–98, Table 10.2
  family context of adaptation, 181–88,
    192–94, Table 10.2, Figure 10.1
  family stressors and resources, 184–90,
    192–94, Table 10.2
  health and functioning, 179–80, 182
  risk and resistance factors, 180, 182,
    187–88, 190–91, 193, Figure 10.3
  sample description, 182
Children of depressed parents, 189
  comparison with children of alcoholic
    parents, 191–93
  comparison with control children, 189–
    90
  parent remission and children's
    functioning, 190–91
Children's health problems. *See* Stressors
Community controls, 18. *See also*
    Remitted patients
  children of, 182
  sample description, 138–39
  spouses of, 161, 163
  value of, 137
Community-Oriented Programs
    Environment Scale (COPES). *See
    also* Treatment environment
  comparing the programs, 34–35
  description of, 23, 28–29
    subscales or dimensions, 28–29,
      Table 2.3
  enriching treatment environments, 207–
    8
  gender differences and program
    environment. *See* Gender
  Ideal Form (Form I), 203, Figure 11.1
  monitoring change in halfway house
    program, 203–5, Figures 11.1–11.2
  monitoring change in milieu-oriented
    program, 33, Figure 2.4
  monitoring change in psychiatric
    programs, 201–2
  norms, 29
  as an objective portrait of social
    climate, 126
  profiles for five programs, 30–35,
    Figures 2.1–2.4
  promoting change in treatment
    programs, 208–10
  Real Form (Form R), 207
  typology of program environments, 206

Community reinforcement approach, 230–
    31
Coping responses, 224
  active behavioral, 105–6, 117, 140
    measurement of, 106
    and treatment outcome, 111, 123
  active cognitive, 106, 117, 140
    measurement of, 105–6
    and treatment outcome, 111, 123
  and adaptation, 107
  appraisal, 104
  avoidance coping, 106, 117, 140
    measurement of, 106
    and treatment outcome, 123
  cognitive appraisal, 91
  and depression, 131–32
  and drinking, 105
  efficacy, 106–7
  family and work contexts, 107–8
  focus of coping, 105
    appraisal-focused, 105
    emotion-focused, 106
    problem-focused, 105–6
  gender differences, 106–7
  and life contexts, 107–8, 111, Figure 7.1
  measurement of, 117
  mediators of relationship to outcome,
    130–32
  predictors of, 126–27
  and recovery process, 104–5, 108
  and relapse, 104–5, 108, 124
  relation to spouse functioning, 168–74,
    Tables 9.3–9.4
  situational specificity, 106–7
  skills training, 229–30
  and smoking cessation, 130–31
  social resources, 110–11, Figure 7.1
  and stable personality tendencies, 123
  stressors, 110–11, Figure 7.1
  and treatment, 111, Figure 7.1
  and treatment outcome, 123–32, 224,
    Tables 7.2–7.3, Figures 7.1–7.2
Cost analysis, 242
Costs of alcoholism to society, 3

Data collection procedures, 22–23. *See
    also* follow-up
  posttreatment data, 23, 111–12, 138–39
  pretreatment data, 22
  treatment data, 22–23
Demographic characteristics. *See* Social
    background characteristics
Depression. *See also* Mood and health
    status
  change pretreatment to six-month
    follow-up, 38, 40, Figure 3.2
  and coping, 131–32
  and family environment, 97–98
  measurement of
    pretreatment, 37, 112
    at six-month follow-up, 37

SUBJECT INDEX

relation to other areas of functioning, 41–43, 112–13
and social resources, 131–32
and stressors, 131–32
Diagnosis
of alcoholism, 226–28
biopsychosocial approach, 227, 232
diagnosis-related group, 231
need for comprehensive assessment, 227–28
Difficulty of follow-up, 46. *See also* Follow-up effort
patient characteristics and, 48–49
relation to six-month outcome, 47–49
Disease concept of alcoholism
as etiologic theory, 6
match with traditional outcome-oriented evaluation, 6
Disulfiram. *See* Antabuse
Disulfiram implant, 25
Divorce rate, 163, 165
Doctor visits. *See* Health services utilization
Drinking history
and gender, 74
and marital status, 74
of six-month follow-up sample, 21–22, Table 2.1
Dropping out of treatment, 234–35
and integration in a program, 234–35
and life context factors, 234–35
and Salvation Army treatment environment, 66
DSM-III-R, 7
role of psychosocial stressors, 7
Duration of treatment. *See* Length of treatment

Effectiveness of treatment programs
and black-box approach to evaluation, 8–9
relative effectiveness of five programs, 53–57, Figures 4.2–4.3
treatment pessimism, 4, 26
Evaluation research
implications of expanded paradigm, 231–42
perceived utility by clinicians, 4
theory-driven approach, 231–42
Expanded evaluation paradigm, 4
broad applicability, 12
description, 9, 52–53, 109–11, Figure 1.2, Figure 4.1, Figure 7.1
utility of, 9–10, 231–48
Extratreatment factors, 8. *See also* Stressors; Social resources; Life context factors; Coping
and decay of treatment outcome, 8
and effect on outcome relative to treatment, 8

Family arguments
measurement of, 117, 139
relation to treatment outcome, Tables 7.2–7.3
Family environment. *See also* Family Environment Scale
and adaptation of children, 184–94, Figure 10.2
and adaptation to remission, 146, 175–76
and adaptive function of drinking, 96, 102, 176
of black versus white alcoholics, 97
and broader social context, 196
and coping responses, 107
and depression, 97–98
determinants of, 194–96
disagreement about, 91–92, 139
enrichment of, 212–16, Figures 11.3–11.4
of family of origin, 96–97
and life stressors, 98, 196
as moderator of life stressors, 97–98
parental functioning as predictor of, 195–96
and psychiatric treatment outcome, 132
relation to spouse functioning, 168–74, Tables 9.3–9.4
and remission/relapse, 143–44, 184–85, Table 8.2, Figure 10.2
resources, 125–26, 132
spouses of remitted/relapsed patients, 162–66, Tables 9.1–9.2
stability of, 121
and substance abuse, 96–97
and treatment outcome, 120–22, 201
and work environment, 102, 104, 196–98
Family Environment Scale (FES), 91–92, 116, 131, 139, 161, 167, Table 6.1. *See also* Family environment
description of, 91–92
subscales or dimensions, 92, Table 6.1
development of, 92
family resources, 92, 125
family stressors, 92
Ideal Form (Form I), 212
incongruence, 91–92, 139
norms, 92
profile, high conflict family, 93–94, Figure 6.1
profile, incongruent family, 95–96, Figure 6.3
profile, structured religious family, 94–95, Figure 6.2
profiles, pre- and posttherapy, 212–14, Figures 11.3–11.4
Real Form (Form R), 212
reliability, 92
typology, 96

Family functioning. *See also* Family environment
  determinants of, 194–96
  measurement of, 139
  paradigm, 194
  and remission/relapse, 142–43, 149, 162–66, Tables 8.2–8.3, Table 8.5, Tables 9.1–9.2
  role performance, 139
  and work setting, 197–98
Family-oriented treatment. *See* Implications for treatment
Family resources. *See also* Family environment
  and depression, 131
  measurement of, 125–26
  predictors of, 126
  and treatment outcome, 127–28, 132
Family sample, 13, 18, 111–12, 137
  compared to nonfamily patients, 112
Family therapy, 228–29
Financing alcoholism services. *See* Implications for treatment
First admission patients, 22, Table 2.1
  relation of length of treatment to outcome, 62
Follow-up
  effort
    description at six months, 47
    locating patients, 47–48
    persuading patients, 47–48
    in relation to six-month functioning, 47–51, Table 3.2
    total effort measure, 48
  rates
    of community controls, 138
    of patient and family samples, 23, 37–38, 111
Follow-up functioning. *See* Outcome functioning
Follow-up Information Form (FIF), 22, 23, 37, 47, 50
For-profit programs
  patient characteristics compared with nonprofit, 21–22, 54, 110, 126, Table 2.1
  patient intake functioning compared with nonprofit, 38, 54, Figures 3.1–3.2
  six-month outcome compared with nonprofit, 38, 110
  treatment effectiveness compared with nonprofit, 56–57, Figures 4.2–4.3
Formative evaluation, 209

Gender
  and Alcoholics Anonymous, 79–80
  and coping, 106–7
  and drinking behavior, 74, 77, 81, Table 5.1, Table 5.3
  and drinking context (or drinking "pattern"), 83–84
  and drinking history, 74, 76
  and intake functioning, 77, Table 5.1
  interaction with marital status
    in relation to drinking behavior, 74
    in relation to drinking history, 76
    in relation to intake functioning, 77, Table 5.1
    in relation to living with a heavy drinker, 80, Table 5.1
    in relation to participation in outpatient aftercare, 80, 84–86, 222, Table 5.2
    in relation to participation in treatment, 76–77, Table 5.2
    in relation to psychiatric treatment outcome, 86, 222
    in relation to treatment outcome, 76–77, 82–83, Table 5.2
  and living with a heavy drinker, 76, 79–80, Table 5.2
  men-to-women ratio in programs, 84
  and outpatient aftercare, 79–80, 84–86, Table 5.2
  and perceptions of program environment, 77–80, 82, 84, Table 5.2
  and posttreatment experiences, 80, Table 5.2
  and psychological adjustment, 74
  in remission/relapse, 140
  and response to treatment, 61, 74, 81–84, 86, 222, Table 5.3
  and response to treatment environment, 75, 81–82, 84, 86, Table 5.3
  and role strain, 83
  and treatment outcome, 74–75, 77, Table 5.1

Halfway house patients
  characteristics, 21–22
  intake functioning, 38–40
  six-month follow-up functioning, 38–40
Halfway house program
  components and outcome, 59
  description, 19–20, 31–32
    COPES profile, 31–32, Figure 2.2
    resident characteristics, 21–22
    staff, 20
  length of treatment and outcome, 61
  outcome, 56–57, Figure 4.2
Halfway house treatment and abstinence rates, 39
Health and Daily Living (HDL) Form, 116, 131, 139, 161
Health services utilization
  measurement of, 139
  and remission/relapse, 140–41, 149, Table 8.1, Table 8.5
  and spouses of remitted/relapsed patients, 162–64, Tables 9.1–9.2
Hospital-based patients
  characteristics, 21–22

SUBJECT INDEX

intake functioning, 38–40
six-month follow-up functioning, 38–40
Hospital-based program
components and outcome, 58–59
description, 19, 30
COPES profile, 30–31, Figure 2.1
patient characteristics, 21–22
staff, 19
length of treatment and outcome, 61
outcome, 56–67, Figure 4.2
Hospitalization. *See* Health services utilization

Implementation of treatment programs
analysis, 206–7
assessment, 25, 220–21
program integrity, 25
program strength, 25
enriching treatment environments, 207–8
five programs, 26–34, Table 2.2
implications for developing and improving programs, 245
as a precursor to outcome studies, 35, 240–41
standards, 26, 201, 206
ideal program, 26, 28
normative conditions, 26
and program development, 206
theoretical analysis or expert judgment, 26
and treatment pessimism, 26
treatment quality, 28–29, 34
treatment quantity, 26–28, 34
Implications of the research for treatment, 226–31
community-oriented treatment programs, 230–31
comprehensive assessment and diagnosis, 227–28
coping skills training, 229–30
family-oriented treatment, 228–29
financing alcoholism services, 231
Improvement of patients following treatment, 221
associations among changes from pretreatment to six-month follow-up, 42, 113
associations among changes from pretreatment to two-year follow-up, 113
associations among changes from pretreatment to 10-year follow-up, 113
pretreatment to six-month follow-up, 38–41, Figures 3.1–3.2
relation of improved drinking to other areas of functioning, 41–43, 112–13
role of treatment at six-month follow-up, 40–41
Income, 21, Table 2.1

Intake functioning
measures, 37, 112, 125
prognostic importance, 43–45, Table 3.1
related to six-month outcome, 69
related to treatment program, 126–27
related to two-year and 10-year outcome, 118, 120–21, 124–28, 132, Tables 7.2–7.3
Intensity of treatment, 65, 67
measurement, 65, 67
and outcome, 69–70
predictors of, 68
program comparisons, 27–28, 68, 126, Table 2.2

Lectures and films and treatment outcome, 58–60, Table 4.1
Length of treatment
in five programs, 27
and outcome, 61–62
for first admission patients, 62
for repeat admission patients, 62
Life context factors, 224, 226, 241–48. *See also* Stressors; Social resources
and etiology of alcohol abuse, 90
relation to spouse functioning, 168–75, Tables 9.3–9.4
and remission/relapse, 143–46, 149–52, Table 8.3, Table 8.5
of spouses of remitted/relapsed patients, 162–66, Tables 9.1–9.2
and treatment outcome, 76, 85, 89, 116–25, 127–30, 224, Tables 7.2–7.3, Figures 7.1–7.2
Life stressors. *See* Stressors
Long-term outcome. *See* Outcome functioning
Low-bottom alcoholics, 57

Marital status, 73
and Alcoholics Anonymous, 79–80
and drinking behavior, 74
and drinking history, 76–77
and gender in relation to drinking behavior, 74
and intake functioning, 77, Table 5.1
and living with a heavy drinker, 79–80, 82–83, Table 5.2
and mental health, 74
and outpatient aftercare, 79–80, Table 5.2
and program components, 77, 79, Table 5.2
and program environment, 79–80, Table 5.2
and response to treatment, 81–82, Table 5.3
and treatment outcome, 77, 81, Table 5.1, Table 5.3
in relation to work environment, 122–23, 145

Matching
  families with interventions, 215–16
  patients with treatments, 73, 86, 242–45
    role of life contexts, 244–45
    role of theory, 243
Medications
  and remission/relapse, 140–41, 149, Table 8.1, Table 8.5
  and treatment outcome, 60
  used in treatment, 28
Methodology of evaluation research. *See* Research design
Milieu-oriented patients
  characteristics, 21–22
  intake functioning, 38–40
  six-month follow-up functioning, 38–40
Milieu-oriented program
  components and outcome, 59–60
  description of, 20, 33
    COPES profile, 33–34, Figure 2.4
    resident characteristics, 21–22
    staff, 20
  outcome, 57, Figure 4.3
Moderate drinkers, 145
Monitoring program development, 201–7. *See also* Community-Oriented Programs Environment Scale
Mood and health status
  measurement of, 139
  and remission/relapse, 140–42, 148–52, Table 8.1, Table 8.5
  of spouses of remitted and relapsed patients, 161–66, Tables 9.1–9.2
Mortality, 223
  patients versus controls, 146
Multiphasic Environmental Assessment Procedure (MEAP), 216–17

Naturalistic study. *See* Research design
Nonprofit programs. *See* For-profit programs

Objectives of the research, 17–18
Occupational functioning
  change pretreatment to six-month follow-up, 40, Figure 3.2
  measurement
    pretreatment, 37, 112
    at six-month follow-up, 37
    at two-year and 10-year follow-up, 139
  relation to other areas of functioning, 41–43, 112–13
  and remission/relapse, 142–43, Table 8.2
Outcome functioning
  assessment
    matching with program components, 57, 71, 241–42
    timing, 241
  changes between intake and six-month follow-up, 38–42, Figures 3.1–3.2
  changes between six-month and two-year follow-up, 114, Table 7.1
  changes between two-year and 10-year follow-up, 114, Table 7.1
  interrelationships at six months, 41–43, 51
  interrelationships at two and 10 years, 112–13
  means at six months, two years, and 10 years, 114, Table 7.1
  measures
    at six months, 37
    at two years, 112
    at 10 years, 112
  multidimensional orientation, 36–37, 51, 241
  stability over time, 113–16, Table 7.1
Outcome variance
  accounted for
    by coping responses, 123, 128–29, Tables 7.2–7.3, Figure 7.2
    by life context factors, 117–21, 124–25, 127–29, Tables 7.2–7.3, Figure 7.2
    for men and women patients, 82
    by pretreatment factors, 44, 68–72, 118, 120–21, 124–28, 222, 224, Table 3.1, Table 4.2, Tables 7.2–7.3, Figure 4.4, Figure 7.2
    by program factors, 68–72, 126–27, 222, Table 4.2, Figure 4.4, Figure 7.2
  at six-month follow-up, 44–45, 51, 68–72, 127, 222, 224, Table 3.1, Table 4.2, Figure 4.4
  at two-year follow-up, 117–18, 120–21, 123–25, 128–29, 224, Tables 7.2–7.3, Figure 7.2
  at 10-year follow-up, 117–18, 120–21, 123–25, 129, 224, Table 7.3
Outpatient treatment
  and gender, 79–80
  and marital status, 79–80
  and six-month outcome, 62

Paraprofessional staff and treatment quality, 34–35
Participation in treatment, 27–28, Table 2.2 *See also* Program components; Process analysis; Salvation Army program
Part-time jobs and outcome, 58, 64, Table 4.1
Patient characteristics. *See also* Social background characteristics; Intake functioning
  for each program prior to treatment, 21–22, Table 2.1
  related to treatment, 68, 110, 126
  relation to treatment outcome, 8, 43–44, 66–71, 127, 132, Table 3.1, Table 4.2, Figure 4.4. *See also* Prognostic indicators

SUBJECT INDEX

and treatment variables as outcome predictors, 8, 66–71, 127, 128
Patient sample, 12, 18
Person-environment transactions, 110
Personal resources, 65–66, 71
Physical symptoms. *See also* Mood and health status
   change pretreatment to six-month follow-up, 38, 40, Figure 3.1
   measurement
     pretreatment, 37, 112
     at six-month follow-up, 37
   relation to other areas of functioning, 41–43, 112–13
Pretreatment factors. *See* Intake functioning; Patient characteristics; Social background characteristics
Pretreatment functioning. *See* Intake functioning; Patient characteristics
Primary sample. *See* Patient sample
Prognostic indicators
   patient background characteristics versus functioning, 44–45
   in relation to six-month outcome, 43–45
Program comparisons
   in intake functioning and six-month outcome, 38–41, 68, Figures 3.1–3.2
   in intensity of treatment, 27–28, 68, Table 2.2
   in patient characteristics, 21–22, Table 2.1
   in treatment components and orientation, 18–20, 58
   in treatment environment, 30–35, Figures 2.1–2.4
   in treatment experiences, 26–28, 58, Table 2.2
Program components
   assessing quantity and quality, 26–35, 220–21, Table 2.2
   and compensatory influence of other program elements, 60
   and gender and marital status, 77, 79
   measurement, 26
   and outcome, 58–61, 221, Table 4.1
   relative effectiveness for patient subgroups, 61, 66
Program effects
   on intensity of treatment, 68
   on outcome, 54–57, 69, 72, 221
   on the treatment environment, 68, 126
Program environment. *See* Treatment environment; Community-Oriented Programs Environment Scale
Program evaluation. *See* Evaluation research

Quality assurance, 210–11

Recovery. *See also* Remission
   natural recovery process, 226

Relapse. *See also* Relapsed patients
   and alcohol consumption, 142
   and coping, 129–30
   and depression, 153
   and other substance abuse, 152–53
   prevention, 229–30
   rate
     compared to other studies, 147–48
     and social resources, 129–30
     at two years, 138, 148, Table 8.4
     at 10 years, 147–48, Table 8.4
   and social resources, 129–30
   and stressors, 11, 120, 129–30
     compared to remitted and control groups, 136–37
   theories, 237
Relapsed patients. *See* Remitted patients
Relapse prevention, 229–30
Remission. *See also* Remitted patients
   and coping, 129–30
   definition
     at two years, 138
     at 10 years, 147
   and depression, 153
   and other substance abuse, 152–53
   process of remission/relapse, 150–54
   rate, 223
     compared to other studies, 147–48
     at two years, 138, 148, Table 8.4
     at 10 years, 147–48, Table 8.4
   and social resources, 129–30
   and stressors, 11, 129–30
   validity of definition, 147
Remitted patients
   compared to controls and relapsed patients, 223
     on divorce rate, 163
     on mood, health, and alcohol consumption, 140–42, 148–52, Table 8.1, Table 8.5
     on occupational, social, and family functioning, 142, 149–152, Table 8.2, Table 8.5
     on life stressors, social resources, and coping, 143–46, 149–52, Table 8.3, Table 8.5
Research design
   and estimating treatment effects, 54, 240–41
   experimental, 24, 238–40
   match with research questions posed, 18, 24–25, 239
   naturalistic, 25, 54, 61, 240–41
   nonexperimental, 239
Risk factors, 145
   for children, 187–88, 190–91, 193, Figure 10.3
   for spouses, 175

Salvation Army patients
   characteristics, 21–22
   intake functioning, 38–40

six-month follow-up functioning, 38–40
Salvation Army Program, 63
  description, 19, 30–31, 63–65, Figure 2.1
  COPES profile, 30–31, 64, Figure 2.1
  length of treatment and outcome, 61
  outcome, 54–56, 64, Figure 4.2
  participation and outcome, 65–66
  program components and outcome, 58, 64–66, Table 4.1
  resident characteristics, 21–22
  staff, 19
  treatment environment, 64
  treatment orientation, 63–64
Sedatives and treatment outcome, 60
Self-confidence
  measurement of, 139
  and remission and relapse, 140–42, 151, Table 8.1
Self-report data
  accuracy of, 23–24
  and confidentiality, 24
  correspondence with collateral data, 24
Sex differences. See Gender
Social activities. See Social functioning
Social background characteristics
  and intake functioning, 110
  and life context factors, 111
  measurement of, 125
  prognostic importance, 43–45, Table 3.1
  related to six-month outcome, 43–44, 69
  related to treatment program, 21–22, 110, 126–27, Table 2.1
  related to two-year and 10-year outcome, 118, 120–21, 124–28, 132, Tables 7.2–7.3
  of six-month follow-up sample, 21–22, Table 2.1
  and six-month follow-up functioning, 43–44, 68–70, Table 3.1, Table 4.2, Figure 4.4
  and stressors and social resources, 111
  and treatment factors, 68
Social climate scales. See also Community-Oriented Programs Environment Scale; Family Environment Scale; Multiphasic Environmental Assessment Procedure; Ward Atmosphere Scale; Work Environment Scale
  and process of program change, 207–10
  promoting change in social contexts, 208–19
Social functioning
  change pretreatment to six-month follow-up, 40, Figure 3.2
  measurement
    pretreatment, 37
    at six-month follow-up, 37
  relation to other areas of functioning, 41–43, 112–13

and remission and relapse, 142–43, Table 8.2
Social resources, 65–66, 71, 75, 224
  and coping responses, 111
  and depression, 131
  etiology of alcohol abuse, 90
  as mediators of treatment outcome, 130
  and patient social background characteristics, 111
  and personal resources, 65, 71
  and reaction to stressors, 11
  relation to spouse functioning, 168–74, Tables 9.3–9.4
  and smoking cessation, 130, 152–53
  and spouses of remitted and relapsed patients, 162–64, Tables 9.1–9.2
  and treatment outcome, 111, 116–25, 127–33, 224, Tables 7.2–7.3, Figures 7.1–7.2
Sociodemographic characteristics. See Social background characteristics
Spouse drinking, 96
  as an adaptive function for the family, 96
  of moderate drinkers, 145
Spouses of alcoholic patients, 225
  dysfunction
    measurement of, 116
    in relation to patient outcome, 116–20, Tables 7.2–7.3
  functioning
    measurement of, 167–68
  perspectives on functioning, 158
    coping perspective, 159–60, 165–66
    personality perspective, 158–59, 165, 175
    stress perspective, 159, 165–66
  predictors of spouse functioning, 120, 168–74
    measurement of, 167–68
    risk factors, 175
  of remitted and relapsed patients, 160–66, 225, Tables 9.1–9.2
  sample description, 161, 163
  stress and coping model of functioning, 166–67, 172–75, Figure 9.1
  two-year adaptation, 161
Spouses of depressed partners, 176
Staff and treatment environment, 35
Stress and coping theory, 10–12, 91
  description, 10–11
  as etiologic theory of alcohol abuse, 10, 237
  in matching patients to treatment, 243
  as perspective to study other disorders, 12
  and relapse, 237
  in relation to biopsychosocial perspective, 10
Stressors, 224
  children's health problems
    measurement of, 116–17

SUBJECT INDEX

relation to treatment outcome, 116–20, Tables 7.2–7.3
and coping responses, 111
and depression, 131
etiology of alcohol abuse, 90
and family environment, 196
life events
  measurement of, 116, 139
  relation to treatment outcome, 117–20, 127–30, Tables 7.2–7.3
life stressors
  measurement of, 125
  predictors of, 126
  mediators of relationship to outcome, 110–11, 130
  and patient social background characteristics, 111
  relation to spouse functioning, 168–74, Tables 9.3–9.4
spouse dysfunction
  measurement of, 116
  relation to treatment outcome, 117–20, 127–30, Tables 7.2–7.3
  and spouses of remitted/relapsed patients, 162–64, Tables 9.1–9.2
  and treatment outcome, 110–11, 117–20, 127–32, 224, Tables 7.2–7.3, Figures 7.1–7.2
  and recovery, 91, 104–5, 120, 129–30
  and relapse, 11, 104–5, 120, 129–30
Systems model, 6, 197, 243. *See also* Biopsychosocial perspective

Tension-reduction effect of alcohol, 11
Theories to guide evaluations, 231–32, 237–38
  of nature and course of disorder, 237–38
  of treatment process, 236–37
  of treatment selection, 232–36, 240
Therapy sessions and treatment outcome, 58–59, Table 4.1
Traditional evaluation paradigm, 7–8, 89
Treatment for alcoholism. *See* Alcoholism treatment
Treatment components. *See* Program components
Treatment entry. *See* Treatment selection
Treatment environment. *See also* Community-Oriented Programs Environment Scale
  enrichment of, 207–8
  measure, 67, 125
  and outcome, 70, 201, 221
  predictors of, 68, 126
  and staffing, 35
Treatment experiences. *See also* Program components; Intensity of treatment
  measurement of, 22, 58, 125
  and outcome, 67–70

predictors of, 68, 126
Treatment Experiences Form (TEF), 22, 58
Treatment implementation. *See* Implementation of treatment programs
Treatment outcome. *See* Outcome functioning
Treatment programs studied
  description, 18–20
  and intensity of treatment, 68
  two tiers of treatment system, 38
Treatment quality. *See* Implementation of treatment programs
Treatment quantity. *See* Implementation of treatment programs
Treatment selection, 54, 68, 232–36
Two-tiered system of treatment, 18, 21–22, 38

Utility of treatment evaluation, 3, 245–48

Variance accounted for. *See* Outcome variance

Ward Atmosphere Scale (WAS)
  monitoring change in psychiatric programs, 202, 206
Work environment. *See also* Work Environment Scale
  and alcohol abuse, 90–91
  and coping, 108
  and depression, 103–4, 116, 131
  enrichment of, 210–11
  and family settings, 102, 104, 196–98
  modifying stressful environments, 211
  and morale, 103
  and performance, 103
  and remission/relapse, 144
  resources, 100
    and functioning, 103–4, 116
  stressors, 100
    and functioning, 103–4, 116
  and treatment outcome, 116, 122–23, 201
  in relation to marital status, 122–23
Work Environment Scale (WES), 98–100, 116, 131, 139, 161, 196, Table 6.2. *See also* Work environment
  description, 98–100, Table 6.2
  subscales or dimensions, 98–99, Table 6.2
  norms, 99–100
  profiles, cohesive task-oriented, 100–1, Figure 6.4
  profiles, highly demanding, 101–2, Figure 6.5
  reliability, 100
Worship services and outcome, 58, 64–65, Table 4.1